Clinical
of Adol
Substance Abuse
Treatment

D0282925

Clinical Manual of Adolescent Substance Abuse Treatment

Edited by
Yifrah Kaminer, M.D., M.B.A.
Ken C. Winters, Ph.D.

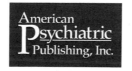

American Psychiatric Publishing, Inc.

Washington, DC
London, England

Copyright © 2011 American Psychiatric Publishing, Inc.
ALL RIGHTS RESERVED

Manufactured in the United States of America on acid-free paper
14   13   12   11   10   5   4   3   2   1
First Edition

Typeset in Adobe AGaramond and Formata.

American Psychiatric Publishing, Inc.
1000 Wilson Boulevard
Arlington, VA 22209-3901
www.appi.org

Library of Congress Cataloging-in-Publication Data
Clinical manual of adolescent substance abuse treatment / edited by Yifrah Kaminer, Ken C. Winters. — 1st ed.
        p. ; cm.
    Includes bibliographical references and index.
    ISBN 978-1-58562-381-5 (pbk. : alk. paper)
    1. Teenagers—Substance use. 2. Substance abuse—Treatment. I. Kaminer, Yifrah, 1951– II. Winters, Ken C.
    [DNLM: 1. Substance-Related Disorders—diagnosis. 2. Substance-Related Disorders—therapy. 3. Adolescent. 4. Comorbidity. WM 270 C64135 2011]
    RJ506.D78C65 2011
    616.86′060835--dc22

                                                                          2010015528

British Library Cataloguing in Publication Data
A CIP record is available from the British Library.

Contents

Yifrah Kaminer, M.D., M.B.A.
Ken C. Winters, Ph.D.

1 **Prevalence and Clinical Course of Adolescent Substance Use and Substance Use Disorders. . . 1**

Tammy Chung, Ph.D.
Christopher S. Martin, Ph.D.

4 **Biomarker Testing for Substance Use in Adolescents** **83**

Janelle E. Arias, M.D.
Albert J. Arias, M.D.
Yifrah Kaminer, M.D., M.B.A.

5 **Placement Criteria and Treatment Planning for Adolescents With Substance Use Disorders.** **113**

Marc Fishman, M.D.

6 **Adolescent Behavioral Change:**
   Process and Outcomes 143

Ken C. Winters, Ph.D.
Yifrah Kaminer, M.D., M.B.A.

7 **Pharmacotherapy of Adolescent**
   Substance Use Disorders 163

Yifrah Kaminer, M.D., M.B.A.
Lisa A. Marsch, Ph.D.

8 Club Drug, Prescription Drug, and Over-the-Counter Medication Abuse: Description, Diagnosis, and Intervention 187

Christian Hopfer, M.D.

9 Brief Motivational Interventions, Cognitive-Behavioral Therapy, and Contingency Management for Youth Substance Use Disorders 213

Yifrah Kaminer, M.D., M.B.A.
Anthony Spirito, Ph.D., A.B.P.P.
William Lewander, M.D.

12 Attention Deficit–Disruptive Behavior Disorders and Substance Use Disorders in Adolescents 283

K.A.H. Mirza, M.B., F.R.C.P.C.
Oscar G. Bukstein, M.D., M.P.H.

13 Assessment and Treatment of Internalizing Disorders: Depression, Anxiety Disorders, and Posttraumatic Stress Disorder 307

Yifrah Kaminer, M.D., M.B.A.
Julian D. Ford, Ph.D.
Duncan Clark, M.D., Ph.D.

14 Assessment and Treatment of Suicidal Behavior.....................349

David B. Goldston, Ph.D.
John F. Curry, Ph.D.
Karen C. Wells, Ph.D.
Michelle Roley, B.A.

Appendixes

List of Tables and Figures

Tables

Figures

Contributors

Albert J. Arias, M.D.
Assistant Professor, Department of Psychiatry, University of Connecticut School of Medicine, Farmington, Connecticut

Janelle E. Arias, M.D.
Assistant Clinical Professor, Department of Psychiatry, University of Connecticut School of Medicine, Farmington, Connecticut

Oscar G. Bukstein, M.D., M.P.H.
Professor of Psychiatry, Western Psychiatric Institute and Clinic, University of Pittsburgh School of Medicine, Pittsburgh, Pennsylvania

Richard F. Catalano, Ph.D.
Bartley Dobb Professor for the Study and Prevention of Violence; Director, Social Development Research Group, School of Social Work, University of Washington, Seattle, Washington

Tammy Chung, Ph.D.
Associate Professor of Psychiatry, Western Psychiatric Institute and Clinic, Pittsburgh Adolescent Alcohol Research Center, Pittsburgh, Pennsylvania

Duncan Clark, M.D., Ph.D.
Associate Professor of Psychiatry, University of Pittsburgh School of Medicine, Western Psychiatric Institute and Clinic, Pittsburgh, Pennsylvania

John F. Curry, Ph.D.
Professor of Medical Psychology, Duke University School of Medicine, Durham, North Carolina

Gayle A. Dakof, Ph.D.
Research Associate Professor, Center for Treatment Research on Adolescent Drug Abuse, University of Miami Miller School of Medicine, Miami, Florida

Anne C. Duffy, M.D., F.R.C.P.C.
Professor, Department of Psychiatry, Dalhousie University; Senior Clinical Research Scholar and Program Head, Mood Disorders Clinical Research Program; Program Head, Flourish Clinical and Research Program, Halifax, Nova Scotia, Canada

Jenna Elgin, M.Ed.
Research Assistant, Social Development Research Group, School of Social Work, University of Washington, Seattle, Washington

Marc Fishman, M.D.
Assistant Professor, Department of Psychiatry, Johns Hopkins University School of Medicine; Medical Director, Maryland Treatment Centers, Baltimore, Maryland

Julian D. Ford, Ph.D.
Associate Professor of Psychiatry, University of Connecticut Health Center, Farmington, Connecticut

Susan H. Godley, Rh.D.
Senior Research Scientist and Director, EBT Coordinating Center, Chestnut Health Systems, Normal, Illinois

David B. Goldston, Ph.D.
Associate Professor of Medical Psychology, Duke University School of Medicine, Durham, North Carolina

Kevin P. Haggerty, M.S.W.
Assistant Director, Social Development Research Group, School of Social Work, University of Washington, Seattle, Washington

J. David Hawkins, Ph.D.
Founding Director, School of Social Work, Social Development Research Group, University of Washington, Seattle, Washington

Christian Hopfer, M.D.
Associate Professor, Division of Substance Dependence, Department of Psychiatry, University of Colorado, Denver, Colorado

Steven L. Jaffe, M.D.
Professor Emeritus of Child and Adolescent Psychiatry, Emory University; Clinical Professor of Psychiatry, Morehouse School of Medicine; Psychiatric Consultant, Metro-Atlanta Serenity House, Atlanta Insight Enthusiastic Sobriety Program and the Nelson Price Adolescent Substance Abuse Program, Atlanta, Georgia

Yifrah Kaminer, M.D., M.B.A.
Professor of Psychiatry and Pediatrics, Alcohol Research Center, University of Connecticut Health Center, Farmington, Connecticut

John F. Kelly, Ph.D.
Associate Professor in Psychiatry, Harvard Medical School; Director, Addiction Recovery Management Service and Associate Director, Center for Addiction Medicine, Department of Psychiatry, Massachusetts General Hospital, Boston, Massachusetts

John R. Knight, M.D.
Associate Professor of Pediatrics, Harvard Medical School; Director, Center for Adolescent Substance Abuse Research, Children's Hospital Boston, Boston, Massachusetts

Sharon Levy, M.D., M.P.H.
Assistant Professor of Pediatrics, Harvard Medical School; Division of Developmental Medicine, Children's Hospital Boston, Boston, Massachusetts

William Lewander, M.D.
Professor of Emergency Medicine, The Warren Alpert Medical School of Brown University, Rhode Island Hospital, Providence, Rhode Island

Lisa A. Marsch, Ph.D.
Director, Center for Technology and Health, National Development and Research Institutes, New York, New York

Christopher S. Martin, Ph.D.
Associate Professor of Psychiatry, Western Psychiatric Institute and Clinic, Pittsburgh Adolescent Alcohol Research Center, Pittsburgh, Pennsylvania

Robert Milin, M.D., F.R.C.P.C.
Director, Adolescent Day Treatment Unit, Royal Ottawa Mental Health Centre; Associate Professor, Department of Psychiatry, University of Ottawa, Ottawa, Ontario, Canada

K.A.H. Mirza, M.B., F.R.C.P.C.
Honorary Senior Lecturer and Consultant Psychiatrist, University Department of Child and Adolescent Psychiatry and South London and Maudsley NHS Trust, Institute of Psychiatry, Kings College, London, England

Peter B. Rockholz, M.S.S.W., L.C.S.W.
Yale School of Medicine, Yale Child Study Center, New Haven, Connecticut; Academic Connections, Ridgefield, Connecticut

Michelle Roley, B.A.
Research Assistant, Duke University School of Medicine, Durham, North Carolina

Jane Ellen Smith, Ph.D.
Professor and Chair, Department of Psychology, University of New Mexico, Albuquerque, New Mexico

Anthony Spirito, Ph.D., A.B.P.P.
Professor, Department of Psychiatry and Human Behavior, Center for Alcohol and Addictions Studies, The Warren Alpert Medical School of Brown University, Providence, Rhode Island

Selena Walker, M.A.
Program Evaluation Coordinator, Youth Psychiatry Program, Royal Ottawa
Mental Health Centre, Ottawa, Ontario, Canada

Karen C. Wells, Ph.D.
Associate Professor of Medical Psychology, Duke University School of Medicine, Durham, North Carolina

Ken C. Winters, Ph.D.
Professor, Department of Psychiatry, University of Minnesota Medical
School, Minneapolis, Minnesota

The following contributors to this book have indicated a financial interest in or other affiliation with a commercial supporter, a manufacturer of a commercial product, a provider of a commercial service, a nongovernmental organization, and/or a government agency, as listed below:

Oscar G. Bukstein, M.D., M.P.H.—*Research support:* Ortho-McNeil-Janssen, Shire

Gayle A. Dakof, Ph.D.—Dr. Dakof's chapter is partly about a substance abuse treatment called multidimensional family therapy (MDFT). The author gets paid as a consultant by organizations to train them in MDFT. In the past 12 months (as of December 2009), Dr. Dakof was paid by the following for MDFT training: Asian American Recovery Services, South San Francisco, CA; Advanced Behavioral Health, Middletown, CT. Dr. Dakof is married to Howard Liddle, who is the developer of MDFT.

Marc Fishman, M.D.—*Salary and equity interest* from a substance abuse treatment program; *Past grant support:* Center for Substance Abuse Treatment; *Current grant support:* National Institute on Drug Abuse (through a subcontract); *Consultation to:* International Center for Health Concerns.

Susan H. Godley, Rh.D.—Dr. Godley is the lead author on the adolescent community reinforcement approach treatment manual and directs a training center to help others use it. Agencies and the federal government pay for these training services.

Steven L. Jaffe, M.D.—*Speaker:* McNeil Pediatrics.

Robert Milin, M.D., F.R.C.P.C.—*Speaker:* Janssen-Ortho, Shire: *Advisory capacity:* Shire; *Research grant:* AstraZeneca Canada (as co-investigator).

Jane Ellen Smith, Ph.D.—Dr. Smith is a paid consultant with the Chestnut Health Systems contract with the Center for Substance Abuse Treatment. The project involves the training of therapists to properly use the adolescent community reinforcement approach (A-CRA), which is one of the treatments discussed in the author's chapter. Dr. Smith is coauthor of a book about the adult version of this treatment and receives royalties for it.

The following contributors to this book have no competing interests to report:

Albert J. Arias, M.D.

Janelle E. Arias, M.D.

Richard F. Catalano, Ph.D.

Tammy Chung, Ph.D.

Duncan Clark, M.D., Ph.D.

John F. Curry, Ph.D.

Anne C. Duffy, M.D., F.R.C.P.C.

Jenna Elgin, M.Ed.

Julian D. Ford, Ph.D.

Kevin P. Haggerty, M.S.W.

J. David Hawkins, Ph.D.

Christian Hopfer, M.D.

Yifrah Kaminer, M.D., M.B.A.

John F. Kelly, Ph.D.

John R. Knight, M.D.

Sharon Levy, M.D., M.P.H.

William Lewander, M.D.

Lisa A. Marsch, Ph.D.

Christopher S. Martin, Ph.D.

Peter B. Rockholz, M.S.S.W., L.C.S.W.

Michelle Roley, B.A.

Anthony Spirito, Ph.D., A.B.P.P.

Selena Walker, M.A.

Karen C. Wells, Ph.D.

Ken C. Winters, Ph.D.

Introduction

Despite some inroads made with prevention and intervention efforts, substance use among young people in the United States is still common and of great health significance (Johnston et al. 2008; Krohn et al. 1997). The onset of substance use during adolescence negatively impacts cognitive, physical, and psychosocial development; increases the progression to more serious addiction and psychopathology; and increases the risk of medical problems (Clark and Winters 2002). National surveys show that approximately 85% of adolescents experiment with substances before graduating from high school, and individuals who begin drug use during adolescence have an increased risk of progression to substance use disorders (SUDs) compared with individuals who delay use until adulthood (Winters and Lee 2008). Increased high-risk behaviors of youth (e.g., drug use, reckless driving, aggression, suicidal behavior, irresponsible sexual behavior)—that is, behaviors that are impulsive, disinhibited, not consequence driven, and devoid of the effective use of executive functions—are significantly associated with developmental dysregulation, particularly in the prefrontal cortex, that occurs throughout adolescence and into young adulthood (up to mid-20s) (Chambers et al. 2003). These findings underscore the importance of clinicians' knowledge of risk factors that predict progression from experimentation to SUD, as well as the challenges of developing age-appropriate intervention and treatment strategies to reduce and eliminate substance use and SUD.

Not all adolescents who use substances escalate their use to levels of abuse or dependence (Schulenberg et al. 2001). For those adolescents who show escalating use, several full cycles of use and abuse spanning many years may be the norm rather than the exception (Chung and Maisto 2006). Nonetheless, emerging research on developmental psychopathology and adolescent development has implications for how we view current prevention, intervention, and treatment paradigms. The field can benefit from a greater understanding of how varying levels of substance use severity are viewed within etiological paradigms and optimally treated with different levels and intensities of prevention, intervention, treatment, and aftercare strategies.

The past 20 years have been characterized by a rapid growth of research in the development of screening and assessment tools (Winters and Kaminer 2008), interventions and treatment approaches, and continued care manuals (Kaminer and Napolitano 2010). Some of these interventions have achieved recognition as evidence-based practices—that is, as recommended interventions to treat adolescents with SUD (Waldron and Turner 2008; Winters et al. 2009).

As recently as 1997, fewer than two dozen adolescent treatment studies and no treatment manuals had been published (Williams and Chang 2000). Since then, the number of published studies has doubled, and over two dozen treatment manuals have been published (for a list of Center for Substance Abuse Treatment protocols, see Chestnut Health Systems 2010). Advances include improvement in assessment, implementation, and treatment, including greater understanding of issues related to the treatment process (Grella et al. 2004; see also Chapter 6, "Adolescent Behavioral Change: Process and Outcomes"), psychiatric comorbidity (Kaminer and Bukstein 2008), outcomes (Winters et al. 2009), and methodological issues (Dennis and Kaminer 2006).

This rapid expansion of knowledge is important to clinical researchers and clinicians in the field. Thus, the purpose of this book is to provide an updated, comprehensive, and clinically oriented text. The aim is to inform clinicians (e.g., pediatricians, family physicians, mental health professionals, substance abuse specialists), applied researchers, and public health officials who will benefit from an updated contemporary knowledge pertaining to the identification, assessment, prevention, and treatment of adolescents who are at risk for or who have problems associated with substance abuse.

The substantive content of the book begins with a review of the prevalence and course of adolescent substance use and SUDs (Chapter 1). This review is followed by chapters on prevention approaches (Chapter 2), screening and brief interventions in the clinic office setting (Chapter 3), and use of biomarker testing to detect substance use (Chapter 4).

Chapters 5–11 address treatment issues more directly. Placement criteria and treatment planning are discussed in Chapter 5. An overview of treatment process and outcome for adolescent substance abusers is provided in Chapter 6. Next are chapters on various treatment approaches: pharmacotherapy for SUDs in adolescents (Chapter 7); clinical issues in dealing with relatively new "exotic" classes of substances of abuse, including club drugs and prescription and over-the-counter medications (Chapter 8); brief motivational interventions, cognitive-behavioral therapy, and contingency management reinforcement approaches (Chapter 9); family therapy approaches and a related community-based strategy (Chapter 10); and the 12-step model (Chapter 11).

The next four chapters focus on assessing and treating youth with comorbid psychiatric disorders and problems. Externalizing-related disorders are addressed in Chapter 12, internalizing-related disorders in Chapter 13, suicidal behavior in Chapter 14, and bipolar disorders, schizophrenia, and drug-induced psychosis in Chapter 15. We conclude with an overview of clinical issues pertaining to youth with SUDs in the juvenile justice system (Chapter 16).

This book also includes a handful of appendixes. We provide a summary of screening and comprehensive tools for assessing youth suspected of problems associated with substance use (Appendix A); a listing of printed and web resources on clinical assessment tools, as well as the national website for evidence-based treatment programs (Appendix B); a select list of websites for parents who are seeking advice and resources to learn more about drug prevention and intervention (Appendix C); and a list of websites for general information about self-help, including how to find Alcoholics Anonymous or Narcotics Anonymous meetings in an individual's neighborhood (Appendix D).

We have assembled some of the most prominent authors in the field. These experts were selected because they excel in bridging the knowledge gap between research and the application of clinical practice. These contributors from the United States, Canada, and the United Kingdom review the state of the art from an international data–based literature, with the goal of advancing clinical work and research with adolescent substance abusers. We trust that our applied approach to this book will serve the needs of both researchers and clinicians.

Yifrah Kaminer, M.D., M.B.A.
Ken C. Winters, Ph.D.

References

Chambers RA, Taylor JR, Potenza MN: Developmental neurocircuitry of motivation in adolescence: a critical period of addiction vulnerability. Am J Psychiatry 160:1041–1052, 2003

Chestnut Health Systems: CSAT protocols. Available at: http://www.chestnut.org/li/apss/CSAT/protocols. Accessed January 11, 2010.

Chung T, Maisto SA: Relapse to alcohol and other drug use in treated adolescents: review and reconsideration of relapse as a change point in clinical course. Clin Psychol Rev 26:149–161, 2006

Clark D, Winters KC: Measuring risks and outcomes in substance use disorders prevention research. J Consult Clin Psychol 70:1207–1223, 2002

Dennis ML, Kaminer Y: Introduction to special issue on advances in the assessment and treatment of adolescent substance use disorders. Am J Addict 15 (suppl 1):1–3, 2006

Grella CE, Joshi V, Hser YI: Effects of comorbidity on treatment processes and outcomes among adolescents in drug treatment programs. J Child Adolesc Subst Abuse 13:13–31, 2004

Johnston LD, O'Malley PM, Bachman JG: Monitoring the Future: National Results on Adolescent Drug Use. Overview of Key Findings, 2007. Ann Arbor, University of Michigan Institute for Social Research, 2008

Kaminer Y, Bukstein OG (eds): Adolescent Substance Abuse: Psychiatric Comorbidity and High-Risk Behaviors. New York, Routledge/Taylor & Francis Group, 2008, pp 53–86

Kaminer Y, Napolitano C: Brief Telephone Continuing Care Therapy for Adolescents. Center City, MN, Hazelden, 2010

Krohn MD, Lizotte AJ, Perez CM: The interrelationship between substance use and precocious transitions to adult statuses. J Health Soc Behav 38:87–103, 1997

Schulenberg J, Maggs JL, Steinman KJ, et al: Development matters: taking the long view on substance abuse etiology and intervention during adolescence, in Adolescents, Alcohol, and Substance Use: Reaching Teens Through Brief Interventions. Edited by Monti PM, Colby SM, O'Leary TA. New York, Guilford, 2001, pp 19–57

Waldron H, Turner C: Evidence-based psychosocial treatments for adolescent substance abuse: a review and meta-analysis. J Clin Child Adolesc Psychol 37:1–24, 2008

Williams RJ, Chang SY: Addiction Centre Adolescent Research Group: a comprehensive and comparative review of adolescent substance abuse treatment outcome. Clinical Psychology: Science and Practice 7:138–166, 2000

Winters KC, Kaminer Y: Screening and assessing adolescent substance use disorders in clinical populations. J Am Acad Child Adolesc Psychiatry 47:740–744, 2008

Winters KC, Lee CY: Likelihood of developing an alcohol and cannabis use disorder during youth: association with recent use and age. Drug Alcohol Depend 92:239–247, 2008

Winters KC, Botzet AM, Fahnhorst T, et al: Adolescent substance abuse treatment: a review of evidence-based research, in Handbook on the Prevention and Treatment of Substance Abuse in Adolescence. Edited by Leukefeld C, Gullotta T, Staton Tindall M. New York, Springer, 2009, pp 73–96

1

Prevalence and Clinical Course of Adolescent Substance Use and Substance Use Disorders

Tammy Chung, Ph.D.

Christopher S. Martin, Ph.D.

Adolescence is a critical developmental period that involves pubertal maturation, continuing brain development, changes in social roles (e.g., initiation of dating, obtaining a driver's license) and contexts (e.g., transition to high school, college, and employment), and an increase in risky behavior, such as substance use (Brown et al. 2008). Although experimentation with alcohol and tobacco may be considered developmentally normative, some adolescents progress to a more regular pattern of substance use and, in some cases, substance

The preparation of this manuscript was supported by National Institute on Alcohol Abuse and Alcoholism grants R01 AA014357, R21 AA017128, and R01 AA13397.

1

use disorders (SUDs). Among youth who report substance-related problems, some show a developmentally limited course, whereas others experience more chronic and severe substance-related problems that persist into adulthood. In this chapter, we review adolescence as a developmental period of peak risk for onset of substance use and substance-related problems, describe the prevalence and course of adolescent substance use, cover developmental considerations in the assessment of SUDs in adolescents, and summarize the literature on the prevalence and course of SUDs in youth.

Adolescence as Critical Developmental Period for Initiation of Substance Involvement

Developmental contexts and transitions unique to adolescence influence the emergence and progression of substance involvement in youth (Masten et al. 2008). In particular, continuing brain development during adolescence, which involves synaptic pruning and continuing myelination, results in a developmentally normative delay in the maturation of behavioral inhibitory systems relative to neural systems associated with reward (e.g., sensation seeking) (Ernst et al. 2009). This normative delay in the maturation of behavioral inhibition results in a greater propensity for reward-seeking and risk-taking behaviors in adolescents than in adults (Ernst et al. 2009). The relative priority of reward-related behaviors during adolescence promotes the adoption of adult social roles (e.g., romantic relationships) and independence, but is also thought to underlie the adolescent increase in risk-taking behavior, such as substance use (Ernst et al. 2009).

In addition, animal models suggest that compared with adults, adolescents have lower sensitivity to the sedative effects of some substances (e.g., alcohol), resulting in consumption of a relatively high quantity of a substance (Spear 2000). High-quantity consumption of a substance, in the context of continuing brain development through adolescence, may have adverse effects on neurodevelopment and may increase risk for addiction. Specifically, heavy substance use during adolescence has been associated with neurocognitive deficits (e.g., Tapert et al. 2004), may alter the development of neural systems that modulate reward and inhibitory behavior (Spear 2000), and may delay social maturation and derail the achievement of academic milestones (Masten et al. 2008). Thus, initiation of substance use peaks at a time when the developing brain may be particularly vulnerable to substance dependence–related neuro-adaptation and possible neurotoxic effects of heavy, chronic substance use, highlighting the importance of early intervention to reduce substance use and risk for SUD in adolescence.

Substance Use Prevalence in Adolescents

Substance involvement has been characterized along a continuum that spans abstinence, experimental use, emerging substance-related problems, and SUDs (i.e., abuse and dependence). Two national surveys, Monitoring the Future (MTF) and the National Survey on Drug Use and Health (NSDUH), provide estimates of the prevalence of adolescent substance use in the United States (for websites, see Suggested Readings at end of chapter). The MTF collects substance use data annually from students in grades 8, 10, and 12, and the NSDUH collects annual data on rates of substance use and SUDs from respondents age 12 and older. These two national surveys provide complementary sources of information on the prevalence of adolescent substance use.

Patterns of Substance Use Onset

The prevalence of substance use increases steadily over ages 12–21 (Johnston et al. 2009; Substance Abuse and Mental Health Services Administration 2008c). The substances used most often by adolescents (ages 12–18) include alcohol, tobacco, and cannabis; rates of other illicit drug use (e.g., cocaine, opiates) are relatively low (Johnston et al. 2009; Substance Abuse and Mental Health Services Administration 2008c). Two primary periods of risk for substance use initiation are early adolescence (around ages 13–14, coincident with pubertal maturation) and the transition from late adolescence to early adulthood (Faden 2006; Tucker et al. 2005).

The sequence of initiation to substance use generally begins with use of alcohol and tobacco, which is then typically followed by first use of cannabis, which in turn is followed by first use of other illicit drugs (Kandel 2002). To explain the fairly predictable sequencing of drug use initiation across drug classes, the gateway hypothesis proposes that use of a substance early in the sequence causes use of the next substance in the sequence (Kandel 2002). Other models, which focus on drug availability and a general propensity to engage in substance use, have been proposed to explain regularity in the sequence of drug use initiation (e.g., Macoun 2006). Regardless of the model used to explain the sequencing of initial drug use episodes, however, the progression of use within a drug class, as well as across drug classes, is probabilistic and not inevitable.

Alcohol, Tobacco, and Cannabis Use

Adolescents tend to engage in a risky pattern of alcohol use (e.g., episodic heavy drinking, defined as consuming five or more drinks in a row) that is associated with alcohol-related problems (Miller et al. 2007). During the past decade, the prevalence of episodic heavy drinking among adolescents has slowly declined (Johnston et al. 2009). Among students ages 12–17 in the 2007 NSDUH, 9.7% reported episodic heavy drinking ("binge alcohol use") in the past month (Substance Abuse and Mental Health Services Administration 2008c). In the 2008 MTF survey, prevalence of alcohol use increased with grade, such that 5.4% of eighth graders, 14.4% of tenth graders, and 27.6% of twelfth graders reported being drunk in the past month (Johnston et al. 2009).

Similar to alcohol, the prevalence of cigarette use in the past month has shown a slow decline over the past decade (Johnston et al. 2009). Tobacco use in the past month was reported by 12.4% of students ages 12–17 in the 2007 NSDUH; 9.8% of adolescents reported use of cigarettes, the most popular form of tobacco, and 2.4% used smokeless tobacco (Substance Abuse and Mental Health Services Administration 2008a). According to the 2008 MTF survey, 6.8% of eighth graders, 12.3% of tenth graders, and 20.4% of twelfth graders reported cigarette use in the past month (Johnston et al. 2009).

From 2002 to 2007, the prevalence of illicit drug use in the past month among students ages 12–17 in the NSDUH decreased from 11.6% to 9.5% (Substance Abuse and Mental Health Services Administration 2008c). Overall, cannabis was the illicit drug most commonly used by students in this age range; however, the type of illicit drug most commonly used in the past month differed by age (Substance Abuse and Mental Health Services Administration 2008c). Among those ages 12–13 years, 1.4% reported nonmedical use of prescription medications (e.g., pain relievers, tranquilizers, stimulants) and 0.9% reported cannabis use (Substance Abuse and Mental Health Services Administration 2008c). Among students ages 14–17 years, cannabis was the illicit drug used most often in the past month (5.7% among those ages 14–15, and 13.1% among those ages 16–17), followed by nonmedical use of prescription medication (3.4% among those ages 14–15, and 4.9% among those ages 16–17)

(Substance Abuse and Mental Health Services Administration 2008c). In the 2008 MTF, which does not ask specifically about nonmedical prescription drug use, cannabis was the illicit drug used most often in the past 30 days: 5.8% of eighth graders, 13.8% of tenth graders, and 19.4% of twelfth graders reported cannabis use in the past month (Johnston et al. 2009). Although findings from both the NSDUH and MTF indicated that cannabis is the illicit drug used most often by adolescents, NSDUH data suggest that nonmedical use of prescription medication warrants careful assessment, particularly among younger adolescents (i.e., ages 12–13) who may have access to these medications in their homes.

Differences in Substance Use Prevalence by Gender and Ethnicity

In recent years, the gender gap in rates of adolescent substance use has narrowed (Johnston et al. 2009). For example, although slightly more males than females ages 12–17 years reported heavy episodic drinking in the past month (10.6% vs. 8.8%), similar rates of past-month cigarette use were found for adolescent males and females (10.0% and 9.7%, respectively) (Substance Abuse and Mental Health Services Administration 2008c). The narrowing gender gap in rates of substance use is even clearer in the MTF surveys. For example, starting in 2002, eighth-grade girls had higher 30-day prevalence of alcohol use than their male counterparts, a difference that continued through 2008 (Johnston et al. 2009). Furthermore, beginning in 2005 and continuing through data collected in 2008, tenth-grade girls and boys had equivalent 30-day prevalence of alcohol use (Johnston et al. 2009). With regard to cigarettes, among eighth and tenth graders, males and females in the 2008 MTF had similar 30-day prevalence of cigarette use, although among twelfth graders, males had slightly higher rates of cigarette smoking compared with females (Johnston et al. 2009). The narrowing gender gap in rates of substance use, with females catching up to or surpassing males at some ages and for certain substances, points to the need to identify and address gender-specific risk and protective factors when intervening with adolescents.

With regard to ethnic differences in substance use, MTF data indicate that among the three largest ethnic groups (i.e., Caucasians, African Americans, Hispanics) in the survey, African American students had lower rates of use for most substances than Caucasians, including lower rates of any illicit drug use and cigarette use (Johnston et al. 2009). According to MTF data, Hispanic students had rates of use that were generally lower than those of Caucasians but generally higher than those of African Americans (Johnston et al. 2009). Hispanic students, however, did have some of the highest rates of use for certain drugs (e.g., crack, crystal methamphetamine) in twelfth grade (Johnston et al. 2009). These examples of ethnic differences in substance use suggest the potential benefit of culturally sensitive and tailored interventions to delay initiation of substance use and to prevent the escalation of substance involvement during adolescence (e.g., Gil et al. 2004).

Trajectories of Substance Use During Adolescence

Cross-sectional prevalence data provide a snapshot of substance use at a given point in time but do not provide information on changes over time in an individual's pattern of substance use. Longitudinal studies beginning in adolescence and extending into young adulthood have identified prototypical trajectories of alcohol, cigarette, cannabis, and substance use more generally (e.g., Schulenberg et al. 2001). Trajectories capture, at the level of the individual, differences in earlier versus later onset of use, changes in level of substance use over time, and turning points in substance involvement (Brown et al. 2008). The most common trajectory types that have emerged in research based on community samples of youth include stable low, chronic high, developmentally limited, and later-onset, increasing trajectories of substance use. In community samples, the developmentally normative and modal trajectory for alcohol, cigarette, and cannabis use involved light (i.e., experimental) to moderate use of alcohol and tobacco, and no use to light use of cannabis; the least prevalent trajectory type generally involved heavy and chronic substance use (e.g., Schulenberg et al. 2001; Tucker et al. 2005). Adolescents with trajectories involving low to no substance use through young adulthood tend to have the best outcomes, whereas individuals with more chronic and severe trajectories across substances, including trajectories of increasing use in the transition to adulthood, tend to have worse young adult outcomes (e.g., Tucker et al. 2005).

Diagnosis of Substance Use Disorders

Although substance involvement may be optimally represented by a continuum of severity in use and problems, diagnosis or the categorical determination of the presence or absence of a disorder serves important functions. Valid diagnosis provides a method for case identification in the service of clinical and research goals, facilitates communication among clinicians and researchers, and can be used to help educate patients and families regarding key features of the disorder and likely prognosis (American Psychiatric Association 2000). The *Diagnostic and Statistical Manual of Mental Disorders*, 4th Edition (DSM-IV; American Psychiatric Association 1994), and its text revision, DSM-IV-TR (American Psychiatric Association 2000), recognize two SUDs: abuse and dependence. Each SUD is operationally defined by a list of criteria, of which no single symptom is necessary or sufficient, and an algorithm that is used to determine the presence or absence of a diagnosis. In addition, clinically significant impairment in functioning or subjective feelings of distress must be present for an SUD diagnosis to be made.

DSM-IV substance abuse, which is considered a milder SUD than dependence, requires meeting one of four criteria. Criteria for substance abuse cover certain recurrent psychosocial consequences related to substance use (e.g., school grades dropped due to substance use, interpersonal relations damaged due to substance use, substance-related legal problems) and hazardous substance use (e.g., driving when intoxicated). Relative to substance abuse, DSM-IV substance dependence is usually considered a more severe SUD and requires meeting three of seven criteria within the same 1-year period. Dependence criteria include physical symptoms (i.e., a high level of tolerance, withdrawal), symptoms indicating high salience of substance use behavior (i.e., much time spent using, prioritization of drug-related activities as indicated by reducing other activities because of substance use), and impaired control over substance use (i.e., more frequent or longer use than intended, difficulty cutting down or abstaining from use, use despite adverse physical and psychological consequences of substance use). The seven dependence criteria are applied to all substances, with the exception that withdrawal is not used to determine a diagnosis of dependence for cannabis and hallucinogens (i.e., for these two substances, three of six dependence criteria need to be met within the same 1-year period). Notably, the criteria used to diagnose substance abuse and dependence do not overlap, a diagnosis of nicotine "abuse" is not included in DSM-IV, and a diagnosis of dependence precludes the diagnosis of the milder disorder of abuse.

DSM-IV SUD Prevalence in Adolescent Samples

The most common SUDs among youth ages 12–17 involve alcohol, cannabis, and tobacco (Substance Abuse and Mental Health Services Administration 2008a, 2008c). Among adolescent substance users, a pattern of polysubstance use, which often involves alcohol, tobacco, and cannabis, is frequently observed (Kaminer and Bukstein 2008), and suggests a concentration of substance-related problems within a relatively small proportion of adolescents who may experience problems in multiple areas of functioning (e.g., home, school, relationships with peers) due to substance use.

From 2002 to 2007, the prevalence of past-year DSM-IV alcohol abuse or dependence was relatively stable among individuals ages 12–17 years (5.9% in 2002 and 5.4% in 2007), although past-year diagnosis of abuse of or dependence on illicit drugs decreased from 5.6% in 2002 to 4.3% in 2007, mostly due to a decline in cannabis diagnoses (Substance Abuse and Mental Health Services Administration 2008b). Cross-sectional survey data indicate that the prevalence of SUD increases with age through adolescence and peaks in young adulthood. In the 2007 NSDUH, prevalence of past-year DSM-IV SUD was 7.7% among individuals ages 12–17 years (5.4% had an alcohol diagnosis, 4.3% had a cannabis diagnosis), 20.7% among individuals ages 18–25 years, and 7.2% among adults age 26 and older (Substance Abuse and Mental Health Services Administration 2008b). Among past-month cigarette users ages 12–17 years, 36.4% were estimated to have nicotine dependence (Substance Abuse and Mental Health Services Administration 2008a). For some adolescents, the transition from initial use to SUD may occur within 3 years of first use of a substance (Substance Abuse and Mental Health Services Administration 2009), emphasizing the importance of early detection and intervention for substance-related problems.

In addition to adolescents who meet criteria for a DSM-IV SUD diagnosis, some youth report one or two dependence symptoms but do not meet criteria for an SUD. In the 2001 NSDUH survey, 4% of students ages 12–17 reported one or two alcohol dependence symptoms but did not have an alcohol use diagnosis (Harford et al. 2005). One review found that these subthreshold cases, known as "diagnostic orphans," represented up to an additional 17% of teens who reported alcohol-related problems in community surveys (Chung et al. 2002). Adolescents with subthreshold symptoms of dependence are at higher risk for SUD in young adulthood (e.g., Wu et al. 2008), highlighting the importance of early detection and intervention in adolescence to halt the progression of substance involvement and to reduce the peak rates of SUD that occur in young adulthood.

Data from the 2007 NSDUH indicate similar rates of past-year SUD for males and females ages 12–17 years (7.7% for both genders), again pointing to a narrowing of the gender gap, particularly among adolescents, in rates of substance involvement (Harford et al. 2005; Substance Abuse and Mental Health Services Administration 2008c). Likewise, the prevalence of DSM-IV nicotine dependence was similar for adolescent males and females in one community survey (Kandel et al. 2005). Similar to ethnic differences that are observed in the prevalence of substance use, Caucasian adolescents had higher rates of past-year SUD (alcohol or illicit drugs) compared with African American and Hispanic youth (9%, 5%, and 7%, respectively); the higher rate of SUD among Caucasian youth is due mainly to the higher prevalence of alcohol use disorders in this subgroup (Substance Abuse and Mental Health Services Administration 2008b). Caucasian youth also had higher rates of DSM-IV nicotine dependence compared with African American and Hispanic youth in a school-based survey (Kandel et al. 2005). Little is known regarding gender and ethnic differences in SUD prevalence among adolescents, although ethnicity and gender may influence the timing and type of substance-related symptoms reported (Wagner et al. 2002).

SUD Diagnosis and Treatment Utilization

Very few adolescents who meet criteria for a DSM-IV SUD reported receiving treatment. Only 0.6% of teens ages 12–17 reported receiving treatment for alcohol or other drugs in the past year, although 8% met criteria for a past-year DSM-IV SUD diagnosis (Substance Abuse and Mental Health Services Administration 2008b). Among admissions to publicly funded substance use treatment programs, adolescents (ages 12–19) represented 11% of all admissions in 2007 (Substance Abuse and Mental Health Services Administration 2009).

Of adolescents ages 15–19 who were admitted, 35% reported cannabis as their primary substance upon treatment admission (Substance Abuse and Mental Health Services Administration 2009). Among adolescents ages 12–17 in publicly funded addiction treatment, most were referred by the criminal justice system, with smaller proportions referred by schools or family (Dennis et al. 2003). Treatment utilization statistics for adolescents suggest a high level of unmet treatment need, as well as the importance of increasing adolescents' readiness to change their substance use behavior, because most youth do not refer themselves to treatment for substance use.

Limitations of DSM-IV SUDs

Although DSM-IV SUDs have demonstrated some validity in adolescents against independent external validators, such as level of substance involvement and impairment in psychosocial functioning (e.g., Crowley et al. 2001), limitations of these diagnoses also have been identified (Martin et al. 2008). For example, research does not support the validity of the DSM-IV distinction between abuse and dependence diagnoses in terms of the relative severity of the diagnoses, or the symptoms used to define abuse and dependence (e.g., Chung and Martin 2005). Specifically, DSM-IV substance abuse and dependence symptoms have generally been found to represent a single continuum of illness severity rather than separate dimensions representing abuse and dependence (e.g., Harford et al. 2009). The total number of symptoms, rather than type of symptom, appears to provide the basis for identifying more homogeneous groups of adolescents with substance-related problems (e.g., Chung and Martin 2005). Furthermore, in one study of adolescents, subthreshold cases of dependence did not differ from cases of substance abuse on various external validators (Pollock and Martin 1999).

At the symptom level, certain symptoms, such as substance-related legal problems, also appear to be more likely to be endorsed by certain subgroups, such as males and youth with conduct problems. Another limitation at the symptom level is that DSM-IV SUD criteria focus on failed attempts to quit or cut down, and may not capture individuals with frequent, heavy substance use who have not yet made an attempt to cut down on substance use, resulting in a possible underestimation of individuals with substance-related problems. These limitations of DSM-IV SUD diagnoses, which apply to adults as well as adolescents, need to be considered in the context of developmentally informed assessment of substance involvement.

Developmentally Informed SUD Assessment

Because of adolescent substance users' relatively short histories of use and developmental context (e.g., living with parents), SUD constructs and criteria need to be adapted to minimize false-positive and false-negative diagnostic and symptom assignments, and to increase overall validity of SUD diagnoses in adolescents. Developmentally informed SUD symptom assessment involves 1) consideration of how SUD constructs (e.g., tolerance) may manifest or be interpreted differently in adolescents and adults, 2) identification of substance-related problems that are relevant to youth, and 3) efforts to scale symptom and diagnostic thresholds to optimize performance in adolescents. Comprehensive reviews of measures used to assess SUDs in adolescents are available (e.g., Winters et al. 2008a).

Certain SUD symptoms may manifest differently in adolescents and adults, or may be interpreted differently by adolescents, due to the developmental context in which a symptom occurs. For example, the frequent endorsement by adolescents of the dependence symptom "spending much time trying to obtain alcohol, drinking, or getting over its effects" was due to their difficulties in obtaining alcohol related to their status as minors rather than to a compulsive pattern of use, which is the intended meaning of the item (Harford et al. 2005). As another example, some adolescents endorsed "using more or longer than intended" because they drank more than the usual amount needed to become intoxicated, rather than due to the intended meaning of the symptom, which involves a failed attempt to cut down on drinking. Differences between adolescents and adults in their interpretation of certain SUD symptoms may lead to biased estimates of SUD in youth (Harford et al. 2005). These differences emphasize the importance of careful construction of symptom queries and of probing adolescents' responses to ensure that the interviewer and respondent have a shared understanding of the phenomenon being queried.

Some SUD criteria represent relatively abstract and complex constructs (e.g., a high level of tolerance to drug effects, impaired control over substance use). To improve validity of the assessment of more complex constructs, a brief description of the phenomenon of interest (e.g., failed attempt to cut down on use) could be provided to the adolescent to ensure a common understanding of the construct being queried. In addition, providing specific examples of how the symptom may manifest in relation to the adolescent's own experiences, or with family, at home, or at school, may facilitate recall of substance-related problems. Some SUD criteria (e.g., using more or longer than intended) need to be split into separate questions to better assess complex constructs. Follow-up probes can be used to reduce false-positive symptom assignments. For example, clarification could be obtained to determine whether much time spent obtaining alcohol reflects a compulsive pattern of use (the intended meaning of the criterion) or difficulties in obtaining alcohol due to minor status (possible false positive).

In addition to improvements in the assessment of certain SUD symptoms, possible revisions to DSM-IV SUD criteria need to be considered to improve the validity of SUD diagnoses in youth. For example, SUD criteria could be expanded to include symptoms such as recurrent substance-related risky sexual behavior, repeated alcohol-related blackouts, and passing out from substance use, which may be of particular relevance to adolescent substance use patterns. Average quantity, frequency, and patterns of substance use also need to be considered when SUDs are being assessed in adolescents, particularly in relation to tobacco use, because adolescents sometimes endorse symptoms of dependence despite low levels of tobacco use (Kandel et al. 2005). Another consideration in revising SUD criteria for use with adolescents involves the need to appropriately scale certain symptoms (e.g., high level of tolerance to drug effects) to efficiently distinguish between normative and clinically significant levels of substance use that are associated with a compulsive pattern of use. Developmentally based assessment can improve diagnostic validity and increase understanding of the development and course of adolescent-onset SUD.

Course of Adolescent-Onset SUDs

Studies of clinical course, which document changes in severity and patterns of substance involvement over time, provide information on factors associated with the onset, maintenance, and remission of substance involvement. Multiple etiological models have been proposed to explain the onset and maintenance of SUD, including individual differences in sensitivity and response to drug effects, deviance proneness, and the use of substances to regulate affect (e.g., to "get high," to reduce negative mood) (Brown et al. 2008). In the following subsections, we review research on SUD symptom development, course of SUD in community and treatment samples, and predictors of SUD course among treated adolescents.

SUD Symptom Development

Although individuals vary in the probability of symptom progression and the speed of symptom development, some regularity exists in the emergence of SUD symptoms in adolescents. Among adolescent regular drinkers, alcohol-related interpersonal problems tend to emerge first, within the first 2 years of regular drinking, followed by other alcohol-related consequences and symptoms of dependence, and withdrawal generally emerges last (Wagner et al. 2002). Among adolescent cannabis users, an indicator of impaired control over cannabis use (i.e., used more than intended) tends to emerge within the first year of regular use, followed by the emergence of cannabis-related physical or psychological problems within another year (Rosenberg and Anthony 2001). Among adolescent cigarette smokers, the first symptoms to emerge involve impaired control over cigarette use (e.g., strong craving), typically within the first year of monthly smoking (DiFranza et al. 2002). The early emergence of symptoms indicating impaired control over use for cannabis and tobacco may reflect greater addiction liability for these substances relative to alcohol, but also needs to be interpreted with some caution due to methodological issues in the assessment of complex constructs such as impaired control over substance use in relatively inexperienced, adolescent substance users.

SUD Symptom Profiles in Youth

Symptom profiles at the level of the individual can help to identify more homogeneous subgroups of youth that may have a common etiology, course, and treatment response. The DSM-IV SUD symptoms that are most often endorsed by adolescents are tolerance and using more or longer than intended (e.g., Chung et al. 2002). For alcohol and other drugs, a milder symptom profile includes endorsement of symptoms such as substance-related interpersonal problems, impairment in meeting major role obligations (e.g., at school or work) due to substance use, and tolerance to drug effects (Chung and Martin 2005). The more severe symptom profile involves endorsement of symptoms in the milder profile in addition to symptoms such as using more or longer than intended, much time spent using, and reducing other activities to engage in substance use. Among the symptoms assessed, withdrawal is generally reported infrequently by teens in relation to alcohol, cocaine, and opiate use (Chung and Martin 2005). Information on adolescents' symptom profiles can provide a focus for intervention by targeting the types of symptoms reported most often by adolescent substance users.

SUD Course in Community Samples

Of adolescents with an alcohol use disorder, 55%–62% had an alcohol diagnosis when followed up as young adults (Clark et al. 2003), suggesting a developmentally limited course of alcohol involvement for some, but a more chronic course for others. Epidemiological data on the course of adolescent-onset cannabis use disorders in the United States are scarce. Longitudinal studies of adolescents in Europe and Australia indicate that adolescent regular cannabis users are more likely to have a chronic cannabis use disorder through young adulthood (i.e., at age 24; Swift et al. 2008), and that rates of remission from cannabis use disorder are relatively low overall, until at least the mid-30s (Perkonigg et al. 2008). These epidemiological studies suggest that risk for more chronic cannabis and alcohol use disorders is concentrated primarily among individuals who establish more regular patterns of substance use during adolescence, although developmentally limited patterns also have been observed.

Posttreatment Course of Substance Involvement

Several models of substance use treatment for adolescents (e.g., group cognitive-behavioral therapy) are in use (for a review, see Wagner 2008), and a recent meta-analysis indicated that no single type of treatment for adolescent substance use is clearly superior to any other (Waldron and Turner 2008). Treated adolescents generally show reductions in substance involvement, compared with pretreatment levels, along with concurrent improvements in psychosocial functioning over short- and longer-term follow-up (Chung and Maisto 2006). However, considerable variability exists in the course of adolescents' posttreatment substance involvement.

Studies of short-term posttreatment course (i.e., ≤18-month follow-up) have identified multiple prototypical trajectories of substance involvement that include stable low and stable high levels of use, and increasing and decreasing patterns of use (e.g., Chung et al. 2005; Waldron et al. 2005). Similar trajectory types have been identified for alcohol and cannabis following treatment (Waldron et al. 2005). Although most studies have focused on level of substance use, one study identified stable low, moderate, and severe levels of alcohol-related symptoms in the year following treatment (Chung et al. 2005). The alcohol symptoms most often reported over 1-year follow-up included interpersonal problems due to drinking, and symptoms involving impaired control over alcohol use (Chung et al. 2005).

Studies of longer-term posttreatment clinical course in treated adolescents provide the opportunity to examine how specific developmental factors (e.g., high school graduation) and changes in social context (e.g., living independently) are associated with changes in pattern of substance use following treatment. Most research has examined changes in level of substance use following treatment (e.g., Winters et al. 2008b), although some studies have documented posttreatment changes in SUD symptoms (e.g., Chung et al. 2008). Across studies, similar trajectory types were identified despite differences in type of substance examined (e.g., alcohol, cannabis, other illicit drugs), differences in definition of substance involvement (e.g., frequency of use, substance-related problems), and regional differences in study location.

The longer-term posttreatment trajectories most commonly identified across studies include stable abstinence, infrequent use, gradually decreasing substance involvement ("slow improvers"), and persistent high substance involvement. Although the actual proportion represented by each trajectory type differed across studies, the relative proportions were similar, with most youth classified as slow improvers or infrequent users, and smaller proportions classified in stable abstinence and persistent high substance involvement trajectories. Analyses of longer-term concurrent patterns of change for alcohol, marijuana, and other drugs indicated a moderate level of cross-drug concordance in posttreatment pattern of change (Chung et al. 2008). The similarity in posttreatment patterns of change across drugs suggests that reductions in the use of one substance may be associated with parallel reductions in the use of other substances, rather than providing support for drug substitution effects, and that treatment has a general positive effect in reducing substance involvement for many youth.

Posttreatment Trajectories of Substance Involvement and Psychosocial Outcomes

As may be expected, adolescents in stable abstinence and low substance involvement trajectories following treatment generally have better emotional, interpersonal, and family functioning in young adulthood compared with those continuing chronic heavy substance involvement (e.g., Brown et al. 2001). Changes in different areas of psychosocial functioning occur at different rates, with improvement in school functioning occurring within 1 year after treatment but improvements in family functioning becoming evident only 2 years after treatment (Brown et al. 2001). More chronic and severe trajectories of substance involvement also may reflect the impact of co-occurring psychopathology (e.g., conduct problems) on the course of recovery from SUD. Despite significant reductions in substance involvement and improvements in areas of school performance, interpersonal relations, and other areas, treated teens continued to show greater problem severity compared with a community comparison sample (Winters et al. 2008b). In one study, treated adolescent substance users were at higher risk for adverse outcomes (e.g., poverty, death) over 30-year follow-up (Hodgins et al. 2009). These studies document how adolescent-onset SUD, in combination with co-occurring psychopathology, can delay or derail achievement of adolescent developmental milestones, with effects that persist into adulthood.

Predictors of SUD Course: Before, During, and After Treatment

The most robust pretreatment characteristics that have been associated with more persistent trajectories of substance involvement include temperament and co-occurring psychopathology. During treatment, factors associated with better outcomes include longer duration of treatment, greater readiness to change substance use behavior, and family involvement in treatment (see review by Waldron and Turner 2008). Importantly, posttreatment factors generally account for more of the variance in outcome over 1-year follow-up than pretreatment and during-treatment factors (Hsieh et al. 1998). Treatment may help initially to increase an adolescent's motivation to reduce substance use; however, the posttreatment environment (e.g., family, peers) is essential to supporting and maintaining treatment gains (Dennis et al. 2003). Posttreatment factors associated with better outcomes include aftercare involvement (e.g., Winters et al. 2000), low levels of peer substance use (e.g., Winters et al. 2000), and continued commitment to abstain (King et al. 2009). Adolescent substance users may require more than one episode of treatment to solidify treatment gains and to make progress toward more stable recovery (Dennis et al. 2003). Dynamic models of posttreatment change in substance use and environmental context need to be investigated, because the importance of a course predictor may differ with the transition from adolescence to young adulthood (e.g., shift in the importance of family vs. peer influence).

Co-occurring Psychopathology and SUD Course

Co-occurring psychopathology refers to two or more psychiatric conditions that may occur simultaneously or sequentially in an individual. Comorbid conditions, such as conduct problems and depression, may affect the timing of onset, rate of development, severity, and duration of SUD (Kaminer and Bukstein 2008). The conditions most commonly associated with adolescent substance involvement include conduct problems, mood disorders (e.g., depression), attention-deficit/hyperactivity disorder, and physical or sexual trauma (Armstrong and Costello 2002). A review of community-based studies found that a majority (~60%) of adolescent substance users had a comorbid psychiatric condition (Armstrong and Costello 2002). Among adolescents in substance use treatment, more than half are estimated to have a co-occurring mental illness (Dennis et al. 2003). Some studies of adolescents with SUD have found that females were more likely than males to exhibit internalizing (e.g., depression, anxiety) symptoms and trauma syndromes (e.g., Kaminer and Bukstein 2008). Little is known about ethnic differences in SUD and co-occurring psychiatric conditions. Dual diagnosis programs for adolescent substance users are still relatively rare (Kaminer and Bukstein 2008), although some youth in substance use treatment indicate a need for intervention that addresses co-occurring psychiatric conditions. (For additional reviews of the literature on co-occurring externalizing and internalizing psychopathology, see Chapters 12 and 13, respectively.)

Conclusion

The use of a developmental framework to assess adolescent substance involvement recognizes the unique features of adolescence, such as continuing brain development and a normative increase in risk-taking behavior, that may influence levels of substance involvement and the types of substance-related problems most often experienced by youth. Although some decline has occurred in the prevalence of adolescent substance use in the past decade, cause for concern still exists with regard to the narrowing gender gap in substance use, particularly during adolescence. Multiple trajectories of substance involvement have been identified, with most youth showing no to low levels of use, or developmentally limited patterns of substance use and related problems. Developmentally informed assessment of adolescent substance involvement is essential to understanding etiology and the factors influencing clinical course. For many youth referred to substance use treatment, the treatment generally results in some reduction in substance use compared with preintervention levels. However, multiple episodes of treatment may be needed for some adolescents, and co-occurring psychopathology complicates the course of recovery from adolescent-onset SUD. Research indicates that treatment for substance use may initially increase adolescents' readiness to change substance use behavior, but family, peers, and the larger community play important roles in supporting and maintaining stable recovery for adolescent substance users.

Key Clinical Concepts

- A developmental framework for adolescent substance use assessment incorporates unique features of adolescence, such as the continuing maturation of the brain into young adulthood, a normative increase in risk-taking behavior, and the increasing importance of peer relationships during adolescence, when patterns and problems related to substance use are being queried.

- Developmentally informed assessment and intervention require querying about substance-related problems that are relevant to the adolescent's developmental stage and environmental context, and addressing emerging symptoms prior to the onset of substance use disorder.

- Initiation of substance use peaks at a time when the developing brain may be particularly vulnerable to the neurotoxic effects of heavy substance use, highlighting the importance of efforts to prevent substance use.

- The gender gap in rates of substance involvement has narrowed in recent years, with females catching up to or surpassing males in rates of use for certain substances, such as tobacco.

- On average, adolescents tend to show a reduction in substance use following treatment; however, posttreatment course is variable, aftercare helps to maintain treatment gains, and more than one episode of treatment may be needed for some adolescents with more severe substance involvement.

References

American Psychiatric Association: Diagnostic and Statistical Manual of Mental Disorders, 4th Edition. Washington, DC, American Psychiatric Association, 1994

American Psychiatric Association: Diagnostic and Statistical Manual of Mental Disorders, 4th Edition, Text Revision. Washington, DC, American Psychiatric Association, 2000

Armstrong TD, Costello EJ: Community studies on adolescent substance use, abuse, or dependence and psychiatric comorbidity. J Consult Clin Psychol 70:1224–1239, 2002

Brown SA, D'Amico EJ, McCarthy DM, et al: Four-year outcomes from adolescent alcohol and drug treatment. J Stud Alcohol 62:381–388, 2001

Brown SA, McGue M, Maggs J, et al: A developmental perspective on alcohol and youths 16 to 20 years of age. Pediatrics 121 (suppl 4):S290–S310, 2008

Chung T, Maisto SA: Relapse to alcohol and other drug use in treated adolescents: review and reconsideration of relapse as a change point in clinical course. Clin Psychol Rev 26:149–161, 2006

Chung T, Martin CS: Classification and short-term course of cannabis, hallucinogen, cocaine, and opioid disorders in treated adolescents. J Consult Clin Psychol 73:995–1004, 2005

Chung T, Martin CS, Armstrong TD, et al: Prevalence of DSM-IV alcohol diagnoses and symptoms in adolescent community and clinical samples. J Am Acad Child Adolesc Psychiatry 41:546–554, 2002

Chung T, Maisto SA, Cornelius JR, et al: Joint trajectory analysis of treated adolescents' alcohol use and symptoms over 1 year. Addict Behav 30:1690–1701, 2005

Chung T, Martin CS, Clark DB: Concurrent change in alcohol and drug problems among treated adolescents over three years. J Stud Alcohol 69:420–429, 2008

Clark DB, DeBellis M, Lynch K, et al: Physical and sexual abuse, depression and alcohol use disorders in adolescents: onsets and outcomes. Drug Alcohol Depend 69:51–60, 2003

Crowley TJ, Mikulich S, Ehlers K, et al: Validity of structured clinical evaluations in adolescents with conduct and substance problems. J Am Acad Child Adolesc Psychiatry 40:265–273, 2001

Dennis ML, Dawud-Noursi S, Muck RD, et al: The need for developing and evaluating adolescent treatment models, in Adolescent Substance Abuse Treatment in the United States: Exemplary Models From a National Evaluation Study. Edited by Stevens SJ, Morral AR. Binghamton, NY, Haworth, 2003, pp 3–34

DiFranza JR, Savageau JA, Rigotti NA, et al: Development of symptoms of tobacco dependence in youths: 30 month follow-up data from the DANDY study. Tob Control 11:228–235, 2002

Ernst M, Romeo RD, Andersen SL: Neurobiology of the development of motivated behaviors in adolescence: a window into a neural systems model. Pharmacol Biochem Behav 93:199–211, 2009

Faden V: Trends in initiation of alcohol use in the United States 1975 to 2003. Alcohol Clin Exp Res 30:1011–1022, 2006

Gil AG, Wagner EF, Tubman JG: Culturally sensitive substance abuse intervention for Hispanic and African American adolescents: empirical examples from the Alcohol Treatment Targeting Adolescents in Need (ATTAIN) project. Addiction 99 (suppl 2):S140–S150, 2004

Harford TC, Grant B, Yi H-Y, et al: Patterns of DSM-IV alcohol abuse and dependence criteria among adolescents and adults: results from the 2001 National Household Survey on Drug Abuse. Alcohol Clin Exp Res 29:810–828, 2005

Harford TC, Yi H-Y, Faden VB, et al: The dimensionality of DSM-IV alcohol use disorders among adolescent and adult drinkers and symptom patterns by age, gender, and race/ethnicity. Alcohol Clin Exp Res 33:868–878, 2009

Hodgins S, Larm P, Molero-Samuleson Y, et al: Multiple adverse outcomes over 30 years following adolescent substance misuse treatment. Acta Psychiatr Scand 119:484–493, 2009

Hsieh S, Hoffmann NG, Hollister CD: The relationship between pre-, during-, posttreatment factors, and adolescent substance abuse behaviors. Addict Behav 23:477–488, 1998

Johnston LD, O'Malley PM, Bachman JG, et al: Monitoring the future national results on adolescent drug use: overview of key findings 2008 (NIH Publ No 09-7401). Bethesda, MD, National Institute on Drug Abuse, 2009

Kaminer Y, Bukstein O (eds): Adolescent Substance Abuse: Psychiatric Comorbidity and High Risk Behaviors. New York, Routledge/Taylor & Francis, 2008, pp 53–86

Kandel DB: Stages and Pathways of Drug Involvement: Examining the Gateway Hypothesis. Cambridge, England, Cambridge University Press, 2002

Kandel D, Schaffran C, Griesler P, et al: On the measurement of nicotine dependence in adolescence: comparisons of the mFTQ and a DSM-IV-based scale. J Pediatr Psychol 30:319–332, 2005

King KM, Chung T, Maisto SA: Adolescents' thoughts about abstinence curb the return of marijuana use during and after treatment. J Consult Clin Psychol 77:554–565, 2009

Macoun RJ: Competing accounts of the gateway effect: the field thins, but still no clear winner. Addiction 101:470–476, 2006

Martin CS, Chung T, Langenbucher JW: How should we revise diagnostic criteria for substance use disorders in DSM-V? J Abnorm Psychol 117:561–575, 2008

Masten AS, Faden VB, Zucker RA, et al: Underage drinking: a developmental framework. Pediatrics 121 (suppl 4):S235–S251, 2008

Miller JW, Naimi TS, Brewer RD, et al: Binge drinking and associated health risk behaviors among high school students. Pediatrics 119:76–85, 2007

Perkonigg A, Goodwin R, Fiedler A, et al: The natural course of cannabis use, abuse and dependence during the first decades of life. Addiction 103:439–449, 2008

Pollock NK, Martin CS: Diagnostic orphans: adolescents with alcohol symptoms who do not qualify for DSM-IV abuse or dependence diagnoses. Am J Psychiatry 156:897–901, 1999

Rosenberg MF, Anthony JC: Early clinical manifestations of cannabis dependence in a community sample. Drug Alcohol Depend 64:123–131, 2001

Schulenberg J, Maggs JL, Steinman KJ, et al: Development matters: taking the long view on substance abuse etiology and intervention during adolescence, in Adolescents, Alcohol, and Substance Use: Reaching Teens Through Brief Interventions. Edited by Monti PM, Colby SM, O'Leary TA. New York, Guilford, 2001, pp 19–57

Spear LP: The adolescent brain and age-related behavioral manifestations. Neurosci Biobehav Rev 24:417–463, 2000

Substance Abuse and Mental Health Services Administration, Office of Applied Studies: The NSDUH report: nicotine dependence: 2006. Rockville, MD, Substance Abuse and Mental Health Services Administration, 2008a

Substance Abuse and Mental Health Services Administration, Office of Applied Studies: The NSDUH report: trends in substance use, dependence, or abuse, and treatment among adolescents: 2002 to 2007. Rockville, MD, Substance Abuse and Mental Health Services Administration, 2008b

Substance Abuse and Mental Health Services Administration, Office of Applied Studies: Results from the 2007 National Survey on Drug Use and Health: national findings (NSDUH Series H-34, DHHS Publ No SMA 08-4343). Rockville, MD, Substance Abuse and Mental Health Services Administration, 2008c

Substance Abuse and Mental Health Services Administration, Office of Applied Studies: Treatment Episode Data Set (TEDS). Highlights—2007: national admissions to substance abuse treatment services (DASIS Series S-45; DHHS Publ No SMA-09-4360). Rockville, MD, Substance Abuse and Mental Health Services Administration, 2009

Swift W, Coffey C, Carlin J, et al: Adolescent cannabis users at 24 years: trajectories to regular weekly use and dependence in adulthood. Addiction 103:1361–1370, 2008

Tapert SF, Schweinsburg AD, Barlett VC, et al: Blood oxygen level dependent response and spatial working memory in adolescents with alcohol use disorders. Alcohol Clin Exp Res 28:1577–1586, 2004

Tucker JS, Ellickson PL, Orlando M, et al: Substance use trajectories from early adolescence to emerging adulthood: a comparison of smoking, binge drinking, and marijuana use. J Drug Issues 5:307–332, 2005

Wagner EF: Developmentally informed research on the effectiveness of clinical trials: a primer for assessing how developmental issues may influence treatment responses among adolescents with alcohol use problems. Pediatrics 121 (suppl 4):S337–S347, 2008

Wagner EF, Lloyd DA, Gil AG: Racial/ethnic and gender differences in the incidence and onset age of DSM-IV alcohol use disorder symptoms among adolescents. J Stud Alcohol 63:609–619, 2002

Waldron H, Turner C: Evidence-based psychosocial treatments for adolescent substance abuse: a review and meta-analysis. J Clin Child Adolesc Psychol 37:1–24, 2008

Waldron H, Turner C, Ozechowski T: Profiles of drug use behavior change for adolescents in treatment. Addict Behav 30:1775–1796, 2005

Winters KC, Latimer WW, Stinchfield RD, et al: Examining psychosocial correlates of drug involvement among drug clinic–referred youth. J Child Adolesc Subst Abuse 9:1–17, 2000

Winters KC, Stinchfield R, Bukstein O: Assessing adolescent substance use and abuse, in Adolescent Substance Abuse: Psychiatric Comorbidity and High Risk Behaviors. Edited by Kaminer Y, Bukstein O. New York, Routledge, 2008a, pp 53–86

Winters KC, Stinchfield R, Latimer WW, et al: Internalizing and externalizing behaviors and their association with the treatment of adolescents with substance use disorder. J Subst Abuse Treat 35:269–278, 2008b

Wu L-T, Ringwalt C, Mannelli P, et al: Prescription pain reliever abuse and dependence among adolescents: a nationally representative study. J Am Acad Child Adolesc Psychiatry 47:1020–1029, 2008

Suggested Readings

Brown SA, McGue M, Maggs J, et al: A developmental perspective on alcohol and youths 16 to 20 years of age. Pediatrics 121 (suppl 4):S290–S310, 2008

Masten AS, Faden VB, Zucker RA, et al: Underage drinking: a developmental framework. Pediatrics 121 (suppl 4):S235–S251, 2008

Wagner EF: Developmentally informed research on the effectiveness of clinical trials: a primer for assessing how developmental issues may influence treatment responses among adolescents with alcohol use problems. Pediatrics 121 (suppl 4):S337–S347, 2008

Waldron H, Turner C: Evidence-based psychosocial treatments for adolescent substance abuse: a review and meta-analysis. J Clin Child Adolesc Psychol 37:1–24, 2008

Relevant Websites

Monitoring the Future (national school-based survey of alcohol and substance use): http://www.monitoringthefuture.org

National Institute on Alcohol Abuse and Alcoholism (NIAAA): http://www.niaaa.nih.gov

NIAAA's informational website for young teens on resisting peer pressure to drink: http://www.thecoolspot.gov

National Institute on Drug Abuse (NIDA): http://www.nida.nih.gov

Students and young adults: http://www.nida.nih.gov/students.html

Parents and teachers: http://www.nida.nih.gov/parent-teacher.html

National Survey on Drug Use & Health (formerly National Household Survey on Drug Abuse) (an annual national survey of substance use): http://www.oas.samhsa.gov/nhsda.htm

2

Prevention of Substance Use and Substance Use Disorders

Role of Risk and Protective Factors

Richard F. Catalano, Ph.D.

Kevin P. Haggerty, M.S.W.

J. David Hawkins, Ph.D.

Jenna Elgin, M.Ed.

Most young people who initiate the use of alcohol, tobacco, or other substances do not go on to develop a problem with abuse or dependence (Thombs 2006). In fact, nearly two-thirds of young people who try a substance do not develop a chronic problem (Hingson et al. 2003). However, about one-third of young people begin a journey down the road to abuse and dependence. What is the difference between those whose use becomes abusive or dependent and those who do not develop these problems? In this chapter, we summarize and update work we have done in examining factors in individuals and their environment that put young people at risk for substance abuse and dependence, as well as factors that promote healthy development or protect against risk exposure (see, e.g., Arthur et al. 2002; Hawkins et al. 1992a). We then discuss findings from controlled trials of prevention approaches that demonstrate what can be done to reduce risk, enhance promotive or protective factors, and reduce adolescent substance abuse.

Nature and Extent of the Problem

Preventing alcohol, tobacco, and other drug use among adolescents is a national priority (Centers for Disease Control and Prevention 2004; U.S. Department of Health and Human Services 2006). The estimated annual cost of abuse and dependence to U.S. society, including health care, law enforcement, crime, and other costs, exceeds $530 billion (National Institute on Drug Abuse 2007).

The epidemiology of drug use suggests that although use is widespread during adolescence, abuse is not. For example, although more than 58% of students in tenth grade have initiated use of alcohol, only 29% report using it monthly, 16% report having had five or more drinks in a row in the past 2 weeks, and only 1% report daily use (Johnston et al. 2008). Johnston et al. (2008) also reported that in 2008, about 30% of students in tenth grade had initiated marijuana use, 14% had used it in the past month, and 2.7% used it daily. As shown in Figure 2–1, one of the strongest predictive relationships of later abuse and dependence is age at first use (DeWit et al. 2000; Grant and Dawson 1997; Pitkänen et al. 2008; Windle and Wiesner 2004).

Although no certainty exists as to who among those who try alcohol, tobacco, or marijuana at age 15 or 16 will become addicted, longitudinal studies and experimental trials have identified a number of individual and environmental factors that are associated with a higher likelihood of abuse and dependence. However, there is no single cause that, if changed, would stop progression to abuse and dependence. There are many sources of increased risk, and many avenues lead to acquisition of substance abuse problems.

Early efforts to prevent substance abuse were largely ineffective, and reviews of these efforts found few programs that had strong evaluations. In fact, some

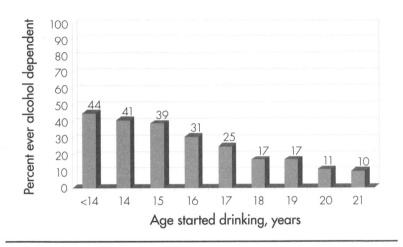

Figure 2–1.   Percentage of lifetime dependence by age of initiation.

Source.   Reprinted from Grant BF, Dawson DA: "Age at Onset of Alcohol Use and Its Association With DSM-IV Alcohol Abuse and Dependence: Results From the National Longitudinal Alcohol Epidemiologic Survey." *Journal of Substance Abuse* 9:103– 110, 1997, with permission from Elsevier.

programs were actually found to increase drug use (Tobler 1986). Thus, in the 1980s, clear evidence was lacking that problems like drug abuse could be prevented.

In response, prevention researchers advocated taking a public health approach (Catalano et al. 1998). The public health framework suggests that to prevent a problem before it happens, one must change the factors that predict it. In part as a response to the ineffectiveness of prevention efforts at the time, prevention researchers began to increasingly explore through longitudinal studies the predictors of adolescent substance abuse. Through increasing investment in research, a set of longitudinal predictors of substance use—often called risk and protective factors—was identified in the individual, family, school, peer group, and community. The findings of this research began to be summarized in the 1980s and 1990s (see, e.g., Hawkins et al. 1985, 1992a); public health approaches have been developed and tested using longitudinal research methods, and a wide range of effective prevention approaches have been found (Elliott and Mihalic 2004; Hawkins et al. 2008).

Role of Risk Factors

Risk factors are those predictors associated with an increased likelihood of substance use and/or abuse or other behavioral disorders (Hawkins et al. 1992a; Kraemer et al. 1997; National Research Council and Institute of Medicine 2009; Newcomb and Felix-Ortiz 1992). Risk factors have been found in the individual (e.g., genetic predisposition) and in the environments in which young people are socialized, including the family (e.g., family conflict), the school (e.g., school failure), the peer group (e.g., friends who use substances), and the community (e.g., availability of alcohol and drugs).

Longitudinal research has identified risk factors for a wide range of youth health and behavior problems (Biglan et al. 2004). Many of the risk factors for substance abuse also predict other problems, including delinquency, teen pregnancy, dropping out of school, violence, depression, and other behavior problems (Howell et al. 1995). Table 2–1 illustrates the predictive relationship between various risk factors and different types of problem behaviors. As can be seen in the table, many of the same risk factors predict multiple problems (Hawkins et al. 2002). For example, the risk factor of "low neighborhood attachment and community disorganization" has been shown to predict youth substance abuse, delinquency, and violence. Because risk factors have been shown to predict future problem behaviors, those risk factors that are amenable to change are potential targets for preventive action. Changing the risk factor of "low neighborhood attachment and community disorganization" has the potential to impact all three undesirable outcomes.

Patterns of Risk Exposure

Two common patterns of risk exposure are apparent. In some children, risks begin to accumulate early, because early developmental challenges without protection lead to increasing challenges as youth are exposed to new environments (e.g., school, peers). This has been referred to as a "snowball" pattern of risk (Mitchell et al. 2001). For example, a mother's smoking during pregnancy might impact fetal and early childhood development, which may lead to cognitive delays. Such delays may in turn lead to poor school adjustment and greater association with other poorly achieving youth in school settings. These factors may then lead to greater vulnerability to early substance use and abuse.

For children who do not have early life risk exposures, a second pattern of risk develops. In adolescence, some youth are exposed to friends who use drugs and to positive norms about drug use. Over time, this exposure, when not countered with protective influences, may lead some to succumb to this "snowstorm" pattern of risk (Toumbourou and Catalano 2005). For example, greater exposure to drug availability, favorable attitudes toward use, peer use, and weakening protection from the family during a time of increasing independence may lead some youth, even those without earlier patterns of risk, to develop substance use problems.

Risk Factor Domains

Community Factors

Multiple factors at the community level have been associated with substance use and abuse. Perceived or actual availability of drugs, community laws or norms favorable to drug use, media portrayals of alcohol use, high levels of transitions and mobility, low neighborhood attachment, and extreme economic deprivation may affect substance use (Beyers et al. 2004; Hawkins et al. 1995a; Wagenaar and Perry 1994).

Availability of substances. The more drugs that are available in a community, the more likely it is that youth will use them. This maxim applies to the number of liquor outlets as well as crack houses (Duncan et al. 2002; Freisthler et al. 2005). Perceived availability is also associated with increased risk of use. In schools where students think drugs are more available, there is a higher rate of drug use (Johnston et al. 2008; Maddahian et al. 1988).

Community laws and norms favorable to use. Laws and norms favorable to substance use, such as low tax rates on liquor or cigarettes, have been shown to increase overall use among young people (Carpenter and Cook 2008; Wagenaar et al. 2009). Community beer tasting events that are sponsored by beer companies are an example of a community norm that may promote use. These laws and norms increase the likelihood of use by reinforcing the social norm that substance use by young people is acceptable (Hawkins et al. 1992a; Wagenaar and Perry 1994).

Media portrayals of alcohol use. Exposure to actors using alcohol in movies significantly increases the risk of early drinking initiation, and predicts alcohol

Table 2–1.   Risk factors for adolescent problem behaviors

Risk factors	Substance use	Delinquency	Teen pregnancy	School dropout	Violence	Depression and anxiety
Community						
Availability of drugs	✓					
Availability of firearms		✓			✓	
Community laws and norms favorable toward drug use, firearms, and crime	✓	✓			✓	
Media portrayals of violence					✓	
Transitions and mobility	✓	✓		✓		✓
Low neighborhood attachment and community disorganization	✓	✓			✓	
Extreme economic deprivation	✓	✓	✓	✓	✓	
Family						
Family history of the problem behavior	✓	✓	✓	✓	✓	✓
Family management problems	✓	✓	✓	✓	✓	✓
Family conflict	✓	✓	✓	✓	✓	✓
Favorable parental attitudes and involvement in the problem behavior	✓	✓			✓	

Table 2–1. Risk factors for adolescent problem behaviors *(continued)*

Risk factors	Substance use	Delinquency	Teen pregnancy	School dropout	Violence	Depression and anxiety
School						
Academic failure beginning in late elementary school	✓	✓	✓	✓	✓	✓
Lack of commitment to school	✓	✓	✓	✓	✓	
Individual/peer						
Early and persistent antisocial behavior	✓	✓	✓	✓	✓	✓
Alienation and rebelliousness	✓	✓		✓		
Friends who engage in the problem behavior	✓	✓	✓	✓	✓	
Favorable attitudes toward the problem behavior	✓	✓	✓	✓		
Early initiation of the problem behavior	✓	✓	✓	✓	✓	
Constitutional factors	✓	✓			✓	✓

Note. A check indicates that at least two longitudinal studies have demonstrated that a particular risk factor predicts the specific problem.

abuse over time (Wills et al. 2009). Interestingly, even low levels of exposure to movie alcohol use have a significant effect on alcohol initiation and use (Hanewinkel and Sargent 2009). Exposure to movie alcohol use leads to positive alcohol use expectancies, more favorable images of young people who use alcohol, and increases in the number of friends who drink, which in turn predict increased willingness to drink and a subsequent increase in alcohol use (Dal Cin et al. 2009).

Transitions and mobility.   Communities that have high rates of mobility also have a higher incidence of drug and crime problems. Whether mobility occurs within communities or from one to another, communities with high rates of mobility also have higher incidences of drug and crime problems (Sampson and Lauritsen 1994).

Low neighborhood attachment and community disorganization.   Another risk factor for drug abuse involves low neighborhood attachment and community disorganization (Beyers et al. 2003). Neighborhoods with high population density, low levels of attachment to neighborhood, a lack of natural surveillance of public places, and high rates of adult crime have high rates of juvenile crime and illegal drug trafficking. Neighborhood disorganization contributes to deterioration in the ability of socializing units, such as churches, schools, and families, to pass on positive values to children. Neighborhood disorganization can be characterized by weak social institutions and lack of shared norms and values, which can result in diminished ties between individuals or between individuals and neighborhood organizations (Elliott et al. 1996; Sampson et al. 1997). These conditions often make it more difficult for residents to identify, monitor, or be willing to regulate young people's drug use (Sampson and Groves 1989) or to reinforce the expectation that substance use is not acceptable.

Extreme economic deprivation.   Nearly 18% of children under age 5 years are living in poverty (Fass and Cauthen 2006). Young people who live in deteriorating conditions, characterized by extreme poverty and high unemployment, are at risk for alcohol and substance use. Moreover, nonwhite children are at greater risk of living in poverty than white children. In 2005, about 10% of white children were living in poverty, compared with nearly 28% of Latino and 35% of African American children (Fass and Cauthen 2006). In addition, children living in poverty who display a high degree of behavior or adjustment problems earlier in life, including difficulty with self-regulation and impulsivity, are even more likely to develop problems with drugs (Elliott et al. 1989; Sampson and Lauritsen 1994; Takeuchi et al. 1991).

Family Factors

Family history of abuse and dependence.   Substantial evidence indicates that children whose parents abuse alcohol or drugs are at greater risk of developing abuse and dependence (Haggerty et al. 2007). Genetic studies have shown a substantial genetic influence on the use and abuse of tobacco and alcohol (Agrawal and Lynskey 2006; Kendler et al. 2003). Evidence also suggests that vulnerability to substance use is generalized across substances in adolescence (Young et al. 2006). Additionally, the developmental progression from initial experimentation through regular use to abuse and dependence appears to be accompanied by a decrease in the influence of shared environmental factors (family and peers) and a corresponding increase in the role of genetic and unique environmental vulnerability (Pagan et al. 2006). Persistent, progressive, and generalized substance use, abuse, and dependence likely represent a heritable phenotype with a close association with antisocial behavior (Kendler et al. 2003).

Family management problems.   Poor family management practices that elevate risk for substance use and problem behavior include parents' failure to set clear expectations for children's behavior; failure to supervise and monitor children; and excessively severe, harsh, or inconsistent punishment (Haggerty et al. 2007; Hawkins et al. 1992a; Kosterman et al. 2000). Children exposed to such poor family management practices are at increased risk for substance abuse and other problem behaviors (Brewer et al. 1995; Loeber and Hay 1997; Patterson and Dishion 1985). Family management that includes setting guidelines about substance use, monitoring behavior to see if it meets the guidelines, and setting consistent moderate consequences for violating the guidelines and positive recognition for following the guidelines is likely to lead to less substance abuse. Good family management is important throughout children's development, not only for young children. For example, parental monitoring during high school has been shown to reduce the risk of marijuana use among college students (White et al. 2006).

Family conflict. Children raised in an environment of conflict among family members—between parents or between parents and children—are more likely to engage in drug use and exhibit problem behaviors than are children raised in families without significant conflict (Maggs et al. 2008; National Research Council and Institute of Medicine 2009; Sartor et al. 2007). Family conflict, including violence or neglect, may lead young people to use drugs to cope with stress or anxiety (Flay et al. 1998; Hawkins et al. 1995b). When such conflict leads to family violence or neglect, young people are placed at greater risk of developing a substance abuse disorder (Kilpatrick et al. 2000).

Favorable parental attitudes toward drug use. Although studies have indicated that parental and adolescent drug use are related, parental attitudes that are favorable to drug use also play an important role in determining adolescent drug abuse (Peterson et al. 1994). Furthermore, parental approval of drinking (Barnes and Welte 1986) and drug use (Brook et al. 1986) significantly predicts the amount of alcohol and drug use by teenagers. This relationship has been shown for European American, Hispanic, African American, Native American, and Asian American youth (Gillmore et al. 1990; Glaser et al. 2005; Jessor et al. 1980).

School Factors

Academic failure. Beginning in late elementary school, academic failure increases the risk of later substance use as well as other problem behaviors. The experience of failure, regardless of the source, apparently increases the risk of these problems (Najaka et al. 2001). Young people fail for many reasons; they may lack stimulating teachers, they may not have the ability, they may have few friends and withdraw from school, or there may be a combination of reasons. Whatever the cause of academic failure, the experience itself is related to increased risk of substance use and abuse.

Low commitment to school. When a young person no longer considers the role of student as meaningful and rewarding, or lacks investment or commitment to school, he or she is at elevated risk for substance use and abuse (Gottfredson 2001; Kosterman et al. 2000). For example, students who have lower educational expectations and those who do not expect to attend college are more likely to be on a trajectory for heavy use (Karlamangla et al. 2006).

Individual Factors

Early and persistent antisocial behavior. One of the most stable distal predictors of later substance abuse and dependence is early antisocial behavior (Englund et al. 2008; Sher et al. 1991). An individual with a greater variety, frequency, and seriousness of antisocial behavior in childhood has a greater likelihood of future abuse and dependence.

Rebelliousness. A relationship exists between rebellious behavior and substance abuse and dependence (Zucker 2008). Research has found that young people who have a high tolerance for deviance are more likely to be involved with drug use (Jessor and Jessor 1977; Shedler and Block 1990).

Friends who use drugs. Peer use of substances is a consistent predictor of substance use among youth (Elliott et al. 1985). Studies of peer influence on drug use have demonstrated that involvement with antisocial peers is a strong predictor of tobacco, alcohol, and other drug use, as well as criminality and risky sexual behavior (Ary et al. 1999; Dishion et al. 1991; Oxford et al. 2001). For example, Guo et al. (2001) followed a longitudinal sample of students from elementary school to emerging adulthood and found that the association with antisocial peers during adolescence was one of the strongest predictors of alcohol abuse and dependence at age 21. In addition, some evidence suggests that peer influence may be moderated by youth perceptions of peers' attitudes toward academic achievement. Those who perceive that their peers are doing well in school are less likely to use cigarettes and tobacco (Bryant and Zimmerman 2002). Even children who grow up without other risk factors but associate with those who use drugs, are delinquent, are violent, are dropouts, or are pregnant are at a higher risk of the specific problem behavior (Toumbourou and Catalano 2005). The good news, however, is that children who grow up with fewer risk factors are not as likely to associate with these types of peers during adolescence, because individuals are typically found in the company of peers with similar behaviors and attitudes. For example, children who grow up with parents who are good family managers, who set guidelines for not using drugs, and who consistently monitor their children's behavior are less likely to have antisocial peers (Oxford et al. 2000).

Favorable attitudes toward alcohol and other drugs. The more favorable a young person's attitude is toward use of a substance, the more likely he or she is to use it at an earlier age (Arthur et al. 2002). This risk factor has been validated not only through predictor research but also through successful preventive interventions. For example, school programs that include normative content regarding youth attitudes toward drug use and perceptions of drug use have reduced favorable attitudes toward substance use and the prevalence of alcohol, tobacco, and other drug use in school populations (Botvin et al. 2003; Spoth et al. 2008; Sussman et al. 1998).

Early initiation of substance use.   A number of studies have documented that early substance use is a strong risk factor for later, more serious substance use (e.g., Grant et al. 2001; Zucker 2008). Pitkänen et al. (2008) examined drinking in early adolescence and found that it was highly predictive of heavy drinking at age 42. Likewise, Robins and Przybeck (1985) found that those who tried drugs before age 15 nearly doubled their risk of drug abuse compared with those who first tried drugs after age 19. Early use of tobacco appears to be a particularly strong predictor of later adult abuse and dependence (Brook et al. 2007). Early age of use of a specific drug is associated with the subsequent development of abuse and dependence later in life. This has been documented for tobacco (Costello et al. 1999), alcohol (Fergusson et al. 1995), cannabis (Coffey et al. 2000), and polydrug use (Newcomb and McGee 1991).

Constitutional factors.   Sensation seeking, low harm avoidance, risk taking, and impulsivity predict early-onset alcoholism and frequent marijuana use (Hawkins et al. 1992a; King and Chassin 2008; Merline et al. 2008). Some researchers who have investigated the mechanism for this connection suggest that sensation seeking may be linked biochemically to platelet manoamine oxidase activity, which has been associated with early-onset alcoholism. Some who have investigated the mechanism for this suggest that sensation seeking may be linked biochemically to platelet monoamine oxidase (MAO) activity, which has been associated with early-onset alcoholism (von Knorring et al. 1987; Zuckerman and Kuhlman 2000).

Reliability and Validity of Risk Factors

The reliability and predictive validity of risk factors is strong across genders, ethnicities, communities, and countries (Arthur et al. 2007; Beyers et al. 2004; Glaser et al. 2005). For example, Figure 2–2 depicts the correlation of risk factors to prevalence of 30-day marijuana use for different ethnic groups. This chart illustrates very little difference in the correlation between risk and marijuana use for different ethnic groups. Furthermore, in a cross-country comparison, Beyers et al. (2004) found that the strength of the correlations between risk and protective factors was comparable in the United States and Australia.

Role of Protective and Promotive Factors

Researchers have noted that many children exposed to risks were able to avoid later problems despite their exposure to risk. This led to the investigation of what protects children and youth who have been exposed to multiple risk factors and what motivates them to develop healthy lifestyles and not become involved in problem behaviors. This research led to the identification of factors that promote positive outcomes and protect against the impact of risk exposure (Gorman-Smith et al. 1996, 2005; Guo et al. 2001; Hawkins et al. 1992a; Hill et al. 2005; Hops et al. 1990). Protective factors are those predictors that buffer the effects of risk factors on substance use and abuse. Promotive factors are those predictors that have a direct negative relationship with substance use and abuse.

Longitudinal, prospective research studies have identified seven factors that promote positive social development: high intelligence; resilient temperament; social, emotional, and cognitive competence; opportunities for prosocial involvement; recognition for positive involvement; bonding; and healthy beliefs and standards for behavior. The first three comprise individual characteristics that protect young people, even in the presence of risks. The last four protective factors involve key environmental processes that protect young people.

High Intelligence

Children with higher intelligence are protected from substance use and abuse (Hawkins et al. 1992a; Werner and Smith 1992). They may be better able to negotiate high-risk environments.

Resilient Temperament

Resilience is an individual's capacity for adapting to change and stressful events in healthy and flexible ways. Resilience has been identified in research studies

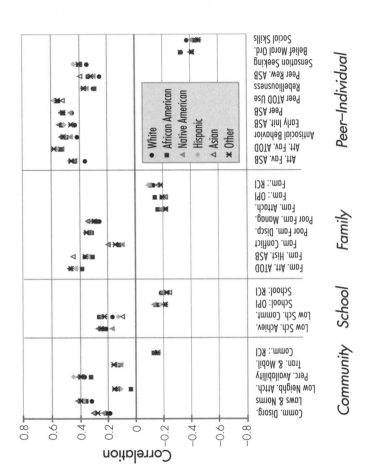

Figure 2–2. Correlations of six state student survey scales by ethnicity: marijuana use (30 day).

Key: Community: Comm. Disorg. = Community Disorganization; Laws & Norms = Laws and Norms Favorable to Substance Abuse; Low Neighb. Attch. = Low Neighborhood Attachment; Perc. Availability = Perceived Availability of Drugs; Tran. & Mobil. = Transitions and Mobility; Comm: RCI = Community Rewards for Constructive Involvement; *School:* Low Sch. Achiev. = Low School Achievement; Low Sch. Commit. = Low School Commitment; School: OPI = School Opportunities for Prosocial Involvement; School: RCI = School Rewards for Constructive Involvement; *Family:* Fam. Att. ATOD = Family; Attitudes Towards Alcohol, Tobacco, or Other Drugs; Fam. Hist. ASB = Family History of Antisocial Behavior; Fam. Conflict = Family Conflict; Poor Fam. Discp. = Poor Family Discipline; Poor Fam. Manag. = Poor Family Management; Fam. Attach. = Family Attachment; Fam.: OPI: Family Opportunities for Prosocial Involvement; Fam.: RCI: Family Rewards for Constructive Involvement; *Peer–Individual:* Att. Fav. ASB = Attitudes Favorable Towards Antisocial Behavior; Att. Fav. ATOD = Attitudes Favorable Towards Alcohol, Tobacco, or Other Drugs; Early Init. ASB = Early Initiation of Antisocial Behavior; Peer ASB = Peer Antisocial Behavior; Peer ATOD Use = Peer Alcohol, Tobacco, or Other Drug Use; Peer Rew. ASB = Peer Rewards for Antisocial Behavior; Belief Moral Ord. = Belief in the Moral Order.

as a characteristic of youth who, when exposed to multiple risk factors, show successful responses to challenge and use this learning to achieve successful outcomes (Masten et al. 1990). Pathways to substance abuse can often be traced back to the earliest years of life. For example, Williams et al. (2000) noted that temperament in early infancy and early childhood was important in protecting young people from substance abuse by age 15.

Social, Emotional, and Cognitive Competence

In the context of this chapter, *competence* refers to the range of interpersonal skills that help youth integrate feelings, thinking, and actions to specific social and interpersonal goals (Masten et al. 1990). These skills include encoding relevant social cues, accurately interpreting those cues, generating effective solutions to interpersonal problems, decision making, realistically anticipating consequences and potential obstacles to one's actions, and translating social decisions into effective behaviors (Consortium on the School-Based Promotion of Social Competence 1994). In experimental studies, the enhancement of competence has led to the prevention of negative outcomes (Botvin et al. 1995).

Opportunities for Prosocial Involvement

Children who have developmentally appropriate opportunities to be meaningfully involved with the family, school, or community are less likely to develop problems (Chalk et al. 1996; Darling and Steinberg 1993). For children to acquire key interpersonal skills in early development, positive opportunities must be available (Hawkins et al. 1987), and during adolescence, when substance use is a more proximal behavior, interactions with positively oriented peers and involvement in roles in which they can make a contribution to their group, whether family, school, neighborhood, peer group, or larger community, are especially important (Dryfoos 1990).

Recognition for Positive Involvement

Parents, teachers, and peers who provide recognition for skillful behavior affect a person's motivation to engage in the same behaviors in the future; behavior is strengthened through rewards and punishments (Akers et al. 1979). Appropriate rewards at age 10 predicted less substance abuse or dependence at age 21 (Guo et al. 2001).

Bonding

Bonding is an important developmental protective and promotive factor (Brook et al. 1990). A number of studies have also shown negative associations between bonding to parents and problem behavior outcomes (Hill et al. 2005; Noller et al. 2001; Rutter 2002), with bonding commonly being assessed as a mixture of attachment, commitment, and positive communication. Additionally, strong family bonds and support during the teen years are associated with lower levels of alcohol and drug use involvement during young adulthood (King and Chassin 2004; Locke and Newcomb 2004; Maggs et al. 1997). Bonding to school and having educational aspirations have consistently been shown to protect against drug use onset, abuse, and dependence (Catalano et al. 2004; Hawkins et al. 1992a). For example, bonding to school at ages 10, 14, and 16 predicted lower alcohol abuse and dependence at age 21 (Guo et al. 2001). Likewise, Crum et al. (1998) found that educational achievement in elementary school predicted fewer alcohol use disorders in the early 30s. In addition, although the role of prosocial peers has been less studied, evidence suggests that strong bonds with prosocial peers can buffer or mitigate the impact of antisocial peer influence on drug use behavior (Kaufmann et al. 2007).

Healthy Beliefs and Standards for Behavior

Clear standards and beliefs that promote healthy and ethical behavior provide protection from substance abuse and dependence (Hawkins et al. 1992b). By communicating clear and consistent expectations about not using drugs, families, schools, and communities help establish a protective buffer against using drugs, even in the presence of risks (Catalano et al. 1996; Peterson et al. 1994). For example, one study found that the stronger a young person's beliefs and standards are at age 10, the lower his or her risk of alcohol abuse and dependence is at age 21 (Guo et al. 2001). Also, the more an older adolescent conforms to acceptable standards of behavior, the less likely he or she is to be involved in alcohol use during the young adult years (Locke and Newcomb 2004). Not surprisingly, the more a young adult conforms to healthy standards for behavior, the less likely he or she is to later experience an alcohol use disorder (Oesterle et al. 2008).

Summary

Some individuals are born with traits, such as high intelligence or a resilient temperament, that help protect them from involvement in substance use and abuse. For young people not born with these traits, families, schools, positive peer groups, and communities need to provide opportunities, recognition, bonding, and healthy beliefs to protect their children from risk. According to our theory of protection, the social development model (Catalano and Hawkins 1996), when young people are provided with opportunities to make a contribution, taught the skills and competencies they need to make a contribution, and given recognition for their contribution, they develop strong connections with and commitment to the families, schools, and communities that provided these opportunities. When those families, schools, and communities to whom a youth is bonded communicate clear standards for behavior, these young people are more likely to follow their standards. These seven factors protect youth from risk and promote positive development (Catalano and Hawkins 2002).

Tested and Effective Programs

The identification of risk and protective factors led to the development of prevention approaches that sought to increase protection while reducing risk. In the 1980s, a new generation of experimental studies of the impact of prevention programs that take this approach began. They focused on changing predictors of a single problem, such as substance use, as a strategy to reduce the selected problem. Tests of this new approach began to have some success. Despite these successes, toward the end of the 1980s and into the 1990s, many conversations were taking place that were critical of this single-behavior-problem approach to prevention. Whether these conversations took place among practitioners, foundations, government agencies, or researchers, they were lively, provocative, and frequently controversial. Groups of scientists, practitioners, and policymakers increasingly came together, and their critiques and recommendations began to converge. Their recommendations suggested that prevention science provided the research base that supports a focus on the individual and the environment, that prevention approaches should address the whole child and not be focused on a single problem behavior, and that prevention programs should address a broad focus on reducing developmentally salient risk factors and promoting protective factors.

Controlled trials over the past 25 years have identified tested and effective prevention programs, policies, and actions that have demonstrated that prevention approaches can reduce risk, increase protection, and reduce problem behaviors (Foxcroft et al. 2003; National Research Council and Institute of Medicine 2009; Substance Abuse and Mental Health Services Administration 2002). An increasing number and range of effective prevention approaches have been identified. Information on these programs is now widely available on a number of Internet sites. The most rigorous of these sites include those of the Campbell Collaboration (http://www.campbellcollaboration.org), the Center for the Study and Prevention of Violence (2010), and the Substance Abuse and Mental Health Services Administration (2010). Wide-ranging types of programs have been found to be effective in controlled trials that compared groups of young people who did and did not receive the intervention (Hawkins and Catalano 2004). In the following subsections, we review several of these programs briefly and provide examples of effective programs. We caution, however, that not all programs using these approaches work. Table 2–2 has a complete list of the types of programs that have been found effective.

School-Based Programs

Early childhood education has demonstrated positive long-term outcomes. For example, one effective strategy is the High Scope Perry Preschool program (Schweinhart 2007). This approach was designed for children born into poverty. The program focuses on social and cognitive development of children, reaches out to parents in their homes to reinforce both cognitive and social development of their children, and works on parenting skills as well as strengthening parent education and occupational goals. Teachers using this approach teach children to learn actively by interacting with ideas and physical objects, and by applying logical thinking to these experiences. By allowing children's active involvement in learning, the program builds bonding to school and teachers at an early age and sets a course for lifelong learning. The program has demonstrated lasting effects on school success, rates of employment, criminal involvement, and emotional problems (Schweinhart 2007).

Effective school-based programs include enhancing instructional and classroom management skills; using classroom curricula that promote social, emotional, and cognitive competence; and tutoring. School programs focused on improving academic performance and bonding to school and reducing class-

Table 2–2.   Effective policies and programs for preventing problem behaviors

1. Prenatal and infancy programs

2. Early childhood education

3. Parent training

4. After-school recreation

5. Mentoring with contingent reinforcement

6. Youth employment with education

7. Organization change in schools

8. Classroom organization, management, and instructional strategies

9. School behavior management styles

10. Classroom curricula for social competence promotion

11. Community and school policies

12. Community mobilization

Source.   Adapted from Hawkins and Catalano 2004.

room management problems have produced reductions in early aggressiveness (Kellam and Anthony 1998; Tremblay et al. 1992), improvements in parent and school bonding and academic performance (Hawkins et al. 1992a), reductions in early substance use (Hawkins et al. 1992a; O'Donnell et al. 1995), and long-term reductions in heavy alcohol use and smoking (Hawkins et al. 1999; Kellam and Anthony 1998). School programs that teach social, emotional, and cognitive competencies and establish norms against substance use have reduced favorable attitudes toward substance use and the prevalence of tobacco and alcohol use in school populations (Pentz et al. 1989; Sussman et al. 1998).

Parenting Programs

Family and parenting programs that focus on children from early infancy through middle school have also had impacts on reducing substance abuse. When family interventions focus on risk and protective factors that can be affected by parents and families, they can produce long-term effects not only on substance abuse and dependence, but on other problem behaviors as well. For example, the Nurse-Family Partnership program works with young, first-time, single mothers during their first pregnancy until their child is age 2 years (Olds et al. 1998). Mothers enrolled in the program are visited by a registered nurse in their home once every week or two. Nurses work with expectant mothers to reduce the mothers' negative behaviors (i.e., smoking, drinking, and drug use) that may lead to poor birth outcomes. After the child is born, nurses continue to visit mothers and teach them how to identify developmental or health problems, create safe environments for their children, and interact with their children in a way that promotes social and emotional competence. The program has long-term positive effects on both mothers and their children. For example, when children of parents who were involved in the program reached age 15, they had 56% fewer days of alcohol consumption than those of parents who did not participate in the program (Olds et al. 1998).

Guiding Good Choices (Hawkins and Catalano 1988) is another example of a parenting program showing long-term reductions in substance use and abuse. The parent training program is intended for parents of children ages 8–14 years. The program's design was guided by the social development model (Catalano and Hawkins 1996). The program provides practical information for parents about the risks for and dangers of early initiation of substance use, and emphasizes 1) creating opportunities for involvement and interaction in the family and rewarding children's participation in the family; 2) establishing clear family rules about substance use, monitoring the behavior of children, and using consistent moderate discipline; 3) teaching children the skills needed to resist peer influences to use drugs; and 4) reducing and managing family conflict (Hawkins and Catalano 1988). Long-term evidence for program efficacy is strong. The program has been found to reduce the growth of alcohol use in adolescent boys and girls (Park et al. 2000) and of substance use (Spoth et al. 2001); to reduce the growth of delinquency (Mason et al. 2003) and depression (Mason et al. 2007); and to reduce substance abuse diagnoses among young women 10 years after the intervention was conducted with their parents (Mason et al. 2009).

Community Programs

Using coalitions to address community issues is a popular approach to prevention. A coalition brings together diverse stakeholders and potentially combines human and financial resources for more effective and sustainable preventive efforts. Early models of coalition-driven prevention provided resources to support community coalitions without a structure or process. These early models were largely ineffective (Hallfors et al. 2002; Klerman et al. 2005; Merzel and D'Afflitti 2003). Later community models, which focused on malleable community-level risk and protective factors, had some success. These strategies often had a normative change approach and either included reducing availability of alcohol and increasing enforcement of underage drinking and drunk driving laws, which had effects among young adults (Holder et al. 2000; Wagenaar et al. 2000), or combined community norm change approaches with school-based curriculum for youth, which had an impact on youth in middle and high schools (Pentz et al. 2006; Perry et al. 2002).

More recently, strategies that build local partnerships or coalitions to promote use of tested and effective programs for addressing community prevention needs have had impacts on reducing community-wide risk, substance use, and delinquency. Communities That Care uses this approach and provides education and tools for community decision making to organize, assess, and prioritize prevention needs; match efficacious programs to prioritized needs; and provide training and technical assistance for implementing efficacious programs with fidelity. Communities That Care, tested in a randomized community trial and a quasi-experimental trial, has shown that it can transform community prevention systems and reduce risk, substance use, and delinquency (Hawkins et al. 2008, 2009).

Other community programs impact risk factors and early substance use initiation. For example, Big Brothers and Big Sisters, a mentoring program that typically works with youth ages 5–18, has been rigorously evaluated. Eight sites used standardized protocols to monitor mentor-youth relationships and required that matches be maintained for a year. The study found that relative to the comparison group, youth receiving the mentoring were 46% less likely to initiate drug use, were 30% less likely to hit someone, and missed 50% fewer days of school (Tierney et al. 1995).

Policy Changes

Community-wide policy changes to reduce availability or changes to norms and laws regarding substance use can have positive impacts on adolescent substance use. For example, policies to restrict availability of tobacco to young people have resulted in decreased cigarette smoking among youths (Forster et al. 1998). Similarly, community-wide policy changes to reduce availability of alcohol to youths, including increasing the drinking age (Cook and Tauchen 1984) and restricting how alcohol is sold (Holder and Blose 1987), have decreased consumption and the frequency of alcohol-related traffic accidents and fatalities. Other examples include a higher minimum age at which one may legally buy alcohol or cigarettes, and zoning ordinances that do not allow a high density of liquor outlets in a neighborhood. For example, one law that has had a profound effect on mortality from alcohol use is raising the legal drinking age to 21. The research evidence supports that this higher legal drinking age was associated with decreased motor vehicle fatalities related to alcohol use (for review, see Wagenaar and Toomey 2002).

Despite this growing research knowledge base for prevention practice, programs that do not work or have not been tested are more widespread in communities than are tested, effective programs (Ennett et al. 2003; Ringwalt et al. 2008, 2009). Two critical issues interfere with the dissemination of effective prevention. First, for programs to be transferable, they must provide a manual or guide describing how to implement the intervention, as well as training and technical support to implement the program with fidelity. Without close replication, these programs are less effective (Dusenbury et al. 2003; Fagan et al. 2008; Mihalic et al. 2004). For example, a number of organizations and states have put in place different approaches to helping new teen mothers through home visitation, similar to the Nurse-Family Partnership model (see Olds et al. 1998). However, in a trial comparing nurses and non-nurse practitioners trained in the same model, effects were found only for the nurse-delivered program (Alper 2002). Installing effective programs in communities requires significant investments in training, technical support, and installation monitoring.

There is good news about the potential for achieving program fidelity. Fagan et al. (2008) have shown that with adequate investments in training and proactive technical support, high fidelity can be achieved in community replications of effective programs. In 12 communities across the United States, The Community Youth Development Study has been able to achieve 90% fidelity to program content, dosage, and quality of delivery (Fagan et al. 2008). With adequate resources, tested and effective programs for preventing substance abuse and dependence can be put in place with fidelity across the United States (Mihalic et al. 2004).

The second critical issue is that a market must be created in local communities for tested and effective programs. Many policies and programs of various types have been tested and proven effective, yet currently they are not widely used (Ennett et al. 2003; Ringwalt et al. 2008, 2009). To increase demand, funders, practitioners, and consumers must be convinced that prevention can make a difference—that is, that tested, effective programs, policies, and practices can reduce individuals' levels of substance use, and that if these tactics reach all for whom they are appropriate, they can result in community-wide reductions in substance use (Hawkins et al. 2009). Many funders have adopted this stance. For example, the Oregon state legislature passed a law requiring that a percentage of interventions provided with state funds must be tested and effective. Increasingly, practitioners are making this transition, but tested, effective programs still compete with usual or "best," but often untested, practices. Little progress, however, has been made in convincing consumers to demand effective prevention programs. To fully transform prevention practice, consumers must ask what evidence indicates that a prevention program or policy is effective. In the medical field, the move toward evidence-based medicine was encouraged by the presence of websites that disseminated medical advice to patients. Armed with this information, patients are frequently asking their doctors why a particular approach is favored over another. Most communities have not yet made the use of tested and effective programs a priority. To increase the use of tested, effective prevention programs and practices, practitioners must educate prevention consumers to ask how the program was tested, to ask whether it was tested in a randomized or controlled trial, and to request a copy of the evaluation. We feel that when this occurs, funding and practice will lead to the widespread use of tested, effective practices. Because the research base exists to reduce substance use and abuse in communities, practitioners need to encourage communities to use policies and programs that have been shown to work, and to empower communities to select programs that are matched to the needs of their youth.

Conclusion

Important prevention implications have emerged from the research on risk and protection and the evaluation of prevention approaches:

1. Preventive approaches should focus on both reducing risk and enhancing protection.
2. For maximum effect, prevention programs should address risk and protective factors early—for example, at the stage of development when the risk factor first emerges in the population.
3. In addition to addressing individual risk and protection, a valuable practice is to assess and diagnose community risk and protection. The level of risk and protective factors at the community level can be assessed by conducting surveys of youth in schools and arraying data on risk and protective factors at the community or neighborhood level (Arthur et al. 2007; Mrazek et al. 2004). This helps communities to diagnose and prioritize which risk factors are elevated and which protective factors are low, thereby obtaining guidance on which risk and protective factors are most pressing to address locally.
4. Preventive interventions that have demonstrated effectiveness should be used to address community profiles of risk and protection.
5. These approaches are most effective when they are implemented as they were designed. The research on these programs shows that if they are not implemented as designed, their effect is weaker, disappearing at some point when less of the intervention is delivered than designed. For example, Botvin et al. (1995) found that Life Skills Training maintains its effects, although diminished, when at least two-thirds of the content is unaltered. The challenge for the early twenty-first century becomes how practitioners (state officials, community members, and agency and school officials) can ensure that they are choosing the most effective programs that meet the needs of children and youth for whom they are responsible.

Current evidence indicates that helping communities address the underlying risk and protective factors that contribute to substance abuse can focus communities on choosing tested and effective programs that meet their needs (Arthur et al. 2003; Harachi et al. 1996; Jenson et al. 1997). When communities implement such programs with a high degree of fidelity, their efforts have been followed by positive changes, not only in reduced risks and increased protection, but more important, in community-wide reductions in youth drug use and delinquency (Feinberg et al. 2005; France and Crow 2005; Hawkins et al. 2008, 2009).

The Institute of Medicine, in a recent report, highlighted the potential for reducing multiple mental health and behavior problems through targeting of risk and protective factors for multiple disorders (National Research Council and Institute of Medicine 2009). The identification of risk and protective factors, the testing of risk reduction and protective factor–enhancing prevention programs and policies, and the development of tools for communities to use to apply this research base to their prevention programming have all contributed to the efforts to reduce substance abuse and dependence, as well as to address other mental health and behavior outcomes.

Key Clinical Concepts

- Epidemiological studies indicate that drug use is widespread during adolescence.
- A set of longitudinal predictors of substance use—often called *risk factors* and *protective factors*—has been identified in the individual, family, school, peer group, and community.
- Current evidence strongly suggests that effective prevention can be realized by helping communities address the underlying risk factors that contribute to substance abuse and protective factors.
- Research has identified tested and effective prevention programs for parents, schools, and communities. When such programs are implemented with a high degree of fidelity, community-wide reductions in substance abuse can be attained.

References

Agrawal A, Lynskey MT: The genetic epidemiology of cannabis use, abuse and dependence. Addiction 101:801–812, 2006

Akers RL, Krohn M, Lanza-Kaduce L, et al: Social learning and deviant behavior: a specific test of a general theory. Am Sociol Rev 44:636–655, 1979

Alper J: The nurse home visitation program, in To Improve Health and Health Care, Vol 5. The Robert Wood Johnson Anthology. Edited by Isaacs SL, Knickman JR. San Francisco, CA, Jossey-Bass, 2002, pp 3–22

Arthur MW, Hawkins JD, Pollard JA, et al: Measuring risk and protective factors for substance use, delinquency, and other adolescent problem behaviors. The Communities That Care Youth Survey. Eval Rev 26:575–601, 2002

Arthur MW, Ayers CD, Graham KA, et al: Mobilizing communities to reduce risks for drug abuse: a comparison of two strategies, in Handbook of Drug Abuse Prevention: Theory, Science, and Practice. Edited by Bukoski WJ, Sloboda Z. New York, Kluwer Academic/Plenum, 2003, pp 129–144

Arthur MW, Briney JS, Hawkins JD, et al: Measuring risk and protection in communities using the Communities That Care Youth Survey. Eval Program Plann 30:197–211, 2007

Ary DV, Duncan TE, Duncan SC, et al: Adolescent problem behavior: the influence of parents and peers. Behav Res Ther 37:217–230, 1999

Barnes GM, Welte JW: Patterns and predictors of alcohol use among 7–12th grade students in New York State. J Stud Alcohol 47:53–62, 1986

Beyers JM, Bates JE, Pettit GS, et al: Neighborhood structure, parenting processes, and the development of youths' externalizing behaviors: a multilevel analysis. Am J Community Psychol 31:35–53, 2003

Beyers JM, Toumbourou JW, Catalano RF, et al: A cross-national comparison of risk and protective factors for adolescent substance use: the United States and Australia. J Adolesc Health 35:3–16, 2004

Biglan A, Brennan PA, Foster SL, et al: Helping Adolescents at Risk: Prevention of Multiple Problem Behaviors. New York, Guilford, 2004

Botvin GJ, Schinke SP, Epstein JA, et al: Effectiveness of culturally focused and generic skills training approaches to alcohol and drug abuse prevention among minority adolescents: two-year follow-up results. Psychol Addict Behav 9:183–194, 1995

Botvin GJ, Griffin KW, Paul E, et al: Preventing tobacco and alcohol use among elementary school students through life skills training. J Child Adolesc Subst Abuse 12:1–17, 2003

Brewer DD, Hawkins JD, Catalano RF, et al: Preventing serious, violent, and chronic juvenile offending: a review of evaluations of selected strategies in childhood, adolescence, and the community, in A Sourcebook: Serious, Violent, and Chronic Juvenile Offenders. Edited by Howell JC, Krisberg B, Hawkins JD, et al. Thousand Oaks, CA, Sage, 1995, pp 61–141

Brook JS, Whiteman M, Gordon AS, et al: Onset of adolescent drinking: a longitudinal study of intrapersonal and interpersonal antecedents. Adv Alcohol Subst Abuse 5:91–110, 1986

Brook JS, Brook DW, Gordon AS, et al: The psychosocial etiology of adolescent drug use: a family interactional approach. Genet Soc Gen Psychol Monogr 116:111–267, 1990

Brook JS, Balka EB, Ning Y, et al: Trajectories of cigarette smoking among African Americans and Puerto Ricans from adolescence to young adulthood: associations with dependence on alcohol and illegal drugs. Am J Addict 16:195–201, 2007

Bryant AL, Zimmerman MA: Examining the effects of academic beliefs and behaviors on changes in substance use among urban adolescents. J Educ Psychol 94:621–637, 2002

Carpenter C, Cook PJ: Cigarette taxes and youth smoking: new evidence from national, state, and local Youth Risk Behavior Surveys. J Health Econ 27:287–299, 2008

Catalano RF, Hawkins JD: The social development model: a theory of antisocial behavior, in Delinquency and Crime: Current Theories. Edited by Hawkins JD. New York, Cambridge University Press, 1996, pp 149–197

Catalano RF, Hawkins JD: Positive youth development in the United States: research findings on evaluations of positive youth development programs. Prevention and Treatment 5:Article 15, June 24, 2002

Catalano RF, Kosterman R, Hawkins JD, et al: Modeling the etiology of adolescent substance use: a test of the social development model. J Drug Issues 26:429–455, 1996

Catalano RF, Arthur MW, Hawkins JD, et al: Comprehensive community and school based interventions to prevent antisocial behavior, in Serious and Violent Juvenile Offenders: Risk Factors and Successful Interventions. Edited by Loeber R, Farrington DP. Thousand Oaks, CA, Sage, 1998, pp 248–283

Catalano RF, Haggerty KP, Oesterle S, et al: The importance of bonding to school for healthy development: findings from the Social Development Research Group. J Sch Health 74:252–261, 2004

Center for the Study and Prevention of Violence, Institute of Behavioral Science, University of Colorado at Boulder: Blueprints for Violence Prevention. Available at: http://www.colorado.edu/cspv/blueprints. Accessed January 14, 2010.

Centers for Disease Control and Prevention: 2004 Surgeon General's report: the health consequences of smoking. 2004. Available at: http://www.cdc.gov/tobacco/data_statistics/sgr/sgr_2004/index.htm. Accessed December 10, 2009.

Chalk R, Phillips DA, National Research Council Institute of Medicine (eds): Youth Development and Neighborhood Influences: Challenges and Opportunities, Summary of a Workshop (Report by the Committee on Youth Development, Board on Children, Youth, and Families, Commission on Behavioral and Social Sciences and Education). Washington, DC, National Academies Press, 1996

Coffey C, Lynskey M, Wolfe R, et al: Initiation and progression of cannabis use in a population-based Australian adolescent longitudinal study. Addiction 95:1679–1690, 2000

Consortium on the School-Based Promotion of Social Competence: The school-based promotion of social competence: theory, research, practice, and policy, in Stress, Risk, and Resilience in Children and Adolescents: Processes, Mechanisms, and Interventions. Edited by Haggerty RJ, Sherrod LR, Garmezy N, et al. New York, Cambridge University Press, 1994, pp 268–316

Cook PJ, Tauchen G: The effect of minimum drinking age legislation on youthful auto fatalities, 1970–1977. J Legal Stud 13:169–190, 1984

Costello EJ, Erkanli A, Federman E, et al: Development of psychiatric comorbidity with substance abuse in adolescents: effects of timing and sex. J Clin Child Psychol 28:298–311, 1999

Crum RM, Ensminger ME, Ro MJ, et al: The association of educational achievement and school dropout with risk of alcoholism: a twenty-five-year prospective study of inner-city children. J Stud Alcohol 59:318–326, 1998

Dal Cin S, Worth KA, Gerrard M, et al: Watching and drinking: expectancies, prototypes, and friends' alcohol use mediate the effect of exposure to alcohol use in movies on adolescent drinking. Health Psychol 28:473–483, 2009

Darling N, Steinberg L: Parenting style as context: an integrative model. Psychol Bull 113:487–496, 1993

DeWit DJ, Adlaf EM, Offord DR, et al: Age at first alcohol use: a risk factor for the development of alcohol disorders. Am J Psychiatry 157:745–750, 2000

Dishion TJ, Patterson GR, Stoolmiller M, et al: Family, school, and behavioral antecedents to early adolescent involvement with antisocial peers. Dev Psychol 27:172–180, 1991

Dryfoos JG: Adolescents at Risk: Prevalence and Prevention. New York, Oxford University Press, 1990

Duncan SC, Duncan TE, Strycker LA: A multilevel analysis of neighborhood context and youth alcohol and drug problems. Prev Sci 3:125–133, 2002

Dusenbury L, Brannigan R, Falco M, et al: A review of research on fidelity of implementation: implications for drug abuse prevention in school settings. Health Educ Res 18:237–256, 2003

Elliott DS, Mihalic S: Issues in disseminating and replicating effective prevention programs. Prev Sci 5:47–53, 2004

Elliott DS, Huizinga D, Ageton SS: Explaining Delinquency and Drug Use. Beverly Hills, CA, Sage, 1985

Elliott DS, Huizinga D, Menard S: Multiple Problem Youth: Delinquency, Substance Use, and Mental Health Problems. New York, Springer, 1989

Elliott DS, Wilson WJ, Huizinga D, et al: The effects of neighborhood disadvantage on adolescent development. J Res Crime Delinq 33:389–426, 1996

Englund MM, Egeland B, Oliva EM, et al: Childhood and adolescent predictors of heavy drinking and alcohol use disorders in early adulthood: a longitudinal developmental analysis. Addiction 103:23–35, 2008

Ennett ST, Ringwalt CL, Thorne J, et al: A comparison of current practice in school-based substance use prevention programs with meta-analysis findings. Prev Sci 4:1–14, 2003

Fagan AA, Hanson K, Hawkins JD, et al: Implementing effective community-based prevention programs in the Community Youth Development Study. Youth Violence Juv Justice 6:256–278, 2008

Fass S, Cauthen NK: Who are America's poor children? The official story. New York, National Center for Children in Poverty, December 2006. Available at: http://www.nccp.org/publications/pub_684.html. Accessed May 6, 2010.

Feinberg M, Greenberg M, Olson J, et al: Preliminary Report: CTC Impact in Pennsylvania: Findings From the 2001 and 2003 PA Youth Survey. University Park, College of Health and Human Development, Pennsylvania State University, 2005

Fergusson DM, Horwood LJ, Lynskey MT: The prevalence and risk factors associated with abusive or hazardous alcohol consumption in 16-year-olds. Addiction 90:935–946, 1995

Flay BR, Hu FB, Richardson J: Psychosocial predictors of different stages of cigarette smoking among high school students. Prev Med 27:A9–A18, 1998

Forster JL, Murray DM, Wolfson M, et al: The effects of community policies to reduce youth access to tobacco. Am J Public Health 88:1193–1198, 1998

Foxcroft D, Ireland D, Lister-Sharp D, et al: Longer-term primary prevention for alcohol misuse in young people: a systematic review. Addiction 98:397–411, 2003

France A, Crow I: Using the "risk factor paradigm" in prevention: lessons from the evaluation of Communities That Care. Children & Society 19:172–184, 2005

Freisthler B, Lascala EA, Gruenewald PJ, et al: An examination of drug activity: effects of neighborhood social organization on the development of drug distribution systems. Subst Use Misuse 40:671–686, 2005

Gillmore MR, Catalano RF, Morrison DM, et al: Racial differences in acceptability and availability of drugs and early initiation of substance use. Am J Drug Alcohol Abuse 16:185–206, 1990

Glaser RR, Van Horn ML, Arthur MW, et al: Measurement properties of the Communities That Care Youth Survey across demographic groups. J Quant Criminol 21:73–102, 2005

Gorman-Smith D, Tolan PH, Zelli A, et al: The relation of family functioning to violence among inner-city minority youths. J Fam Psychol 10:115–129, 1996

Gorman-Smith D, Tolan PH, Henry D: Promoting resilience in the inner city: families as a venue for protection, support, and opportunity, in Resilience in Children, Families, and Communities: Linking Context to Practice and Policy. Edited by Peters RD, Leadbeater B, McMahon RJ. New York, Kluwer Academic/Plenum, 2005, pp 137–155

Gottfredson DC: Schools and Delinquency. Cambridge, UK, Cambridge University Press, 2001

Grant BF, Dawson DA: Age at onset of alcohol use and its association with DSM-IV alcohol abuse and dependence: results from the National Longitudinal Alcohol Epidemiologic Survey. J Subst Abuse 9:103–110, 1997

Grant BF, Stinson FS, Harford TC: Age at onset of alcohol use and DSM-IV alcohol abuse and dependence: a 12-year follow-up. J Subst Abuse 13:493–504, 2001

Guo J, Hawkins JD, Hill KG, et al: Childhood and adolescent predictors of alcohol abuse and dependence in young adulthood. J Stud Alcohol 62:754–762, 2001

Haggerty KP, Skinner ML, MacKenzie EP, et al: A randomized trial of Parents Who Care: effects on key outcomes at 24-month follow-up. Prev Sci 8:249–260, 2007

Hallfors DD, Cho H, Livert D, et al: Fighting back against substance abuse: are community coalitions winning? Am J Prev Med 23:237–245, 2002

Hanewinkel R, Sargent JD: Longitudinal study of exposure to entertainment media and alcohol use among German adolescents. Pediatrics 123:989–995, 2009

Harachi TW, Ayers CD, Hawkins JD, et al: Empowering communities to prevent adolescent substance abuse: process evaluation results from a risk- and protection-focused community mobilization effort. J Prim Prev 16:233–254, 1996

Hawkins JD, Catalano RF: Preparing for the Drug Free Years: Family Guide. South Deerfield, MA, Channing Bete, 1988

Hawkins JD, Catalano RF: Communities That Care: Prevention Strategies Guide. South Deerfield, MA, Channing Bete, 2004

Hawkins JD, Lishner DM, Catalano RF: Childhood predictors and the prevention of adolescent substance abuse. NIDA Res Monogr 56:75–126, 1985

Hawkins JD, Lishner DM, Jenson JM, et al: Delinquents and drugs: what the evidence suggests about prevention and treatment programming, in Youth at High Risk for Substance Abuse (DHHS Publ No ADM-87-1537). Edited by Brown BS, Mills AR. Rockville, MD, National Institute on Drug Abuse, 1987, pp 81–131

Hawkins JD, Catalano RF, Miller JY: Risk and protective factors for alcohol and other drug problems in adolescence and early adulthood: implications for substance abuse prevention. Psychol Bull 112:64–105, 1992a

Hawkins JD, Catalano RF, Morrison DM, et al: The Seattle Social Development Project: effects of the first four years on protective factors and problem behaviors, in Preventing Antisocial Behavior: Interventions From Birth Through Adolescence. Edited by McCord J, Tremblay RE. New York, Guilford, 1992b, pp 139–161

Hawkins JD, Arthur MW, Catalano RF: Preventing substance abuse, in Crime and Justice, Vol 19: Building a Safer Society: Strategic Approaches to Crime Prevention. Edited by Tonry M, Farrington D. Chicago, IL, University of Chicago Press, 1995a, pp 343–427

Hawkins JD, Catalano RF, Brewer DD: Preventing serious, violent, and chronic juvenile offending: effective strategies from conception to age six, in A Sourcebook: Serious, Violent, and Chronic Juvenile Offenders. Edited by Howell JC, Krisberg B, Hawkins JD, et al. Thousand Oaks, CA, Sage, 1995b, pp 47–60

Hawkins JD, Catalano RF, Kosterman R, et al: Preventing adolescent health-risk behaviors by strengthening protection during childhood. Arch Pediatr Adolesc Med 153:226–234, 1999

Hawkins JD, Catalano RF, Arthur MW: Promoting science-based prevention in communities. Addict Behav 27:951–976, 2002

Hawkins JD, Kosterman R, Catalano RF, et al: Effects of social development intervention in childhood fifteen years later. Arch Pediatr Adolesc Med 162:1133–1141, 2008

Hawkins JD, Oesterle S, Brown EC, et al: Results of a type 2 translational research trial to prevent adolescent drug use and delinquency: a test of Communities That Care. Arch Pediatr Adolesc Med 163:789–798, 2009

Hill KG, Hawkins JD, Catalano RF, et al: Family influences on the risk of daily smoking initiation. J Adolesc Health 37:202–210, 2005

Hingson R, Heeren T, Zakocs R, et al: Age of first intoxication, heavy drinking, driving after drinking and risk of unintentional injury among U.S. college students. J Stud Alcohol 64:23–31, 2003

Holder HD, Blose JO: Impact of changes in distilled spirits availability on apparent consumption: a time series analysis of liquor-by-the-drink. Br J Addict 82:623–631, 1987

Holder HD, Gruenewald PJ, Ponicki WR, et al: Effect of community-based interventions on high-risk drinking and alcohol-related injuries. JAMA 284:2341–2347, 2000

Hops H, Tildesley E, Lichtenstein E, et al: Parent-adolescent problem-solving interactions and drug use. Am J Drug Alcohol Abuse 16:239–258, 1990

Howell JC, Krisberg B, Jones M: Trends in juvenile crime and youth violence, in A Sourcebook: Serious, Violent, and Chronic Juvenile Offenders. Edited by Howell JC, Krisberg B, Hawkins JD, et al. Thousand Oaks, CA, Sage, 1995, pp 1–35

Jenson JM, Hartman JC, Smith JR, et al: Evaluation of Iowa's Juvenile Crime Prevention Community Grant Fund Program. Iowa City, University of Iowa, School of Social Work, 1997

Jessor R, Jessor SL: Problem Behavior and Psychological Development: A Longitudinal Study of Youth. New York, Academic Press, 1977

Jessor R, Chase JA, Donovan JE: Psychosocial correlates of marijuana use and problem drinking in a national sample of adolescents. Am J Public Health 70:604–613, 1980

Johnston LD, O'Malley PM, Bachman JG, et al: Various stimulant drugs show continuing gradual declines among teens in 2008, most illicit drugs hold steady. Ann Arbor, MI, University of Michigan News and Information Services, December 11, 2008. Available at: http://www.monitoringthefuture.org/pressreleases/08drugpr_complete.pdf. Accessed December 13, 2009.

Karlamangla A, Zhou K, Reuben D, et al: Longitudinal trajectories of heavy drinking in adults in the United States of America. Addiction 101:91–99, 2006

Kaufmann DR, Wyman PA, Forbes-Jones EL, et al: Prosocial involvement and antisocial peer affiliations as predictors of behavior problems in urban adolescents: main effects and moderating effects. J Community Psychol 35:417–434, 2007

Kellam SG, Anthony JC: Targeting early antecedents to prevent tobacco smoking: findings from an epidemiologically based randomized field trial. Am J Public Health 88:1490–1495, 1998

Kendler KS, Prescott CA, Myers J, et al: The structure of genetic and environmental risk factors for common psychiatric and substance use disorders in men and women. Arch Gen Psychiatry 60:929–937, 2003

Kilpatrick DG, Acierno R, Saunders B, et al: Risk factors for adolescent substance abuse and dependence: data from a national sample. J Consult Clin Psychol 68:19–30, 2000

King KM, Chassin L: Mediating and moderated effects of adolescent behavioral undercontrol and parenting in the prediction of drug use disorders in emerging adulthood. Psychol Addict Behav 18:239–249, 2004

King KM, Chassin L: Adolescent stressors, psychopathology, and young adult substance dependence: a prospective study. J Stud Alcohol Drugs 69:629–638, 2008

Klerman LV, Santelli JS, Klein JD: So what have we learned? The Editors' comments on the coalition approach to teen pregnancy. J Adolesc Health 37:S115–S118, 2005

Kosterman R, Hawkins JD, Guo J, et al: The dynamics of alcohol and marijuana initiation: patterns and predictors of first use in adolescence. Am J Public Health 90:360–366, 2000

Kraemer HC, Kazdin AE, Offord DR, et al: Coming to terms with the terms of risk. Arch Gen Psychiatry 54:337–343, 1997

Locke TF, Newcomb MD: Adolescent predictors of young adult and adult alcohol involvement and dysphoria in a prospective community sample of women. Prev Sci 5:151–168, 2004

Loeber R, Hay D: Key issues in the development of aggression and violence from childhood to early adulthood. Annu Rev Psychol 48:371–410, 1997

Maddahian E, Newcomb MD, Bentler PM: Risk factors for substance use: ethnic differences among adolescents. J Subst Abuse 1:11–23, 1988

Maggs JL, Frome PM, Eccles JS, et al: Psychosocial resources, adolescent risk behaviour and young adult adjustment: is risk taking more dangerous for some than others? J Adolesc 20:103–119, 1997

Maggs JL, Patrick ME, Feinstein L: Childhood and adolescent predictors of alcohol use and problems in adolescence and adulthood in the National Child Development Study. Addiction 103:7–22, 2008

Mason WA, Kosterman R, Hawkins JD, et al: Reducing adolescents' growth in substance use and delinquency: randomized trial effects of a parent-training prevention intervention. Prev Sci 4:203–212, 2003

Mason WA, Kosterman R, Hawkins JD, et al: Influence of a family focused substance use preventive intervention on growth in adolescent depressive symptoms. J Res Adolesc 17:541–564, 2007

Mason WA, Kosterman R, Haggerty KP, et al: Gender moderation and social developmental mediation of the effect of a family focused substance use preventive intervention on young adult alcohol abuse. Addict Behav 34:599–605, 2009

Masten AS, Best KM, Garmezy N: Resilience and development: contributions from the study of children who overcome adversity. Dev Psychopathol 2:425–444, 1990

Merline A, Jager J, Schulenberg JE: Adolescent risk factors for adult alcohol use and abuse: stability and change of predictive value across early and middle adulthood. Addiction 103:84–99, 2008

Merzel C, D'Afflitti J: Reconsidering community-based health promotion: promise, performance, and potential. Am J Public Health 93:557–574, 2003

Mihalic SF, Fagan A, Irwin K, et al: Blueprints for violence prevention (OJJDP Publ No NCJ-204274). Washington, DC, U.S. Department of Justice, Office of Justice Programs, Office of Juvenile Justice and Delinquency Prevention 2004

Mitchell P, Spooner C, Copeland J, et al: The role of families in the development, identification, prevention and treatment of illicit drug problems. 2001. Available at: http://www.nhmrc.gov.au/_files_nhmrc/file/publications/synopses/ds8.pdf. Accessed May 6, 2010.

Mrazek PJ, Biglan A, Hawkins JD: Community-monitoring systems: tracking and improving the well-being of America's children and adolescents. 2004. Society for Prevention Research. Available at: http://www.preventionresearch.org/CMSbook.pdf. Accessed December 13, 2009.

Najaka SS, Gottfredson DC, Wilson DB: A meta-analytic inquiry into the relationship between selected risk factors and problem behavior. Prev Sci 2:257–271, 2001

National Institute on Drug Abuse: Topics in brief: drug abuse prevention. U.S. Department of Health and Human Services, National Institutes of Health. March 2007. Available at: http://www.drugabuse.gov/pdf/tib/prevention.pdf. Accessed December 13, 2009.

National Research Council and Institute of Medicine: Preventing Mental, Emotional, and Behavioral Disorders Among Young People: Progress and Possibilities. Washington, DC, National Academies Press, 2009

Newcomb MD, Felix-Ortiz M: Multiple protective and risk factors for drug use and abuse: cross-sectional and prospective findings. J Pers Soc Psychol 63:280–296, 1992

Newcomb MD, McGee L: Influence of sensation seeking on general deviance and specific problem behaviors from adolescence to young adulthood. J Pers Soc Psychol 61:614–628, 1991

Noller P, Feeney JA, Peterson C: Personal Relationships Across the Lifespan. Hove, East Sussex, UK, Psychology Press, 2001

O'Donnell J, Hawkins JD, Abbott RD: Predicting serious delinquency and substance use among aggressive boys. J Consult Clin Psychol 63:529–537, 1995

Oesterle S, Hill KG, Hawkins JD, et al: Positive functioning and alcohol-use disorders from adolescence to young adulthood. J Stud Alcohol Drugs 69:100–111, 2008

Olds D, Henderson CR Jr, Cole R, et al: Long-term effects of nurse home visitation on children's criminal and antisocial behavior: 15-year follow-up of a randomized controlled trial. JAMA 280:1238–1244, 1998

Oxford ML, Harachi TW, Catalano RF, et al: Early elementary school-aged child attachment to parents: a test of theory and implications for intervention. Prev Sci 1:61–69, 2000

Oxford ML, Harachi TW, Catalano RF, et al: Preadolescent predictors of substance initiation: a test of both the direct and mediated effect of family social control factors on deviant peer associations and substance initiation. Am J Drug Alcohol Abuse 27:599–616, 2001

Pagan JL, Rose RJ, Viken RJ, et al: Genetic and environmental influences on stages of alcohol use across adolescence and into young adulthood. Behav Genet 36:483–497, 2006

Park J, Kosterman R, Hawkins JD, et al: Effects of the "Preparing for the Drug Free Years" curriculum on growth in alcohol use and risk for alcohol use in early adolescence. Prev Sci 1:125–138, 2000

Patterson GR, Dishion TJ: Contributions of families and peers to delinquency. Criminology 23:63–79, 1985

Pentz MA, Brannon BR, Charlin VL, et al: The power of policy: the relationship of smoking policy to adolescent smoking. Am J Public Health 79:857–862, 1989

Pentz MA, Jasuja GK, Rohrbach LA, et al: Translation in tobacco and drug abuse prevention research. Eval Health Prof 29:246–271, 2006

Perry C, Williams CL, Komro KA, et al: Project Northland: long-term outcomes of community action to reduce adolescent alcohol use. Health Educ Res 17:117–132, 2002

Peterson PL, Hawkins JD, Abbott RD, et al: Disentangling the effects of parental drinking, family management, and parental alcohol norms on current drinking by black and white adolescents. J Res Adolesc 4:203–227, 1994

Pitkänen T, Kokko K, Lyyra A-L, et al: A developmental approach to alcohol drinking behaviour in adulthood: a follow-up study from age 8 to age 42. Addiction 103:48–68, 2008

Ringwalt CL, Hanley S, Vincus AA, et al: The prevalence of effective substance use prevention curricula in the nation's high schools. J Prim Prev 29:479–488, 2008

Ringwalt CL, Vincus AA, Hanley S, et al: The prevalence of evidence-based drug use prevention curricula in U.S. middle schools in 2005. Prev Sci 10:33–40, 2009

Robins LN, Przybeck TR: Age of onset of drug use as a factor in drug and other disorders. NIDA Res Monogr 56:178–192, 1985

Rutter M: Family influences on behavior and development: challenges for the future, in Retrospect and Prospect in the Psychological Study of Families. Edited by McHale JP, Grolnick WS. Mahwah, NJ, Erlbaum, 2002, pp 321–351

Sampson RJ, Groves WB: Community structure and crime: testing social-disorganization theory. Am J Sociol 94:774–802, 1989

Sampson RJ, Lauritsen JL: Violent victimization and offending: individual, situational, and community level risk factors, in Understanding and Preventing Violence, Vol 3: Social Influences. Edited by Reiss Albert J Jr, Roth JA. Washington, DC, National Academies Press, 1994, pp 1–114

Sampson RJ, Raudenbush SW, Earls F: Neighborhoods and violent crime: a multilevel study of collective efficacy. Science 277:918–924, 1997

Sartor CE, Lynskey MT, Heath AC, et al: The role of childhood risk factors in initiation of alcohol use and progression to alcohol dependence. Addiction 102:216–225, 2007

Schweinhart LJ: Crime prevention by the High/Scope Perry Preschool Program. Victims and Offenders 2:141–160, 2007

Shedler J, Block J: Adolescent drug use and psychological health: a longitudinal inquiry. Am Psychol 45:612–630, 1990

Sher KJ, Walitzer KS, Wood PK, et al: Characteristics of children of alcoholics: putative risk factors, substance use and abuse, and psychopathology. J Abnorm Psychol 100:427–448, 1991

Spoth RL, Redmond C, Shin C: Randomized trial of brief family interventions for general populations: adolescent substance use outcomes 4 years following baseline. J Consult Clin Psychol 69:627–642, 2001

Spoth RL, Greenberg M, Turrisi R: Preventive interventions addressing underage drinking: state of the evidence and steps toward public health impact. Pediatrics 121 (suppl 4):S311–S336, 2008

Substance Abuse and Mental Health Services Administration: National Registry of Evidence-based Programs and Practices (NREPP), April 15, 2010. Available at: http://nrepp.samhsa.gov/. Accessed May 6, 2010.

Substance Abuse and Mental Health Services Administration: SAMHSA's Prevention Platform. Available at: https://preventionplatform.samhsa.gov. Accessed January 14, 2010.

Sussman S, Dent CW, Stacy AW, et al: One-year outcomes of Project Towards No Drug Abuse. Prev Med 27:632–642, 766 [erratum], 1998

Takeuchi DT, Williams DR, Adair RK: Economic stress in the family and children's emotional and behavioral problems. Journal of Marriage and the Family 53:1031–1041, 1991

Thombs DL: Introduction to Addictive Behaviors, 3rd Edition. New York, Guilford, 2006

Tierney JP, Grossman JB, Resch NL: Making a Difference: An Impact Study of Big Brothers/Big Sisters. Philadelphia, PA, Public/Private Ventures, 1995

Tobler NS: Meta-analysis of 143 adolescent drug prevention programs: quantitative outcome results of program participants compared to a control or comparison group. J Drug Issues 16:537–567, 1986

Toumbourou JW, Catalano RF: Predicting developmentally harmful substance use, in Preventing Harmful Substance Use: The Evidence Base for Policy and Practice. Edited by Stockwell T, Gruenewald PJ, Toumbourou JW, et al. London, Wiley, 2005, pp 53–65

Tremblay RE, Vitaro F, Bertrand L, et al: Parent and child training to prevent early onset of delinquency: the Montreal Longitudinal-Experimental Study, in Preventing Antisocial Behavior: Interventions From Birth Through Adolescence. Edited by McCord J, Tremblay R. New York, Guilford, 1992, pp 117–138

U.S. Department of Health and Human Services: A comprehensive plan for preventing and reducing underage drinking (DHHS Publ No SMA-01-3517). Rockville, MD, U.S. Department of Health and Human Services, Substance Abuse and Mental Health Services Administration, Center for Mental Health Services, National Institute of Health, National Institute of Mental Health, 2006

von Knorring L, Oreland L, von Knorring AL: Personality traits and platelet MAO activity in alcohol and drug abusing teenage boys. Acta Psychiatr Scand 75:307–314, 1987

Wagenaar AC, Perry CL: Community strategies for the reduction of youth drinking: theory and application. J Res Adolesc 4:319–345, 1994

Wagenaar AC, Toomey TL: Effects of minimum drinking age laws: review and analyses of the literature from 1960 to 2000. J Stud Alcohol 14:206–225, 2002

Wagenaar AC, Murray DM, Gehan JP, et al: Communities mobilizing for change on alcohol: outcomes from a randomized community trial. J Stud Alcohol 61:85–94, 2000

Wagenaar AC, Salois MJ, Komro KA: Effects of beverage alcohol price and tax levels on drinking: a meta-analysis of 1003 estimates from 112 studies. Addiction 104:179–190, 2009

Werner EE, Smith RS: Overcoming the Odds: High Risk Children From Birth to Adulthood. Ithaca, NY, Cornell University Press, 1992

White HR, McMorris BJ, Catalano RF, et al: Increases in alcohol and marijuana use during the transition out of high school into emerging adulthood: the effects of leaving home, going to college, and high school protective factors. J Stud Alcohol 67:810–822, 2006

Williams B, Sanson A, Toumbourou J, et al: Patterns and Predictors of Teenagers' Use of Licit and Illicit Substances in the Australian Temperament Project Cohort. Melbourne, Australia, The Ross Trust, 2000

Wills TA, Sargent JD, Gibbons FX, et al: Movie exposure to alcohol cues and adolescent alcohol problems: a longitudinal analysis in a national sample. Psychol Addict Behav 23:23–35, 2009

Windle M, Wiesner M: Trajectories of marijuana use from adolescence to young adulthood: predictors and outcomes. Dev Psychopathol 16:1007–1027, 2004

Young SE, Rhee SH, Stallings MC, et al: Genetic and environmental vulnerabilities underlying adolescent substance use and problem use: general or specific? Behav Genet 36:603–615, 2006

Zucker RA: Anticipating problem alcohol use developmentally from childhood into middle adulthood: what have we learned? Addiction 103:100–108, 2008

Zuckerman M, Kuhlman DM: Personality and risk-taking: common biosocial factors. J Pers 68:999–1029, 2000

Suggested Readings

Hawkins JD, Catalano RF, Arthur MW: Promoting science-based prevention in communities. Addict Behav 27:951–976, 2002

Ringwalt CL, Hanley S, Vincus AA, et al: The prevalence of effective substance use prevention curricula in the nation's high schools. J Prim Prev 29:479–488, 2008

Relevant Website

National Registry of Evidence-based Programs and Practices: http://www.nrepp.samhsa.gov

Screening and Brief Interventions for Adolescent Substance Use in the General Office Setting

Sharon Levy, M.D., M.P.H.

Ken C. Winters, Ph.D.

John R. Knight, M.D.

Use of substances (alcohol and other drugs) by adolescents is ubiquitous and is associated with injuries, both intentional and unintentional, that are the leading causes of death in this age group (Eaton et al. 2008). Before finishing high school, more than 40% of teens have tried marijuana and 72% have drunk alcohol (Johnston et al. 2008). Although these percentages have declined slightly during the past decade, they remain quite high. Of particular concern, use of prescription narcotic medications has risen dramatically since 2001 (Johnston et al. 2008), and many adolescents believe that prescription medi-

65

cations are "safe" even when used without a doctor's prescription (Friedman 2006).

Annual well-care visits provide an opportunity for physicians to screen adolescent patients in a confidential setting and to provide individualized advice about the health risks associated with drug use. Research has demonstrated that even very brief medical advice from a physician can have a significant impact on the behavior of adults and results in significant cost savings (Babor et al. 2007). Preliminary research suggests that brief advice from a primary care provider can significantly decrease drinking by adolescents.

To be practical, screening must be easy to administer and must distinguish accurately between risk groups so that a physician can quickly determine the appropriate level of intervention. In this chapter, we describe a practical framework that can be used for screening and brief intervention for adolescent substance use and then demonstrate how appropriate tools may be used by presenting case vignettes.

Screening

Setting

National guidelines call for routine screening for drug use at each health maintenance visit during adolescence (Elster and Kuznets 1994; Green and Palfrey 2000; Schydlower 2002). Adolescents with a drug abuse or dependence disorder (American Psychiatric Association 2000) may be less likely to present for routine health care than their peers, and research has demonstrated that positive screen rates are higher among patients presenting for urgent care and follow-up visits than among those presenting for well-care visits (Knight et al. 2007b). This finding suggests that substance use screening may be beneficial whenever a teen presents for care of a problem that may be associated with drug use, such as a sexually transmitted infection or trauma.

Physicians should always use a developmentally appropriate and validated screening instrument and avoid relying on clinical impressions alone. Assessors, including physicians, tend to underestimate the level of drug use involvement without the benefit of information from a structured screening tool (Wilson et al. 2004). Both interview and self-administered screening tools are available. We favor self-administered (i.e., written or computerized) tools, because adolescents tend to prefer them to interviews (Knight et al. 2007a), and if the patients are allowed to complete them in a private area of the clinic while waiting to see the provider, these tools improve efficiency for both physician and patient. However, the interview format, with its opportunity for probing, may be preferred when the physician knows the adolescent well and has already established rapport with him or her (Martin and Winters 1998).

Regardless of the format, physicians must ensure that they ask questions about substance use in a private setting (i.e., without parents present), to increase chances of getting honest answers. We recommend that physicians protect confidentiality as long as an adolescent's drug use does not pose a clear safety risk to self or others. For example, heavy binge drinking of potentially lethal volumes of alcohol, driving while intoxicated, and sexual activity while intoxicated should be considered for discussion with parents if the adolescent is unwilling or unable to contract for safety or if the physician believes that the behavior is likely to be repeated.

A related issue pertains to involvement of the parent if a physician determines that an adolescent is in need of specialty treatment for a drug disorder. The physician should consider involving parents in treatment planning and to help facilitate referral. In our experience, adolescents with high-risk drug use identified by screening do not always return for treatment on their own. However, laws in some states allow adolescents to enter drug treatment without parental consent, so adolescents who are motivated to enter treatment on their own should be supported. In each situation, the physician must carefully weigh the risks of breaking confidentiality (loss of therapeutic alliance) with the risks of maintaining it (continued high-risk behavior, failure to engage in treatment, and loss to follow-up).

Tools

Screening for substance use should begin with unambiguous questions about whether the adolescent has used alcohol, marijuana, or another drug in the past 12 months. We recommend three opening questions (see also Table 3–1).

During the *past 12 months*, did you

1. Drink any *alcohol* (more than a few sips)?
2. Smoke any *marijuana or hashish*?
3. Use *anything else* to get high?

Table 3–1.   Opening screening questions on substance use

During the *past 12 months*, did you

1. Drink any *alcohol* (more than a few sips)?
2. Smoke any *marijuana or hashish*?
3. Use *anything else* to get high?

"Anything else" includes

Illegal drugs—such as speed, mushrooms, ecstasy, cocaine, opium, or heroin

Inhalants—such as sniffing or huffing glue, propane, whippets, nitrous oxide, paint thinner, or gasoline

Over-the-counter medications—such as cough syrup, dextromethorphan (DXM), or caffeine pills

Prescription drugs—such as Percocet, OxyContin, Ritalin, Adderall, Dexedrine, Valium, or Klonopin

"Anything else" does NOT include

Tobacco (cigarettes or chewing)

Body-building steroids

Medicine prescribed by your doctor that you take according to the instructions

Adolescents who have not used alcohol or drugs in the past year should be asked whether they have ridden in a car with an intoxicated driver, and those who report this risk should receive counseling to avoid it in the future. If the intoxicated driver is a parent or guardian, providers should offer the teen support and guidance, offer to speak with the parent, and respect the child's privacy if he or she declines. Providers may consider reporting the situation to child protective services if the behavior is ongoing. We recommend that physicians seek assistance from legal or child protection staff in these instances.

Adolescents who report using alcohol or drugs during the past year require additional screening to identify those at high risk. The ideal screening tool would be brief, easy to administer and score, developmentally appropriate, and well validated. To maximize efficiency, we recommend using a tool that can screen for alcohol and drug use risk simultaneously. Various psychometrically sound tools for use with adolescents are available (Winters and Kaminer 2008); a list of recommended tools is presented in Appendix A, and a listing of resources on adolescent drug abuse assessment is provided in Appendix B. The decision regarding which tool to use depends on several factors, including time and training requirements and planned use and breadth of desired information.

Table 3–2.   The CRAFFT

1. Have you ever ridden in a **CAR** driven by someone (including yourself) who was "high" or had been using alcohol or drugs?
2. Do you ever use alcohol or drugs to **RELAX**, feel better about yourself, or fit in?
3. Do you ever use alcohol or drugs while you are by yourself, or **ALONE**?
4. Do you ever **FORGET** things you did while using alcohol or drugs?
5. Do your **FAMILY** or **FRIENDS** tell you that you should cut down on your drinking or drug use?
6. Have you ever gotten into **TROUBLE** while you were using alcohol or drugs?

One of the more efficient tools is the six-item CRAFFT (Knight 1999). It has been validated in medical office settings (Knight et al. 2002), has been endorsed by the American Academy of Pediatrics (2002), and is available in interview and self-administered formats (see Table 3–2). The CRAFFT is very quick to administer, easy to score, and available without cost, making it desirable for use in the medical office setting.

Brief Interventions in Primary Care

All adolescents, whether or not they have used drugs, may benefit from a brief intervention. The goals of brief interventions are threefold: 1) to prevent or delay initiation of drug use for adolescents who have never used alcohol or drugs; 2) to increase quit rates for adolescents who have initiated drug use but have not developed substance dependence; and 3) to reduce acute risk and encourage adolescents with substance dependence to engage in specialty treatment. Universal drug use screening provides an opportunity for office-based intervention for every adolescent, from those who are abstinent to those who are drug dependent.

Adolescents Who Screen Negative for High-Risk Drug Use

Delaying Initiation: Praise, Encouragement, and Advice Not to Start

Adolescence is a particularly vulnerable time for developing substance use disorders. Those who begin drinking alcohol before age 14 years are 5 times more likely to develop an alcohol use disorder than are those who delay initiation until age 21 (Hingson et al. 2006), and similar statistics have been found for marijuana (Winters and Lee 2008). Delaying the onset of alcohol use into their 20s may significantly reduce individuals' lifetime risk of developing a substance use disorder.

Physicians should give praise and encouragement to adolescents who have not initiated substance use (e.g., by saying, "That's a smart decision"). Positive reinforcement, or rewarding a desired behavior, is a fundamental principle of behavior modification (Hancock 2002; Henderlong and Lepper 2002; Sutherland et al. 2002). A private office visit with a physician provides a unique opportunity for approbation from a respected source. Messages that credit an adolescent for making good choices and using good judgment may help build self-esteem and resilience. Emerging research is demonstrating that even very brief encouraging statements may reduce substance initiation rates during the months following the interaction.

Case Vignette

Sarah is a 14-year-old girl who presented for a school physical and answered no to the three opening questions about drug and alcohol use (During the past 12 months, did you drink any alcohol [more than a few sips]? Smoke any marijuana or hashish? Use anything else to get high?) However, she had ridden in a car with her older sister's boyfriend after he had been drinking at a party.

Dr. Smith said to Sarah, "You have made some very good decisions in your choice not to use drugs and alcohol. For the sake of your health, I hope that you will keep it up, and I want you to know that you can always ask me any questions you may have about drugs and alcohol. I do want to talk to you about car safety. Many young people think they are OK to drive after drinking, but the truth is that teenagers should never drive after drinking, even after a single drink. Adolescents often don't notice the early effects of alcohol that can make driving very dangerous. I'd like you to think about alternative ways of getting home. Some kids in my practice have agreed to sleep over at a friend's house if they do not have a safe ride home. Others have agreed with their parents that they can call for a safe ride home anytime, day or night. Parents promise to give the ride with no questions asked and no discussion until the next day. Can you agree never to ride with anyone who has been drinking or using other drugs?"

Increasing Quit Rates: Brief Advice

When adolescents report that they have begun to use alcohol or drugs but have not yet experienced related problems, physicians should advise them to quit. This advice should be supported by health information, including the danger of using drugs while the brain is still developing during adolescence. Adolescents are exposed to a multitude of media and advertising messages that portray use of alcohol and drugs as both normative and fun, with few negative consequences (Strasburger and Donnerstein 1999). Teens who have begun to use substances may be ambivalent about quitting. Accurate, personalized health information from a physician may make a big impact. Physicians can give brief advice quickly; as with praise and encouragement, even very brief statements may increase quit rates during the months after the interaction.

Case Vignette

Marcus is a 16-year-old boy who came to the office after injuring his ankle at football practice. During the exam, Dr. Miller screened him for substance use. The young man said that he had been drunk on several occasions, but not at the time of this injury. He reportedly had never used other drugs, and his CRAFFT score was 0.

Dr. Miller said, "I would recommend that you stop drinking alcohol entirely for the sake of your health. Wait until you are older, when your brain is more fully developed and less likely to be damaged. People often do stupid things when they are drunk that they later regret. Heavy alcohol use can disrupt your sleep and affect your concentration. Over time it can impact your mood and affect your performance on the football field."

Adolescents Who Screen Positive for High-Risk Drug Use

We recommend that physicians assess all adolescents who screen positive for high-risk drug use to rule out a diagnosis of drug dependence. A sufficiently detailed interview may require 10–30 minutes (see Appendix A at the end of this volume for some examples of structured and semistructured interviews). Physicians should ask questions about drug history to determine whether use has been increasing in frequency or quantity as a marker of tolerance. Questions about negative consequences associated with drug use may help to increase an adolescent's motivation to make a behavior change. Physicians should also ask about unsuccessful quit attempts, which are highly suggestive of drug dependence. Asking about reasons for a quit attempt may also provide insight into an adolescent's ambivalence.

Reducing Acute Risk:
Motivational Enhancement Therapy

Adolescents who screen positive for high-risk drug use but are not drug dependent may benefit from an intervention to help them consider the impact of substance use on their future goals. Motivational enhancement therapy, based on motivational interviewing (Miller and Rollnick 2002), is particularly effective and well suited for the general office setting (Fleming 2004). *Motivational interviewing* is a counseling style that encourages patients to explore the discrepancy between current behavior and future goals and to closely examine the benefits and risks of continued drug use versus the benefits and risks of quitting. The motivational interviewing approach uses techniques such as open-ended questions, reflections, and summaries. *Motivational enhancement therapy* refers to directive therapy in which the clinician uses motivational interviewing techniques with a series of concrete tools, such as an activity that formalizes the task of comparing benefits and risks of drug use, called the decisional balance exercise, to explore a specific behavior. (The reader can find an overview of these approaches in Chapter 9, "Brief Motivational Interventions, Cognitive-Behavioral Therapy, and Contingency Management for Youth Substance Use Disorders.")

All adolescents who screen positive for high-risk substance use should receive an intervention, and we recommend a follow-up session to improve results. To improve compliance with return visits, we recommend that the brief intervention be scheduled with the primary care clinician. If this is not possible, the primary care clinician should facilitate the return visit by introducing the adolescent to the clinician who will conduct the session.

In motivational enhancement therapy, treatment goals are determined by the patient and most often achieved incrementally. In many cases, the adolescent's goal will not be to discontinue substance use entirely, especially in the first session. The physician should always be attuned to high-risk situations that the adolescent has reported (e.g., large alcohol binges) and include these in the intervention goals. If the adolescent is unwilling to avoid behaviors that may lead to acute danger, the physician may need to consider breaking confidentiality and involving the parents.

Case Vignette

Katie is a 16-year-old girl who came to the office to discuss emergency contraception. On screening, she said that she drinks alcohol and has tried marijuana twice but has never used other drugs. She answered yes to Relax, Forget, and Trouble questions, giving her a CRAFFT score of 3. Dr. Brown asked follow-up assessment questions.

When asked "Tell me more about your drinking," Katie replied that she started drinking at parties last year. Now she drinks about once a month, four to six drinks, which is enough to get drunk.

Dr. Brown asked, "Have you ever had problems when you were drinking?" Katie said she was suspended for 2 days because she brought a bottle of vodka to a school football game. Her parents were upset and grounded her for 2 weeks after that incident. She told them she would not drink anymore, but she continued to drink with her friends.

Dr. Brown asked, "Have you ever had sexual contact after drinking?" Katie replied that she had had sex while drunk on two occasions. Two days earlier, she had sex with a peer while drunk, and she could not remember whether they had used a condom.

When asked, "Have you ever tried to quit drinking?" Katie said she has not tried to quit drinking. She drinks less than her friends and does not think that her drinking is a problem.

Because Katie experienced serious consequences and risks related to her use of alcohol, Dr. Brown said, "I am worried about your use of alcohol. I understand that you enjoy drinking with your friends, but it seems that you have put yourself in risky situations because of alcohol use. Would you be willing to return for an appointment to talk more about how drinking fits into your life?"

Katie replied that she is not interested in quitting. All of her friends drink and she cannot imagine being the only one not drinking at a party.

Dr. Brown continued, "As your doctor, who cares about your health, I recommend that you quit drinking entirely until you are older. However, you are the only one who can make that decision. For today, I ask only that you schedule another appointment so that we can continue our conversation. OK?" Katie agreed reluctantly. Dr. Brown gave her positive feedback: "Great, agreeing to come back is a really smart decision. Let's plan on spending some time on this when you come back for your postcontraceptive check." Dr. Brown asked Katie to avoid high-risk behaviors. "Before we finish, I want to talk about safety. Having sex when you or your partner is drunk or high is risky because people make bad decisions, like forgetting to use a condom. Can you agree not to have sex when you have had anything to drink?" Katie agreed, and Dr. Brown continued, "Great. One last thing. I am glad that you have not ever ridden with a driver who has been drinking or using drugs. That is a very smart decision. Please keep it up." Katie thanked Dr. Brown on the way out and scheduled a follow-up appointment for 4 weeks later.

Facilitating Referrals

Substance dependence refers to loss of control and preoccupation with substance use despite negative consequences. The disorder is described in the *Diagnostic and Statistical Manual of Mental Disorders*, 4th Edition, Text Revision (DSM-IV-TR; American Psychiatric Association 2000); the diagnosis is made if a patient meets three or more of seven diagnostic criteria (see Table 3–3). Drug dependence, or addiction, has been described for all psychoactive substances, although the presentation varies considerably, leading to the misperception that some psychoactive substances are not addictive. To complicate matters, teens with cannabis dependence often have difficulty establishing causation between cannabis use and associated problems.

Physicians should maintain a high degree of suspicion for cannabis dependence whenever an adolescent reports daily or near-daily use and a decline in functioning. Markers of alcohol use disorders include amnestic periods associated with alcohol use ("blackouts") and episodes of alcohol poisoning. Adolescents with CRAFFT scores of 5 or 6 are also at very high risk of drug dependence (Knight et al. 2002). Adolescents who have developed dependence on any substance may need specialized treatment to learn new self-care behaviors and relapse-prevention skills.

Most adolescents who are substance dependent will need specialized treatment for substance use disorders to achieve and maintain abstinence. The primary goal of an office-based intervention with an adolescent who is substance dependent is to facilitate treatment referral. Some of these adolescents will have recognized their drug problems prior to screening and will be ready to accept a referral to treatment. In such a case, goals for the office-based intervention may include sympathetic listening, identifying an appropriate referral source, facilitating treatment entry, encouraging the adolescent to allow parents or guardians to be involved in treatment, and maintaining a therapeutic relationship with the adolescent during aftercare. Some adolescents with substance dependence will not see their use of substances as problematic and will not be willing to accept a referral to treatment. In our experience, this occurs most frequently with adolescents who are cannabis dependent. In these instances, the physician should use the tools of motivational interviewing to encour-

Table 3–3. DSM-IV-TR criteria for substance dependence

A maladaptive pattern of substance use, leading to clinically significant impairment or distress, as manifested by three (or more) of the following, occurring at any time in the same 12-month period:

(1) tolerance, as defined by either of the following:
   (a) a need for markedly increased amounts of the substance to achieve intoxication or desired effect
   (b) markedly diminished effect with continued use of the same amount of the substance

(2) withdrawal, as manifested by either of the following:
   (a) the characteristic withdrawal syndrome for the substance (refer to Criteria A and B of the criteria sets for withdrawal from the specific substances)
   (b) the same (or a closely related) substance is taken to relieve or avoid withdrawal symptoms

(3) the substance is often taken in larger amounts or over a longer period than was intended

(4) there is a persistent desire or unsuccessful efforts to cut down or control substance use

(5) a great deal of time is spent in activities necessary to obtain the substance (e.g., visiting multiple doctors or driving long distances), use the substance (e.g., chain-smoking), or recover from its effects

(6) important social, occupational, or recreational activities are given up or reduced because of substance use

(7) the substance use is continued despite knowledge of having a persistent or recurrent physical or psychological problem that is likely to have been caused or exacerbated by the substance (e.g., current cocaine use despite recognition of cocaine-induced depression, or continued drinking despite recognition that an ulcer was made worse by alcohol consumption)

Specify if:

With Physiological Dependence: evidence of tolerance or withdrawal (i.e., either Item 1 or 2 is present)

Without Physiological Dependence: no evidence of tolerance or withdrawal (i.e., neither Item 1 nor 2 is present)

Course specifiers (see DSM-IV-TR, pp. 195–197, for definitions):

Early Full Remission, Early Partial Remission, Sustained Full Remission, Sustained Partial Remission, On Agonist Therapy, In a Controlled Environment

Source.   Reprinted from the *Diagnostic and Statistical Manual of Mental Disorders,* 4th Edition, Text Revision. Washington, DC, American Psychiatric Association, 2000. Copyright 2000, American Psychiatric Association. Used with permission.

age treatment entry. Parent guidance and advice on limit setting may be necessary for safety, particularly if an adolescent has access to a car, and may also help create leverage necessary for the adolescent to accept treatment.

Primary care physicians can play a critical role in helping adolescents and their parents understand substance dependence and facilitate appropriate treatment. Adolescents with drug dependence often hear a multitude of negative messages from parents and other adults, and may benefit simply from hearing an empathic message from a physician. Adolescents who have decided to quit using drugs on their own or who are willing to enter treatment should receive affirmation for making these decisions. Physicians may be in an ideal position to encourage teens and parents to participate in treatment together. Family involvement significantly improves outcomes (Liddle et al. 2001; Williams and Chang 2000). The physician should explain that adolescents who are substance dependent have lost control over drug use and need specialized treatment to achieve abstinence. However, a diagnosis of substance dependence should not translate into a "free pass" for drug use, but rather a clear indication for both structure (e.g., limiting free time and financial resources) and support (including emotional support and access to treatment).

Physicians may need to familiarize themselves with local substance abuse treatment resources; adolescents should always be referred to providers experienced in working with adolescents and programs designed specifically for that age group. Various counseling styles and treatment settings have all been shown to be effective; the key elements to successful treatment seem to be engagement and continuation.

An adolescent with substance dependence who refuses to engage in treatment may require parent notification and direction. The primary care physician should express concern over the adolescent's behavior. Parents may be aware of the drug use but may underestimate the extent (Fisher et al. 2006). The physician may ask the adolescent for permission to share screening results and treatment recommendations with parents, without revealing the details (i.e., who, when, and where) of drug use. However, the physician may need to inform parents of need for treatment when an adolescent refuses permission. Safety always comes first.

Parents play an important role in limit setting for adolescents who are dependent on substances, and primary care physicians can provide important guidance. Parents of substance-dependent adolescents should be encouraged to limit resources that enable drug use. In particular, access to cars, cash, credit cards, computers, and cell phones should be removed or strictly supervised. Physicians should advise parents to suspend all driving privileges until the adolescent enters treatment and remains drug free for a period of time. Adolescents should understand that continued drug use may be their choice, but they have to accept all of the associated consequences, including parents' restriction of privileges.

Case Vignette

Eric is a 17-year-old young man who came to the office with flu-like symptoms. On screening, he revealed that he has drunk alcohol, smoked marijuana, and used several other drugs, including oxycodone. He answered yes to all of the CRAFFT questions. After talking about troubles related to his drug use, he said that he thinks he is addicted to opioids and that he would like to quit. Twice in the past he tried to quit on his own, but each time he began using again after a few days, and he thinks he might need help.

Dr. Wilson praised Eric, saying, "I am proud of you for recognizing your drug problem and asking for help. It can be hard to stop using drugs on your own; most people find they need support. I will give you the name of a local treatment center where several of my patients have gotten help for addictions. You may have to wait a few days before you can get an appointment. If you cannot wait, I can send you to the emergency room and the doctors there will help you get into a detoxification program today." Eric said he could wait a few days and decided not to go to a detoxification program. Dr. Wilson asked Eric whether his parents know about his drug problems and offered to facilitate a conversation with them.

Follow-Up

All adolescents should receive follow-up after screening and brief intervention. Adolescents who have not initiated drug use should be rescreened annually or sooner if suggested by medical history. Adolescents who received brief advice should be followed at the next intermittent health care visit to determine whether use has stopped, continued, or progressed.

Adolescents who received a brief intervention should have a specially scheduled appointment to determine whether they have been successful in achieving the goals they set for themselves. Those who have been successful should receive positive feedback. Those who have not been successful may have a more serious substance use problem than initially determined and may benefit from referral to specialized treatment.

The primary care clinician should encourage adolescents who are referred for substance abuse treatment to return to primary care so the physician can follow their progress and assist in coordinating treatment for any co-occurring medical or psychiatric problems. The primary care clinician makes an important statement of caring by continuing to follow adolescents diagnosed with substance dependence and can help decrease feelings of shame.

Conclusion

The standard of care for adolescent medical practice includes screening and brief intervention for substance use. Easy-to-use screening tools and practical brief intervention and referral strategies are available for teenagers with varied levels of drug and alcohol use. Motivational interviewing may help ambivalent teenagers become ready to change substance use behaviors. However, safety is always the priority, and physicians may need to involve parents when adolescents are unable to contract for reducing serious risks.

Key Clinical Concepts

- All adolescents should be screened for alcohol and other drug use at routine health care visits.
- Confidentiality should be ensured unless a teen's behavior poses a safety risk to self or others.
- The use of validated, developmentally appropriate screening tools is important because clinical impressions alone tend to underestimate the problems associated with drug use.
- After every screen, clinicians should provide praise and encouragement for an adolescent who has not used substances, brief advice for an adolescent who reports substance use but screens negative for high-risk use, and a brief intervention for an adolescent who screens positive for high-risk use.
- Adolescents with substance dependence should be referred for specialty treatment.

References

American Academy of Pediatrics: Make time to screen for substance use during office visits (Committee on Substance Abuse). AAP News 21:14, 34, 2002

American Psychiatric Association: Diagnostic and Statistical Manual of Mental Disorders, 4th Edition, Text Revision. Washington, DC, American Psychiatric Association, 2000

Babor TF, McRee BG, Kassebaum PA, et al: Screening, brief intervention, and referral to treatment (SBIRT): toward a public health approach to the management of substance abuse. Subst Abuse 3:7–30, 2007

Eaton DK, Kann L, Kinchen S, et al: Youth risk behavior surveillance—United States, 2007. MMWR Surveill Summ 57:1–131, 2008

Elster A, Kuznets NJ (eds): AMA Guidelines for Adolescent Preventive Services (GAPS): Recommendations and Rationale. Baltimore, MD, Williams & Wilkins, 1994

Fisher SL, Bucholz KK, Reich W, et al: Teenagers are right—parents do not know much: an analysis of adolescent-parent agreement on reports of adolescent substance use, abuse, and dependence. Alcohol Clin Exp Res 10:1699–1710, 2006

Fleming MF: Screening and brief intervention in primary care settings. Alcohol Res Health 2:57–62, 2004

Friedman RA: The changing face of teenage drug abuse—the trend toward prescription drugs. N Engl J Med 14:1448–1450, 2006

Green M, Palfrey J (eds): Bright Futures: Guidelines for Health Supervision of Infants, Children, and Adolescents, 2nd Edition. Arlington, VA, National Center for Education in Maternal and Child Health, 2000

Hancock DR: Influencing graduate students' classroom achievement, homework habits and motivation to learn with verbal praise. Educational Research 1:83–95, 2002

Henderlong J, Lepper MR: The effects of praise on children's intrinsic motivation: a review and synthesis. Psychol Bull 5:774–795, 2002

Hingson RW, Heeren T, Winter MR: Age at drinking onset and alcohol dependence: age at onset, duration, and severity. Arch Pediatr Adolesc Med 7:739–746, 2006

Johnston LD, O'Malley PM, Bachman JG, et al: Monitoring the Future national survey results on adolescent drug use: overview of key findings, 2007 (NIH Publ No 08-6418). Bethesda, MD, National Institute on Drug Abuse, 2008

Knight JR: The CRAFFT Questions: A Brief Screening Test for Adolescent Substance Abuse. Boston, MA, Children's Hospital Boston, 1999

Knight JR, Sherritt L, Shrier A, et al: Validity of the CRAFFT substance abuse screening test among adolescent clinic patients. Arch Pediatr Adolesc Med 6:607–614, 2002

Knight JR, Harris SK, Sherritt L, et al: Adolescents' preference for substance abuse screening in primary care practice. Subst Abuse 4:107–117, 2007a

Knight JR, Harris SK, Sherritt L, et al: Prevalence of positive substance abuse screen results among adolescent primary care patients. Arch Pediatr Adolesc Med 11:1035–1041, 2007b

Liddle HA, Hogue A, Wagner EF, et al: Multidimensional family therapy for adolescent substance abuse, in Innovations in Adolescent Substance Abuse Interventions. Edited by Wagner EF, Waldron HB. New York, Bergman Press/Elsevier Science, 2001, pp 229–261

Martin CS, Winters KC: Diagnosis and assessment of alcohol use disorders among adolescents. Alcohol Health Res World 2:95–105, 1998

Miller WR, Rollnick S: Motivational Interviewing: Preparing People for Change. New York, Guilford, 2002

Schydlower M (ed): Substance Abuse: A Guide for Health Professionals. Elk Grove Village, IL, American Academy of Pediatrics, 2002

Strasburger VC, Donnerstein E: Children, adolescents, and the media: issues and solutions. Pediatrics 1:129–139, 1999

Sutherland KS, Wehby JH, Yoder PJ: Examination of the relationship between teacher praise and opportunities for students with EBD to respond to academic requests. J Emot Behav Disord 1:5–13, 2002

Williams RJ, Chang SY: A comprehensive and comparative review of adolescent substance abuse treatment outcome. Clinical Psychology: Science and Practice 7:138–166, 2000

Wilson CR, Sherritt L, Gates E, et al: Are clinical impressions of adolescent substance use accurate? Pediatrics 114:E536–E540, 2004

Winters KC, Kaminer Y: Screening and assessing adolescent substance use disorders in clinical populations. J Am Acad Child Adolesc Psychiatry 7:740–744, 2008

Winters KC, Lee CY: Likelihood of developing an alcohol and cannabis use disorder during youth: association with recent use and age. Drug Alcohol Depend 92:239–247, 2008

Suggested Readings

Bukstein OG, Bernet W, Arnold V, et al: Practice parameter for the assessment and treatment of children and adolescents with substance use disorders. J Am Acad Child Adolesc Psychiatry 44:609–621, 2005

Winters KC, Kaminer Y: Screening and assessing adolescent substance use disorders in clinical populations. J Am Acad Child Adolesc Psychiatry 47:740–744, 2008

Relevant Website

National Institute on Alcohol Abuse and Alcoholism: Assessing Alcohol Problems: A Guide for Clinicians and Researchers, 2nd Edition: http://pubs.niaaa.nih.gov/publications/Assesing%20Alcohol/.

4

Biomarker Testing for Substance Use in Adolescents

Janelle E. Arias, M.D.

Albert J. Arias, M.D.

Yifrah Kaminer, M.D., M.B.A.

Relying on adolescents' self-reports of drug use is problematic. In particular, youth in community, school, and justice system–related settings may either deny use or underreport the amounts, frequency, and latency of drug used (Buchan et al. 2002). Underreporting may be due to social desirability, concern for legal consequences, and other perceived consequences. In contrast to self-report only, drug testing provides objective information regarding drug use to those who screen and/or treat adolescents who use, abuse, or depend on substances.

In addition to chemically screening samples of patient fluids or tissue for drugs of abuse (or their metabolites), the clinician may gain information about the patient's status by testing other biological markers that correspond to drug and alcohol use. A *biomarker* is any material or substance used as an indicator of a biological state. Biomarkers may range from those that directly detect the substance and/or its metabolites to those that signal end-organ damage from chronic substance use. Biomarkers can be useful in working with adolescent clinical populations by contributing to screening and diagnostic efforts, and by identifying relapse, continued use, and occult use of substances in patients already identified as having substance use disorders. Biomarkers, in conjunction with clinical suspicion and rating scales, aid in the screening and diagnosis of substance use disorders (Center for Substance Abuse Treatment 2006a). In addition to their use by clinicians, biomarker tests can be used in the home setting by parents and are available over the counter.

In this chapter, we review ethical, legal, and practical considerations of drug testing for youth in school, home, and clinical settings. We examine concordance among self-reports, collateral reports, and drug testing. A discussion of available biomarkers is included, as well as an overview of testing by sample source and listing of the Drug Enforcement Administration schedule for selected drugs of abuse. Finally, we provide updated information and directions regarding the available biomarker testing methods for monitoring specific drugs of abuse.

Social Context of Youth Drug Testing

Illegal drug use commonly begins during the teenage years. Some adolescents also begin using tobacco products or drinking alcohol while under the legal age (18 years and 21 years, respectively, in the United States). In many cases, parents either are completely oblivious to drug abuse by their children or have very little knowledge regarding the extent and details of their drug use. Only negative consequences (e.g., legal problems, injuries, health issues) prompt the parents to confront their children's drug problems.

School and home drug testing have been in use for more than a decade. Parents, schools, and the legal system have been struggling with the following questions: What is the purpose of drug testing for youth? Is it legal to conduct drug testing for adolescents? How can testing be done effectively and confidentially? What should be done with the results? What should the consequences be (if any)?

School Drug Testing

The purpose of random student drug testing (RSDT) is preventive in nature and aims to keep U.S. youth safe, healthy, and drug free (Institute for Behavior and Health 2009). More specifically, RSDT programs have four primary goals: to deter and prevent use, to reinforce all other prevention efforts, to identify students who need help getting and staying drug free, and to prepare students for workplace drug testing (Institute for Behavior and Health 2009).

The Institute for Behavior and Health (2009) reported that 11.4% of middle schools and 19.5% of high schools in the United States include some type of drug testing as part of their drug prevention programs. Approximately 7% of U.S. schools (approximately 4,200 schools) conduct RSDT. Although incorporation of RSDT in schools faced two important legal challenges, in 1995 and in 2002, the Supreme Court has ruled that "it is a reasonable means of furthering the School District's important interest in preventing and deterring drug use among its schoolchildren and does not violate the Fourth Amendment" (Institute for Behavior and Health 2009). The Supreme Court also ruled that drug testing for athletes is constitutional. A study of student athlete drug testing found no decrease in sport-activity participation by students when subjected to a random drug testing program; in fact, an 11% increase in participation was reported (Institute for Behavior and Health 2009).

Testing programs are of two types: mandatory and voluntary. Mandatory testing is for students designated into specific groups, such as athletes and drivers. Voluntary testing requires parental consent allowing the student to join the program without penalty. There is a specific manual for RSDT. If a student tests positive for drug use, the test is verified by a medical review officer—that is, a licensed physician who is responsible for reviewing laboratory drug test results and evaluating medical explanations for the results. The student then has an evaluation with a counselor, without any legal involvement or disciplinary consequences. Continued positive tests for drug use may lead to a referral for treatment. Legal use of prescription drugs with parental knowledge is reported by the medical review officer to the school as a negative result (Institute for Behavior and Health 2009).

School-based testing, as well as probation and parole supervision testing, appears appropriate for the detection of any drug use by minors. Cutoff levels are chosen to protect against false positives, which can occur at levels below the specificity of the method of testing (DuPont et al. 2008). The most common drug test panel is the National Institute on Drug Abuse's NIDA-5, which is used to identify the five drugs mandated in federal workplace guidelines: opiates (morphine/codeine), cannabis, cocaine, phencyclidine (PCP), and amphetamine/methamphetamine. Cannabis poses a diagnostic problem in youth because of the latency of cannabis metabolites due to the lipophilic nature of tetrahydrocannabinol (THC), the most active component of cannabis, which is deposited and stored in fatty tissues and released back into blood over time (Buchan et al. 2002). Clinicians need to recognize that an adolescent may report no current drug use and still have a positive drug test for cannabis. Consequently, it is advised to give a 2- to 4-week window before considering a positive drug test for cannabis as valid, as the main psychoactive ingredients can be built up in the body and can take weeks to eliminate in chronic users. Please refer to "Testing for Specific Drugs of Abuse" later in this chapter for more information on testing for cannabis.

Home Drug Testing

Home drug testing is a sensitive issue that involves trust, cooperation, consistency, and enforcement. Parents usually resort to home drug testing after a child has repeatedly violated trust by continued drug use despite promises to quit. Findings of drugs, drug paraphernalia, physical signs of drug use, and "shady" behavior usually signal to parents the need to take some active measures and enforce rules in the household. If the adolescent is in treatment, the counselor, parent, and consenting youth contract for home drug testing. An effective contract includes negotiating negative and positive reinforcers for drug use or nonuse, respectively. These might include curfew hours, car use, or social and entertainment opportunities. A contract should be reviewed periodically (e.g., quarterly). Refusal to give urine for analysis is considered a positive sample, which should activate the contracted consequences. Parents should be consistent and stand firm in light of expected manipulations, acting-out behaviors, or any effort to test their will. If they face difficulty enforcing home drug testing, they should request further consult and support with the counselor/ therapist.

Concordance Among Reports

The assessment of youth with either suspected substance use or known alcohol and other substance use disorder (AOSUD) has been challenging. A common perception is that relying solely on adolescent self-report is certain to result in data with limited reliability. Most adolescents are at least somewhat coerced into screening or assessment of their AOSUD. The majority of these youths do not perceive their levels of use as severe enough to warrant an intervention and consequently are reluctant to cooperate fully (Kaminer 1994). Self-reports may, however, provide reliable and valid information, particularly when no legal contingencies for drug use are pending (Barnea et al. 1987; Buchan et al. 2002; Burleson and Kaminer 2006).

The long-standing and general consensus is that integrated input from both parent and child is ideal for a best-estimate clinical diagnosis of the youth (Leckman et al. 1982; Rutter 1989). To the extent that good agreement exists between the adolescent's and collateral informant's diagnostic information, confidence increases in the validity of the assessment (Cantwell et al. 1997). The limited data available on this topic provide a mixed picture, revealing a considerable range of parent-adolescent agreement. The association among different sources of diagnostic information, however, has often been found to be low (Edelbrock and Achenbach 1986). Parent-child concordance has been shown to vary, for example, as a function of disorder type (Achenbach et al. 1987). Concordance is generally higher for externalizing problems than for internalizing problems, presumably because the former are more easily observable.

Youth have reported significantly more internalizing symptoms and more alcohol and drug abuse than their parents have reported being aware of (Achenbach et al. 1987; Andrews et al. 1993). Cantwell et al. (1997) examined the degree of agreement between parents' and adolescents' reports of the youths' major psychiatric disorders. The κ values for parent-adolescent agreement on the disorders ranged from a low of 0.19 for alcohol abuse/dependence, to 0.41 for substance abuse/dependence, to 0.79 for conduct disorder. Agreement was not influenced by gender, current adolescent age, age at onset of the disorder, or severity of the disorder.

Edelbrock and Achenbach (1986) reported an average mother-child agreement of 63% for AOSUD symptoms, whereas Weissman et al. (1987) reported an average agreement of only 17% for AOSUD symptoms. Winters et al. (2000) reported moderate agreement ($r=0.27$) between mother and child on the drug involvement severity scales. Mothers, however, tended to underreport a child's level of drug involvement and resulting problems compared with the child's self-report.

A Partnership for a Drug-Free America community survey stressed the low levels of agreement between child and parental reports of AOSUD (Center for Substance Abuse Research 1996). Adolescent-reported rates of AOSUD were much higher than parent-reported rates. Similarly, O'Donnell et al. (1998) reported that AOSUD rates varied by informant and were higher when the child, rather than the parent, was the reporter. Parental reports were frequently endorsed by the child's report, whereas the converse was rarely true. One clear methodological limitation of most studies exploring this issue has been lack of objective confirmation of AOSUD, namely via urinalysis.

A more recent study by Burleson and Kaminer (2006) examined the parent-child subjective agreement, as well as agreement with objective results (i.e., drug urinalysis), for adolescents with AOSUD in an outpatient program. Similar to previous reports, the agreement between urinalysis and youth self-report, while moderate, was higher than any agreement with parental assessments. Associations between urinalysis and self-report were highest ($r=0.69$), followed by self-report and collateral informant's report ($r=0.55$), and finally urinalysis and collateral informant's report ($r=0.43$). Separate from the urinalyses, the agreement between parent and youth subjective measures was of similar strength regardless of whether substance use or alcohol use was assessed. Because less agreement might be expected concerning illegal substance use due to associated social admonitions and legal risks, the similarity of substance use agreement and alcohol use agreement is noteworthy.

Results showing that youth report more substance use than their parents perceive are consistent and suggest that parents may often be unaware of the general recent history, as well as the specificity, frequency, and magnitude, of their children's substance use. Between 95% and 100% of cases of adolescent alcohol and other substance abuse are identified by adolescents' reports. Presumably, for these disorders, parents' reports identify very few additional cases (Cantwell et al. 1997). If a clinician had to choose between believing the adolescent and the parent, relying on the adolescent's report would more likely result in a correct diagnosis (Cantwell et al. 1997). Despite the severe deficits in parents' knowledge regarding their children's substance use, Buchan et al. (2002) and Winters et al. (2000) have advocated for use of multiple sources of information. The parents' collateral report remains a desirable source of information that may allow functional assessment of other life domains, legal consequences, and potential treatment outcomes.

Available Biomarkers

Biomarkers may be found in urine, hair, saliva, sweat, and blood. The most common drug test panel is the previously mentioned NIDA-5 panel, used to identify the five drugs mandated in federal workplace testing guidelines. This panel can be tested in each of the aforementioned biomarkers. Screening urine tests consist of immunoassays using monoclonal antibodies against the specific drug or drug metabolite. Immunoassay tests have high sensitivity but lower specificity due to occasional cross-reactivity. Such qualitative tests are often all that is needed in the clinical setting.

All drug-use biomarker tests vary in their sensitivity and specificity based on the method used and the sample source. High specificity within a particular drug class (e.g., benzodiazepines) is not necessarily desirable for a screening test. Confirmation testing of a positive result is performed with chromatography (usually gas chromatography) and mass spectroscopy, which detect the specific substance or its metabolite with high specificity. A test is considered to be highly *sensitive* if it detects as positive most or all of the samples that are actually positive (with few false negatives). A test is considered highly *specific* if it detects as negative most or all of the actual negative samples (with few false positives). In general, screening tests available for office use tend to be reasonably sensitive and specific and are fairly inexpensive. Availability of tests for in-office use and access to regional labs for screening and confirmation have increased in recent years.

In-office screening at the point of care tends to be highly affordable and cost-effective, with most general 5- to 10-panel tests costing less than $10. Although these qualitative screening tests will detect the presence of the substance above a threshold cutoff, they do not give any further quantitative information on the level of specific substances or their metabolites. In general, point-of-care screening kits, combined with occasional use of regional labs for confirmatory testing, are all that is needed for most cases involving clinical management. Sending samples to one of the many widely available regional commercial laboratories is considerably more expensive (often costing between $100 and $300 for a 5- to 10-panel test), but usually includes repeated testing of positively screened samples with gas chromatography–mass spectroscopy or similar confirmatory methods, and results in a report of quantitative levels of substances and relevant metabolites. This testing might be necessary for legal cases, as well as to resolve the discrepancy between self-report and on-site qualitative urine testing by confirming a continued decrease in drug levels for a heavy cannabis user. In such forensic cases, the clinician should consult a medical review officer or a medical toxicologist.

Overview of Testing by Sample Source

Urine tests are the most cost-effective and widely available tests. They can detect a wide range of substances and can be done in the office or at home. However, falsification of urine tests is problematic, especially when sample collection is unobserved (DuPont and Selavka 2008). To minimize the risk for tampering with samples in clinical settings, the patient should provide a urine sample while supervised by someone of the same gender. Urine samples can be retained for about 1 year and can be retested if original results are disputed. The Internet has become a source of information about obtaining adulterants and urine substitutes to produce false-negative results (Greenfield and Hennessy 2008). The period of detection of most substances and their metabolites in urine is relatively short, often only 1–3 days, depending on substance type and acute versus chronic use. The level of the substance or its metabolite in the urine is influenced by fluid consumption, enabling patients to obscure drug use through abrupt drinking of large amounts of fluids to dilute the urine sample (DuPont and Selavka 2008). Parents can easily obtain urine drug screening kits for in-home use at their local drugstore or via the Internet. Some of these tests include indicators for urine tampering by testing for changes in pH and specific weight. Measurement of temperature is another rough measurement for urine tampering (i.e., the cup should feel warm when filled with fresh urine).

Saliva tests can be performed in the office. Saliva collection is easy, cheating is difficult, and the test is cost effective, although more expensive than urine testing. However, there is only a short window of detection (6–12 hours).

Drugs are present in lower concentrations in saliva than in other fluids (except for blood, in which the concentrations are equal to those in saliva) (DuPont and Selavka 2008).

Hair testing, via a 1.5-inch sample, accounts for drug use in the last 90 days. Drug use in the week immediately before the sample is collected cannot be measured in the hair, as hair requires 7 days to grow out of the follicle. Hair testing can discriminate the amount of substance used and the chronicity of use (DuPont and Selavka 2008). Subjects are unable to manipulate results, and despite an alleged racial and hair color bias, none has been scientifically detected (Mieczkowski and Lersch 2002; Mieczkowski and Newel 2000). Perming, bleaching, and straightening treatments may alter drug levels in the hair. Hair testing is more expensive than other means, cannot be completed on-site, is done by relatively few laboratories, and reveals only a limited number of substances (DuPont and Selavka 2008). Companies have begun to market hair testing for cocaine, marijuana, opiates, ecstasy, amphetamine, and PCP so parents can screen for potential substance use in their children by sending a hair sample to the company for analysis.

For sweat testing, a patch is applied to a patient to prospectively test for substance use over a 1- to 3-week period. Substances enter the sweat from the bloodstream via passive diffusion (Cone 1997). As the water, oxygen, and carbon dioxide evaporate from the patch, traces of substance remain. The amount of the substance is not affected by fluid consumption. If the patch is removed or tampered with, it will pucker (DuPont and Selavka 2008). The patch's adhesive film also changes color when removed. The sweat patch ("PharmChek") is available from PharmChem Laboratories (http://www. pharmchem.com) and is FDA approved to test for cocaine, marijuana, opiates, amphetamines, methamphetamines, and PCP. Unlike urine testing, the patch can detect both the parent drug and its metabolite. An immunoassay screening test is followed by confirmation of any positive results via gas chromatography–mass spectrometry. The test is more expensive than urine or saliva testing, but less expensive than hair testing.

Direct testing of many substances can be performed on blood samples via immunoassay or gas chromatography–mass spectroscopy (DuPont and Selavka 2008; Kerrigan and Phillips 2001). Testing blood samples may be a useful method for avoiding tampering (as can occur with urine samples) but is usually more costly. Substances in the blood are usually cleared within 12 hours (DuPont and Selavka 2008).

In the adolescent population, screening tests for episodic drug use (e.g., binge drinking during the weekends) would be particularly useful, as would a biomarker that could indicate low-level but chronic drug use. Because sensitivity and specificity data are calculated from an adult population, the results discussed are indicative of that population, and results must be extrapolated to the adolescent population until more studies are conducted.

Drug Enforcement Administration Schedule for Selected Drugs of Abuse

The Drug Enforcement Administration classifies controlled substances with a five-level system (Schedules I–V), as shown in Table 4–1. Schedule I consists of substances that are considered not legitimate for medical use, such as heroin, illicit fentanyl ("China white"), marijuana, and lysergic acid diethylamide (LSD). Schedule II includes substances with a strong potential for abuse or addiction but with legitimate medical use, such as amphetamine, methamphetamine, methylphenidate, cocaine, and codeine. Schedule III consists of substances that have less potential for abuse or addiction than Schedule I or II drugs and that have a useful medical purpose, such as buprenorphine, ketamine, and gamma-hydroxybutyric acid preparations (Xyrem) that have been approved by the U.S. Food and Drug Administration (FDA). Schedule IV comprises substances that are medically useful with less potential for abuse or addiction than those of Schedules I, II, and III, such as most benzodiazepines, modafinil, and phenobarbital. Schedule V consists of substances that are medically useful with less potential for abuse or addiction than those of Schedules I through IV, such as preparations using codeine, opium, or ethylmorphine (Drug Enforcement Administration 2008).

Testing for Specific Drugs of Abuse

The properties of common biomarker tests for drug and alcohol use are described in Table 4–2 and reviewed below.

Table 4–1. Drug Enforcement Administration schedules for selected drugs of abuse

Schedule I	Schedule II	Schedule III	Schedule IV	Schedule V
Illicit fentanyl ("China white") and its derivatives	Amphetamine and methamphetamine	Anabolic steroids	Most benzodiazepines	Codeine preparations (Cosanyl, Robitussin A-C, Cheracol, Cerose, Pediacof)
GHB	Cocaine	Buprenorphine	Modafinil	
Heroin and synthetic heroin	Codeine	Dronabinol (Marinol)	Phenobarbital	Ethylmorphine preparations
LSD	Fentanyl	FDA-approved GHB drug products (Xyrem)		Opium preparations (Parepectolin, Kapectolin PG, Kaolin Pectin PG)
MDMA, MDA, MDEA	Hydrocodone	Ketamine		
Mescaline, peyote	LAAM			
Morphine	Lisdexamfetamine			
N,N-dimethyl-amphetamine	Meperidine			
Psilocin, psilocybin	Methadone			
Marijuana	Methylphenidate			
	Opium			
	Oxycodone			
	Pentobarbital			
	Phencyclidine (PCP)			

Note. FDA=U.S. Food and Drug Administration; GHM=gamma-hydroxybutyric acid; LAAM=L-α-acetylmethadol; LSD=lysergic acid diethylamide; MDA=methylenedioxyamphetamine; MDEA=methylenedioxyethylamphetamine; MDMA=methylenedioxymethylamphetamine.
Schedule I: Not legitimate for medical use
Schedule II: Strong potential for abuse or addiction but have legitimate medical use
Schedule III: Less potential for abuse or addiction than Schedule I or II drugs and have a useful medical purpose
Schedule IV: Medically useful category of drugs that have less potential for abuse or addiction than those of Schedules I, II, and III
Schedule V: Medically useful category of drugs that have less potential for abuse or addiction than those of Schedules I–IV
Source. Adapted from Drug Enforcement Administration 2008.

Table 4–2.   Properties of common drug screens

Drug of abuse	Sample type	Method of detection[a]	Approximate sensitivity (%)	Approximate specificity (%)	Common detection cutoff (mg/L)	Approximate window of detection for use
Alcohol	Blood	GGT	40–73	63–91		4 weeks
	Urine	CDT	40–63	80–93		3 weeks
		EtG	81	79		3–5 days
Cannabis	Urine	IA screen	73–98	83–99	50	72–96 hours
		CHRM	77	100		
Heavy and chronic use						Up to about 5 weeks
Nicotine						
Cotinine	Urine	IA screen	98	97		3–4 days
	Saliva		93	95		3–4 days
Carbon monoxide	Breath (exhaled)					4–5 hours
Benzodiazepines	Urine	IA screen	77–91	87–97	1,000	Varies based on half-life (often ≥24 hours)
		CHRM	8–23	97–100		
Opioids	Urine	GC-MS				
6-Monoacetyl-morphine[b]						4–6 hours
Morphine		IA screen	84–95	89–99	300	24 hours
		CHRM	41–73	96–100		

Table 4–2. Properties of common drug screens (continued)

Drug of abuse	Sample type	Method of detection[a]	Approximate sensitivity (%)	Approximate specificity (%)	Common detection cutoff (mg/L)	Approximate window of detection for use
Opioids (continued)	Urine					
Buprenorphine						48–56 hours
Norbuprenorphine						
Oxycodone						
Cocaine (via benzoylecgonine)	Urine	IA screen	72–98	88–99	300	8 hours
		CHRM	50–84	99–100	300	48–72 hours
Amphetamines	Urine	IA screen	44–94	84–99	1,000	48 hours
		CHRM	54–71	98–99	500	48–72 hours
MDMA (ecstasy)[c]	Urine	IA screen	99[d]	98[d]	500	1–3 days
		CHRM				

Note. CDT = carbohydrate-deficient transferrin; CHRM = chromatography methods *other than* GC-MS; EtG = ethyl glucuronide; GC-MS = gas chromatography–mass spectrometry; GGT = γ-glutamyltransferase; IA screen = immunoassay-based screening systems; MDMA = methylenedioxymethamphetamine (ecstasy).

[a]GC-MS is the gold standard for identifying substances and is usually assumed to be nearly 100% sensitive and 100% specific because it can detect and differentiate trace amounts of most substances. However, errors are possible due to sample mishandling or to improper operation or maintenance of the GC-MS machines.

[b]Because of its very short half-life, heroin is usually not tested in blood or urine, but its metabolites 6-monoacetylmorphine and morphine can be detected for a brief window of time, allowing heroin use to be differentiated from morphine and codeine use.

[c]MDMA (ecstasy) will cross-react as amphetamines with a number of in-office screening kits (Crouch et al. 2002).

[d]From Loor et al. 2002, using CEDIA (cloned enzyme donor immunoassay) multiplex assay.

Source. Table adapted and compiled from Benowitz 1996; Center for Substance Abuse Treatment 2006a; Cooke et al. 2008; Ferrera et al. 1994; Korzec et al. 2004; Miller et al. 2006; Niemelä 2007; Verstraete 2004; Verstraete and Heyden 2005; Wolff et al. 1999; Wurst et al. 2004.

Alcohol

For detecting alcohol consumption, breath analysis is a highly sensitive test with low cost, yet it is only effective for minutes to hours after drinking based on the amount consumed and the individual's metabolism (Greenfield and Hennessy 2008). Its best purpose is to determine use at a specific point in time rather than as a measure of chronic use.

Biomarkers for detecting use and relapse in alcohol use disorders are numerous, but there are specific limitations to their use. Alcohol biomarkers include serum gamma-glutamyltransferase, aspartate aminotransferase, alanine aminotransferase, mean corpuscular volume, carbohydrate-deficient transferrin, ethyl glucuronide, ethyl sulfate, and phosphatidylethanol.

The most commonly used traditional biomarker is serum gamma-glutamyltransferase (GGT). This biomarker is elevated in individuals who have been drinking at least five drinks per day for several weeks, and it has moderate sensitivity and specificity (Center for Substance Abuse Treatment 2006a). It is not increased in individuals who occasionally binge on alcohol. In individuals who consume 40 g/day of alcohol, elevated GGT levels are found in 20% of males and 15% of females. In individuals who drink more than 60 g/day of alcohol, elevated GGT levels are found in 40%–50% of males and 30% of females. GGT level returns to normal after 4–5 weeks of abstinence (its half-life is between 14 and 26 days) (Sharpe 2001). The test has been found to perform best in adults ages 30–60 (Center for Substance Abuse Treatment 2006a), because GGT levels are rarely elevated in subjects under age 30 (Whitfield et al. 1978). GGT level elevation reflects liver damage secondary to alcoholism, but GGT levels can also be elevated as a result of liver and biliary disease, nicotine use, obesity, and microsomal enzyme–inducing medications (Center for Substance Abuse Treatment 2006a).

Aspartate aminotransferase (AST) and alanine aminotransferase (ALT) indicate heavy alcohol use over several weeks, with moderate sensitivity and specificity. AST and ALT reflect liver damage secondary to alcohol use, with AST being more sensitive than ALT. These tests have been found to perform best in adults ages 30–70. Elevations in levels of AST and ALT due to non-alcohol-related causes are similar to those of GGT, and excessive coffee consumption can lower values (Center for Substance Abuse Treatment 2006a).

Mean corpuscular volume (MCV) can be used to detect heavy drinking that lasts at least a few months (Center for Substance Abuse Treatment 2006a). MCV may be elevated after a month of drinking 60 g/day of alcohol, and MCV returns to baseline after several months of abstinence (Whitehead et al. 1978). It has low sensitivity and moderate-high specificity, without gender effect (Center for Substance Abuse Treatment 2006a), although studies have found that measuring MCV in women may be more sensitive than measuring carbohydrate-deficient transferrin (CDT) or GGT (Sillanaukee et al. 1998). Liver diseases, hemolysis, anemia, folate deficiency, bleeding disorders, and medications reducing folate may also cause elevated MCV (Center for Substance Abuse Treatment 2006a).

Carbohydrate-deficient transferrin was the first biomarker to receive FDA approval (Center for Medicare and Medicaid Services 2001). CDT is elevated when an individual has been drinking 5 drinks per day for about 2 weeks (Center for Substance Abuse Treatment 2006a). Another study showed that CDT levels were elevated in subjects consuming 50–80 g/day of alcohol for at least 1 week; CDT's half-life is 15 days for a decrease in the level (Stibler 1991). Its sensitivity is moderate and specificity is high (Center for Substance Abuse Treatment 2006a). In a primary care setting sample of adult patients with diabetes and hypertension, the sensitivity was found to be 60% and specificity to be 85% in detecting individuals drinking at least 42 g/day of alcohol (Fleming and Mundt 2004). It is less sensitive for women and younger individuals, but is good at detecting relapse to drinking. CDT has been found to perform better at detecting alcohol dependence than at detecting high alcohol consumption without dependence (Mikkelsen et al. 1998). False positives may be caused by carbohydrate-deficient glycoprotein syndrome, fulminant hepatitis C, iron deficiency, and hormonal status in women (Center for Substance Abuse Treatment 2006a).

Ethyl glucuronide (EtG) and ethyl sulfate (EtS) can detect as little as a single drink. They are direct analytes of nonoxidative breakdown of alcohol. Urine EtG sensitivity and specificity for differentiating nondrinkers and light drinkers from heavy drinkers have been estimated at 80.5% and 78.7%, respectively, at a cutoff level of 0.445 mg/L (Wurst et al. 2004). Differences in ethnicity, gender, and age do not affect the test results. The test is inexpensive. Incidental exposure to alcohol contained in foods, cosmetics, hygiene products, and medications may cause false-positive results (Center for Substance Abuse Treatment 2006a).

The Substance Abuse and Mental Health Services Administration issued a clarification in October 2006, warning that EtG should not be used as the sole basis of legal or disciplinary action due to the high sensitivity of the test. This clarification targeted licensure bodies, monitoring organizations, and the criminal justice system (Center for Substance Abuse Treatment 2006b). Therefore, negative results may be more meaningful than positive results. However, it may be possible for patients to dilute urine EtG with excessive water intake (Wojcik and Hawthorne 2007).

EtG is a new biomarker, warranting more research on its usefulness in the clinical setting (Center for Substance Abuse Treatment 2006a). By raising the cutoff point for metabolite detection, false positives can be reduced. Many labs offering the EtG test now offer a variety of cutoff points, which they suggest may eliminate false positives. Further independent investigation into the use of EtG is warranted. The EtG test is most useful in clinical or legal settings that require abstinence. EtG can also be tested in hair samples, with high sensitivity (0.92) and specificity (0.96) at a cutoff level of 27 pg/mg for detecting heavy drinking (>60 g/day of alcohol) (Morini et al. 2009).

EtS has similar properties to EtG. Laboratories have begun to test for EtS; however, such testing is not as widely available as testing for EtG (Center for Substance Abuse Treatment 2006a).

Phosphatidylethanol (PEth) is a phospholipid formed only in the presence of ethanol (Aradottir et al. 2006). PEth is raised when a person has had three or four drinks per day for a few days. It has high sensitivity and unknown specificity. There is little ethnicity, gender, or age effect. Because of the paucity of research on this new biomarker, there are no known sources of false positives (Center for Substance Abuse Treatment 2006a). In a study of adult inpatients and outpatients with alcohol dependence, the sensitivity of PEth was 99% among all patients despite quantity of alcohol use, whereas the sensitivity of CDT and GGT was related to the amount of ethanol intake (Aradottir et al. 2006).

Cannabis

The compound tetrahydrocannabinol, which is found in cannabis, and its metabolite 11-nor-9-carboxy-THC (THC-COOH) have a terminal half-life of 48 hours or longer (Gustafson et al. 2004). Testing for THC-COOH is usually done in urine and serum; THC-COOH is more abundant than THC in these fluids (Johansson and Halldin 1989; Johansson et al. 1989). A urine level of 20–200 ng/mL of THC-COOH corresponds with 10–50 mg of cannabis use (Wall et al. 1983). A urine screen may be positive for 1–3 days. With chronic cannabis use, the range of detection estimated varies from 1 to 11 weeks because of the lipophilic nature of THC, which is stored in fatty tissues and released back into blood over time (Hall and Degenhardt 2005; Schuckit 2000). It can be clinically useful to consider the use of "creatinine-corrected" cannabinoid levels (Musshoff and Madea 2006), which are obtained by measuring the urine creatinine concentration and contrasting the levels as a ratio. Over time, in a now-abstinent previously chronic user, the ratio of urine cannabinoid to creatinine should follow a general linear trend downward.

Cannabis also can be detected in the blood, ranging from 0 to 500 ng/mL. Levels of more than 10–15 ng/mL indicate recent use. The ratio of THC to 9-carboxy-THC can be used to extrapolate time since last use (Hall and Degenhardt 2005).

Saliva testing for cannabis is not sensitive. Cannabis can be detected in hair if use is twice per week for the 90-day period prior to sampling (DuPont and Selavka 2008). Some evidence suggests that pubic hair may contain higher concentrations. Sweat patches can be used to test for cannabis, but, as in saliva, concentrations tend to be lower in sweat than in urine (Hall and Degenhardt 2005).

Nicotine

Cotinine, a metabolite of nicotine, is the preferred biomarker to test for cigarette smoking, and can be found in saliva, urine, and blood (Florescu et al. 2009). Although a number of other biomarkers can be used for detecting cigarette smoking, cotinine is the most commonly tested because it has the most ideal window of detection, at around 3–4 days, and is relatively inexpensive. Hair testing for nicotine is a promising new method for measuring cigarette smoking and exposure to cigarette smoke. To gather information regarding the recency of smoking, particularly for research purposes, one can measure carbon monoxide level by having the individual breathe into a specific instrument. The instrument performing quantitative analysis of carbon monoxide costs approximately $1,500.

Sedatives, Hypnotics, and Anxiolytics

Immunoassay screens for benzodiazepines are readily available; however, the sensitivity and window of detection vary for the different compounds. Because of the variability in cross-reactivity for different benzodiazepines and the large proportion of conjugated benzodiazepines excreted in the urine (which are often not cross-reactive with immunoassays aimed at detecting the actual benzodiazepine molecules), urine drug screening by immunoassay can be difficult to interpret. For example, some screening assays are much less sensitive to detecting clonazepam than alprazolam (DeRienz et al. 2008). When beta-glucuronidase enzyme is added to urine samples and the conjugates are hydrolyzed, sensitivity to benzodiazepines can be improved considerably.

Opiates

Urine tests for opiates detect morphine (the main metabolite of heroin), which can usually be detected 12–36 hours after use. Poppy seed consumption can yield a positive urine test; however, fentanyl may not be detected. In hair sampling, poppy seed use does not lead to positive results for opiates (DuPont and Selavka 2008). Longer-acting opiates may be detected in the urine for up to 4 days. Saliva testing has about the same sensitivity as urine testing (Jaffe and Strain 2005). Regular opioid immunoassay screens are less sensitive for synthetic and semisynthetic opioids, with variable cross-reactivity (Haller et al. 2006). Specific immunoassays must be ordered to detect fentanyl and related compounds. Oxycodone also should be tested for specifically, because many regular opioid screens detect only high levels of oxycodone in the urine, leading to false negatives. Methadone and buprenorphine are not detected by standard opioid screens, so specific immunoassay screens must be used to detect their presence in urine. To more clearly determine adherence to buprenorphine, a quantitative assay demonstrating adequate levels of its major metabolite norbuprenorphine is recommended, because patients not regularly taking the medicine will not have sufficient levels of the metabolite. A study examining the monitoring of opiate use via sweat patches in an adult outpatient sample found sensitivity of 36.5% and specificity of 95.0% based on comparison with urine test results and self-reports over a 1-week period (Chawarski et al. 2007).

Dextromethorphan

Dextromethorphan is an ingredient in commonly abused over-the-counter cough suppressant medications. It has a complex pharmacological mechanism of action, acting as a noncompetitive N-methyl-D-aspartate (NMDA) antagonist, a sigma-1 receptor agonist, and a voltage-gated calcium channel blocker (Werling et al. 2007). Although antitussive effects are thought to be mediated by dextromethorphan's effects on sigma receptors, the psychotropic properties of dextromethorphan are usually attributed to its ability to antagonize NMDA receptors (Boyer 2004; Brown et al. 2004). Dextromethorphan is often abused by adolescents because it is readily available in cough syrups and over-the-counter cough and cold preparations. Overdose and severe toxicity with dextromethorphan can cause death, probably through respiratory depression (Logan et al. 2009). Direct urine testing of dextromethorphan appears to have limited accessibility in the United States. Kim et al. (2006) reported a standardization of a method for the analysis of dextromethorphan and its metabolite dextrorphan in urine, but stated that further experimentation would be needed to generalize results to monitoring illegal use. In our own research into the local availability of such tests, we found that local commercial and hospital labs only offer serum levels, making serial monitoring more cumbersome for the patient. Dextromethorphan may yield a false-positive result on a urine screen for opiates and/or PCP, due to its molecular basis and mode of action, respectively, although this is more likely to occur when large dosages are used.

Cocaine

Cocaine use can be tested using urine, blood, hair, perspiration, and saliva. Cocaine has a short elimination half-life of 1 hour. Benzoylecgonine is a cocaine metabolite with a half-life of 6 hours and is thus used in testing biological fluids for cocaine use (Warner 1993). Acute cocaine use can be monitored in the urine 1–2 days after recent use, and prolonged positive results may be present in chronic, heavy users (>0.5 g/day) (Burke et al. 1990). False-positive results may be caused by high dosages of prilocaine (Baselt and Baselt 1987) and coca tea (Mazor et al. 2006). False-negative results may be caused by the addition of Drano, bleach, and sodium chloride solution (Mikkelsen and Ash 1988).

A study examining the monitoring of cocaine use via sweat patches in an adult outpatient sample found a sensitivity of 95.0% and a specificity of 92.6% based on comparison with urine test results and self-reports over a 1-week period (Chawarski et al. 2007). Hair analysis has been used to probe for chronic use, because the hair matrix absorbs and traps cocaine. Measuring the distance of cocaine concentrations from the hair root can be used to approximate time elapsed since drug use (Mercolini et al. 2008). Other research has found that cocaine and benzoylecgonine can be measured in the hair as early as 1 day after intranasal use, and therefore hair analysis may be able to differentiate between chronic and episodic cocaine use (Ursitti et al. 2001).

Amphetamine and Methamphetamine

Methamphetamine undergoes N-demethylation to its metabolite amphetamine. A considerable portion of the parent compound is excreted into the urine unchanged, with the exact amount varying based on urinary pH level (Hsu et al. 2003; Schepers et al. 2003). Metabolites of amphetamine may be detected in blood, urine, saliva, sweat, and hair. Screening for amphetamine should also include testing for methamphetamine, methylenedioxyamphetamine (MDA), methylenedioxyethylamphetamine (MDEA), and methylenedioxy-methylamphetamine (MDMA) (Verstraete and Hayden 2005). Hsu et al. (2003) described monoclonal antibody tests to differentiate among amphetamine, methamphetamine, and MDMA, because MDMA may require higher concentrations to yield a positive result on amphetamine immunoassays. The Division of Workplace Programs of the Substance Abuse and Mental Health Services Administration (2004) specifies an initial immunoassay-positive drug test for amphetamine at a level ≥ 1,000 ng/mL and confirmatory tests for amphetamine and methamphetamine via gas chromatography–mass spectroscopy at a level ≥ 500 ng/mL. If the methamphetamine test is positive, the sample must also contain amphetamine at a concentration ≥ 200 ng/mL. A study by Verstraete and Heyden (2005) comparing urine immunoassays found that fewer false positives or false negatives can be obtained if the cutoff for detection of amphetamine and MDMA is optimized based on each laboratory's validation and not set at 500 ng/mL.

The amphetamine assay is perhaps the most difficult test to interpret clinically because of the large number of false-positive results due to medications containing amphetamine and medication with similar structures. Some prescribed and over-the-counter medications that can trigger a false positive include amantadine, benzphetamine, bupropion, chlorpromazine, clobenzorex, L-deprenyl, desipramine, dextroamphetamine, ephedrine, fenproporex, isometheptene, isoxsuprine, labetalol, MDMA, methamphetamine, L-methamphetamine (Vick's inhaler), methylphenidate, phentermine, phenylephrine, phenylpropanolamine, promethazine, pseudoephedrine, ranitidine, ritodrine, selegiline, thioridazine, trazodone, trimethobenzamide, and trimipramine (Moeller et al. 2008). Some commonly used immunoassay-based testing kits have fewer false positives (Hsu et al. 2003).

Methods of differentiating illicit amphetamine use from legal use of amphetamine medications based on the enantiomeric ratio of amphetamine have been proposed, but the clinical usefulness of such methods is questionable (Kraemer and Maurer 2002). Diagnostix (http://www.diagnostix.ca) developed a commercially available enzyme-linked immunosorbent assay (ELISA) for methylphenidate and ritalinic acid in urine, but it is expensive and nonquantitative. Lewis et al. (2003) developed an "in-house" quantitative, rapid, and direct ELISA for methylphenidate equivalents in urine that has acceptable performance, allowing its routine use in the laboratory. This test may be helpful to identify those who are abusing others' prescription drugs and cut down on adolescent trafficking of prescription methylphenidate to peers for profit. Clinically, confirmation of methamphetamine in the urine indicates the use of methamphetamine. Selegiline, a monoamine oxidase A inhibitor, is metabolized to methamphetamine in the body. The only other available approved prescription drug in the United States that is metabolized to methamphetamine is benzphetamine, which is used for weight loss. For a patient with attention-deficit/hyperactivity disorder who requires pharmacotherapy, medications other than amphetamine (e.g., atomoxetine, bupropion, modafinil) should be used when there is a concern about possible stimulant abuse, because this may allow for easier detection of illicit amphetamine or designer drug abuse.

Hallucinogens

Most hallucinogens, such as LSD, can be tested in the blood or urine using gas chromatography–mass spectroscopy methods (Burnley and George 2003). Psilocybin and its metabolite psilocin are psychoactive alkaloids found in certain species of mushrooms. Levels can be detected in the serum, with psilocin having a half-life of 163 minutes when given as pure psilocybin by mouth (Passie et al. 2002). Mescaline, a ring-substituted phenethylamine, is a hallucinogenic alkaloid found in peyote cactus. It can be detected in urine and serum via gas chromatography–mass spectrometry (Habrdova et al. 2005).

Phencyclidine and Phencyclidine-Like Substances

Biomarkers for PCP use are thought to be somewhat unreliable because observed individuals with acute psychotic reactions can have an undetectable serum level due to PCP's long duration of action, lipophilicity, and pK_a (Javitt and Zukin 2005). Sweat patches may be used for the detection of PCP.

Rapid screening tests are not readily available for ketamine, which reacts unreliably with urine immunoassays for PCP (Javitt and Zukin 2005).

Inhalants

Most inhalants are difficult to track via biomarkers in bodily fluids. Toluene can be measured directly in the serum. Industry maximum exposure is 100 parts per million, which yields a blood level of 0.5 μg/g, whereas blood levels during intoxication range from 0.8 to 8.0 μg/g. Blood levels can normalize 4–10 hours after exposure. Hippuric acid, a direct metabolite, can be measured in urine. Recent intoxication can be assumed given a ratio of 1 g or more of hippurate to 1 g of creatinine in the urine. False-positive results may occur with concomitant intake of benzoic acid food preservatives (Crowley and Sakai 2005). Red and white blood cell counts, as well as kidney and liver functioning, may be altered due to toxic reactions (Schuckit 2000). Testing for volatile inhalant use must be performed on blood samples using headspace gas chromatography (Broussard 2000).

Anabolic-Androgenic Steroids

The range of normal plasma testosterone levels in men is from 300 to 1,000 ng/dL. The following anabolic steroid compounds can be measured in the urine via gas chromatography–thermionic specific detection and gas chromatography–flame ionization detection: testosterone, 19-noretiocholanolone, oxymetholone, dehydroepiandrosterone, 10-norestosterone, 11-β-hydroxyandrosterone, methandienone, 19-norandrosterone, 16-α-hydroxyetiocholanolone, 17-α-epitestosterone, and stanozolol. Hair can also be tested for anabolic steroids. Changes in liver function, cholesterol, and endocrine measures can be seen in those individuals misusing anabolic-androgenic steroids (Pope and Brower 2005).

Conclusion

Although experts disagree regarding the usefulness of routine drug screening using biomarkers (Gold et al. 2006; Levy et al. 2006), biomarker testing is useful when making initial psychiatric evaluations, for the purpose of establishing diagnostic authority. Clinicians should consider drug testing on occasion for patients with a history of substance misuse or substance use disorder who are receiving controlled substances for co-occurring disorders or other indications (e.g., dextroamphetamine for attention-deficit/hyperactivity disorder) because medications may have potentially lethal interactions with drugs of abuse, and drug testing may also help to ascertain adherence to the treatment regimen and possibility of diversion.

Biomarker testing is clinically useful for the assessment, screening, and monitoring of adolescent substance use in conjunction with rating scales and clinical and diagnostic interviews. Biomarker testing can be used as a tool for outreach testing in settings other than the doctor's office, such as at home and at school. Urine, blood, sweat, hair, and saliva can all be used to test for multiple drugs of abuse. Choosing the most appropriate sample source and test depends on the specific substance(s) of interest, suspected pattern of drug use, and intent or purpose of testing. Affordable, in-office, qualitative screening kits for use with saliva and urine samples are widely available and may be the most convenient and useful form of testing for general clinical and legal management.

Key Clinical Concepts

- Use of objective biomarkers for the detection of drug use is important.
- Testing of minors is legal.
- The choice between qualitative and quantitative tests is based on the purpose of the test and what will be done with the results.
- It is important to be aware of the cutoff point (in particular for cannabis), sensitivity, and specificity of the test used for a specific drug.

References

Achenbach TM, McConaughy SH, Howell CT: Child/adolescent behavioral and emotional problems: implications of cross-informant correlations for situational specificity. Psychol Bull 101:213–232, 1987

Andrews VC, Garrison CZ, Jackson KL, et al: Mother-adolescent agreement on the symptoms and diagnoses of adolescent depression and conduct disorders. J Am Acad Child Adolesc Psychiatry 32:731–738, 1993

Aradottir S, Asanovska G, Gjerss S, et al: Phosphatidylethanol (PEth) concentrations in blood are correlated to reported alcohol intake in alcohol-dependent patients. Alcohol Alcohol 41:431–437, 2006

Barnea A, Rahav G, Teichman M: The reliability and consistency of self-reports of substance use in a longitudinal study. Br J Addict 82:891–898, 1987

Baselt RC, Baselt DR: Little cross reactivity of local anesthetics with Abuscreen, EMIT d.a.u., and TDX immunoassays for cocaine metabolite (letter). Clin Chem 33:747, 1987

Benowitz NL: Cotinine as a biomarker of environmental tobacco smoke exposure. Epidemiol Rev 18:188–204, 1996

Boyer EW: Dextromethorphan abuse. Pediatr Emerg Care 20:858–863, 2004

Broussard LA: The role of the laboratory in detecting inhalant abuse. Clin Lab Sci 13:205–209, 2000

Brown C, Fezoui M, Selig WM, et al: Antitussive activity of sigma-1 receptor agonists in the guinea-pig. Br J Pharmacol 141:233–240, 2004

Buchan BJ, Dennis M, Tims FM, et al: Cannabis use: consistency and validity of self-report, on-site urine testing and laboratory testing. Addiction 97 (suppl 1):98–108, 2002

Burke WM, Ravi NV, Dhopesh V, et al: Prolonged presence of metabolite in urine after compulsive cocaine use. J Clin Psychiatry 51:145–148, 1990

Burleson J, Kaminer Y: Adolescent alcohol and marijuana use: concordance among objective-, self-, and collateral-reports. J Child Adolesc Subst Abuse 16:53–68, 2006

Burnley BT, George S: The development and application of a gas chromatography–mass spectrometric (GC-MS) assay to determine the presence of 2-oxo-3-hydroxy-LSD in urine. J Anal Toxicol 27:249–252, 2003

Cantwell DP, Lewinsohn PM, Rohde P, et al: Correspondence between adolescent report and parent report of psychiatric diagnostic data. J Am Acad Child Adolesc Psychiatry 36:610–619, 1997

Center for Medicare and Medicaid Services: Coverage and administrative policies for clinical diagnostic laboratory services. Fed Regist 66:58788–58890, 2001

Center for Substance Abuse Research: Poll shows that parents seriously underestimate availability and use of drugs among their children, in Partnership for a Drug Free America, Vol 5, Issue 16. College Park, University of Maryland, April 29, 1996

Center for Substance Abuse Treatment: The role of biomarkers in the treatment of alcohol use disorders. Substance Abuse Treatment Advisory, Vol 5, Issue 4, 2006 (DHHS Publ No SMA-06-4223). Rockville, MD, Center for Substance Abuse Treatment, Substance Abuse and Mental Health Services Asministration, 2006a

Center for Substance Abuse Treatment: SAMHSA Advisory: lab test for alcohol abuse. SAMHSA News 14(6):2006b

Chawarski MC, Fiellin DA, O'Connor PG: Utility of sweat patch testing for drug use monitoring in outpatient treatment for opioid dependence. J Subst Abuse Treat 33:411–415, 2007

Cone E: New development in biological measures of drug prevalence. NIDA Res Monogr 167:108–129, 1997

Cooke F, Bullen C, Whittaker R, et al: Diagnostic accuracy of NicAlert cotinine test strips in saliva for verifying smoking status. Nicotine Tob Res 10:607–612, 2008

Crouch DJ, Hersch RK, Cook RF, et al: A field evaluation of five on-site drug-testing devices. J Anal Toxicol 26:493–499, 2000

Crowley TJ, Sakai J: Inhalant related disorders, in Kaplan and Sadock's Comprehensive Textbook of Psychiatry, 8th Edition, Vol 1. Edited by Sadock B, Sadock V. Philadelphia, PA, Lippincott Williams & Wilkins, 2005, pp 1247–1257

DeRienz RT, Holler JM, Manos ME, et al: Evaluation of four immunoassay screening kits for the detection of benzodiazepines in urine. J Anal Toxicol 32:433–437, 2008

Drug Enforcement Administration, Office of Diversion Control, Drug and Chemical Evaluation Section: Lists of: Scheduling Actions, Controlled Substances, Regulated Chemicals. Washington, DC, U.S. Department of Justice, Drug Enforcement Administration, Office of Diversion Control, Drug and Chemical Evaluation Section, April 2008

DuPont RL, Selavka CM: Testing to identify recent drug use, in The American Psychiatric Publishing Textbook of Substance Abuse Treatment, 4th Edition. Edited by Galanter M, Kleber HD. Washington, DC, American Psychiatric Publishing, 2008, pp 655–664

DuPont RL, Skipper DE, White WL: Testing for recent alcohol use. Student Assistance Journal 20:12–18, 2008

Edelbrock C, Achenbach TM: A typology of child behavior profile patterns: distribution and correlates for disturbed children age 6 to 16. J Abnorm Child Psychol 8:441–470, 1986

Ferrera SD, Tedeschi L, Frison G, et al: Drugs-of-abuse testing in urine: statistical approach and experimental comparison of immunochemical and chromatographic techniques. J Anal Toxicol 18:78–291, 1994

Fleming M, Mundt M: Carbohydrate-deficient transferrin: validity of a new alcohol biomarker in a sample of patients with diabetes and hypertension. J Am Board Fam Pract 17:247–255, 2004

Florescu A, Ferrence R, Einarson T, et al: Methods for quantification of exposure to cigarette smoking and environmental tobacco smoke: focus on developmental toxicology. Ther Drug Monit 31:14–30, 2009

Gold MS, Frost-Pineda K, Goldberger BA, et al: Physicians and drug screening. J Adolesc Health 39:154–155, 2000

Greenfield SF, Hennessy G: Assessment of the patient, in The American Psychiatric Publishing Textbook of Substance Abuse Treatment, 4th Edition. Edited by Galanter M, Kleber HD. Washington, DC, American Psychiatric Publishing, 2008, pp 55–78

Gustafson RA, Kim PR, Stout KL, et al: Urinary pharmacokinetics of 11-nor-9-carboxy-delta9-tetrahydrocannabinol after controlled oral delta9-tetrahydrocannabinol administration. J Anal Toxicol 28:160–167, 2004

Habrdova V, Peters F, Theobald D, et al: Screening for and validated quantification of phenethylamine-type designer drugs and mescaline in human blood plasma by gas chromatography/mass spectrometry. J Mass Spectrom 40:785–795, 2005

Hall W, Degenhardt L: Cannabis-related disorders, in Kaplan and Sadock's Comprehensive Textbook of Psychiatry, 8th Edition, Vol 2. Edited by Sadock B, Sadock V. Philadelphia, PA, Lippincott Williams & Wilkins, 2005, Section 11.5

Haller CA, Stone J, Burke V, et al: Comparison of an automated and point-of-care immunoassay to GC-MS for urine oxycodone testing in the clinical laboratory. J Anal Toxicol 30:106–111, 2006

Hsu J, Liu C, Liu CP, et al: Performance characteristics of selected immunoassays for preliminary test of 3,4-methylenedioxymethamphetamine, methamphetamine, and related drugs in urine specimens. J Anal Toxicol 27:471–478, 2003

Institute for Behavior and Health: Commentary: reflections on random student drug testing Supreme Court case: both support and criticsms remain, October 23, 2009. Available at: http://www.ibhinc.org. Accessed April 10, 2010.

Jaffe JH, Strain EC: Opioid-related disorders, in Kaplan and Sadock's Comprehensive Textbook of Psychiatry, 8th Edition. Edited by Sadock B, Sadock V. Philadelphia, PA, Lippincott Williams & Wilkins, 2005, pp 1265–1290

Javitt D, Zukin SR: Phencyclidine (or phencyclidine-like)-related disorders, in Kaplan and Sadock's Comprehensive Textbook of Psychiatry, 8th Edition. Edited by Sadock B, Sadock V. Philadelphia, PA, Lippincott Williams & Wilkins, 2005, Section 11.10

Johansson E, Halldin MM: Urinary excretion half-life of delta 1-tetrahydrocannabinol-7-oic acid in heavy marijuana users after smoking. J Anal Toxicol 13:218–223, 1989

Johansson E, Halldin MM, Agurell S, et al: Terminal elimination plasma half-life of delta 1-tetrahydrocannabinol (delta 1-THC) in heavy users of marijuana. Eur J Clin Pharmacol 37:273–277, 1989

Kaminer Y: Adolescent Substance Abuse: A Comprehensive Guide to Theory and Practice. New York, Plenum, 1994

Kerrigan S, Phillips WH Jr: Comparison of ELISAs for opiates, methamphetamine, cocaine metabolite, benzodiazepines, phencyclidine, and cannabinoids in whole blood and urine. Clin Chem 47:540–547, 2001

Kim EM, Lee JS, Park MJ, et al: Standardization of method for the analysis of dextromethorphan in urine. Forensic Sci Int 161:198–201, 2006

Korzec A, de Bruijn C, van Lambalgen M: The Bayesian Alcoholism Test had better diagnostic properties for confirming diagnosis of hazardous and harmful alcohol use. J Clin Epidemiol 58:1024–1032, 2005

Kraemer T, Maurer HH: Toxicokinetics of amphetamines: metabolism and toxicokinetic data of designer drugs, amphetamine, methamphetamine, and their N-alkyl derivatives. Ther Drug Monit 24:277–289, 2002

Leckman J, Sholomskas D, Thompson W: Best estimate of lifetime psychiatric diagnosis: a methodological study. Arch Gen Psychiatry 39:879–883, 1982

Levy S, Harris SK, Sherrit L, et al: Drug testing of adolescents in general medical clinics, in school and at home: physician attitudes and practices. J Adolesc Health 38:336–342, 2006

Lewis MG, Lewis JG, Elder PA, et al: An enzyme-linked immunosorbent assay (ELISA) for methylphenidate (Ritalin) in urine. J Anal Toxicol 27:342–345, 2003

Logan BK, Goldfogel G, Hamilton R, et al: Five deaths resulting from abuse of dextromethorphan sold over the internet. J Anal Toxicol 33:99–103, 2009

Loor R, Lingenfelter C, Wason PP, et al: Multiplex assay of amphetamine, methamphetamine, and ecstasy drug using CEDIA technology. J Anal Toxicol 26:267–273, 2000

Mazor SS, Mycyk MB, Wills BK, et al: Coca tea consumption causes positive urine cocaine assay. Eur J Emerg Med 13:340–341, 2006

Mercolini L, Mandrioli R, Saladini B, et al: Quantitative analysis of cocaine in human hair by HPLC with fluorescence detection. J Pharm Biomed Anal 48:456–461, 2008

Mieczkowski T, Lersch K: Drug-testing police officers and police recruits: the outcome of hair analysis and urinalysis compared. Policing: An International Journal of Police Strategies & Management 25:581–601, 2002

Mieczkowski T, Newel R: Statistical examination of hair color as a potential biasing factor in hair analysis. Forensic Sci Int 107:13–38, 2000

Mikkelsen SL, Ash KO: Adulterants causing false negatives in illicit drug testing. Clin Chem 34:126–131, 1988

Mikkelsen IM, Kanitz RD, Nilssen O, et al: Carbohydrate-deficient transferring: marker of actual alcohol consumption or chronic alcohol misuse? Alcohol Alcohol 33:646–650, 1998

Miller PM, Spies C, Neumann T, et al: Alcohol biomarker screening in medical and surgical settings. Alcohol Clin Exp Res 30:185–193, 2006

Moeller KE, Lee KC, Kissack JC: Urine drug screening: practical guide for clinicians. Mayo Clin Proc 83:66–76, 2008

Morini L, Politi L, Polettini A: Ethyl glucuronide in hair: a sensitive and specific marker of chronic heavy drinking. Addiction 104:915–920, 2009

Musshoff F, Madea B: Review of biologic matrices (urine, blood, hair) as indicators of recent or ongoing cannabis use. Ther Drug Monit 28:155–163, 2006

Niemelä O: Biomarkers in alcoholism. Clin Chim Acta 377:39–49, 2007

O'Donnell D, Biederman J, Jones J: Informativeness of child and parent reports on substance use disorders in a sample of ADHD probands, control probands, and their siblings. J Am Acad Child Adolesc Psychiatry 37:752–758, 1998

Passie T, Seifert J, Schneider U, et al: The pharmacology of psilocybin. Addict Biol 7:357–364, 2002

Pope HG, Brower KJ: Anabolic-Androgenic Steroid Abuse, in Kaplan and Sadock's Comprehensive Textbook of Psychiatry, 8th Edition. Edited by Sadock B, Sadock V. Philadelphia, PA, Lippincott Williams & Wilkins, 2005, Section 11.13

Rutter M: Isle of Wight revisited: twenty-five years of child psychiatric epidemiology. J Am Acad Child Adolesc Psychiatry 28:633–653, 1989

Schepers RJ, Oyler JM, Joseph RE Jr, et al: Methamphetamine and amphetamine pharmacokinetics in oral fluid and plasma after controlled oral methamphetamine administration to human volunteers. Clin Chem 49:121–132, 2003

Schuckit MA: Drug and Alcohol Abuse: A Clinical Guide to Diagnosis and Treatment, 5th Edition. New York, Kluwer Academic/Plenum, 2000, pp 174–188, 221–229

Sharpe PC: Biochemical detection and monitoring of alcohol abuse and abstinence. Ann Clin Biochem 38:652–664, 2001

Sillanaukee P, Aalto M, Seppä K: Carbohydrate deficient transferrin and conventional alcohol markers as indicators for brief intervention among heavy drinkers in primary health care. Alcohol Clin Exp Res 22:892–896, 1998

Stibler H: Carbohydrate-deficient transferrin in serum: a new marker of potentially harmful alcohol consumption reviewed. Clin Chem 37:2029–2037, 1991

Substance Abuse and Mental Health Services Administration: Mandatory guidelines for federal workplace drug testing programs. Fed Regist 69:19644–19673, 2004

Ursitti F, Klein J, Koren G: Confirmation of cocaine use during pregnancy: a critical review. Ther Drug Monit 23:347–353, 2001

Verstraete AG: Detection times of drugs of abuse in blood, urine, and oral fluid. Ther Drug Monit 26:200–205, 2004

Verstraete AG, Heyden FV: Comparison of the sensitivity and specificity of six immunoassays for the detection of amphetamines in urine. J Anal Toxicol 29:359–364, 2005

Wall ME, Sadler BM, Brine D: Metabolism, disposition, and kinetics of delta-9-tetrahydrocannabinol in men and women. Clin Pharmacol Ther 34:352–363, 1983

Warner EA: Cocaine abuse. Ann Intern Med 119:226–235, 1993

Weissman MM, Wickramaratne P, Warner V: Assessing psychiatric disorders in children: discrepancies between mothers' and children's reports. Arch Gen Psychiatry 44:747–753, 1987

Werling LL, Lauterbach EC, Calef U: Dextromethorphan as a potential neuroprotective agent with unique mechanisms of action. Neurologist 13:272–293, 2007

Whitehead TP, Clarke CA, Whitfield AG: Biochemical and haematological markers of alcohol intake. Lancet 6:978–981, 1978

Whitfield JB, Hensley WJ, Bryden D, et al: Effects of age and sex on biochemical responses to drinking habits. Med J Aust 2:629–632, 1978

Winters KC, Anderson N, Bengston P: Development of a parent questionnaire for use in assessing adolescent drug abuse. J Psychoactive Drugs 32:3–13, 2000

Wojcik MH, Hawthorne JS: Sensitivity of commercial ethyl glucuronide (ETG) testing in screening for alcohol abstinence. Alcohol Alcohol 42:317–320, 2007

Wolff K, Farrell M, Marsden J, et al: A review of biological indicators of illicit drug use, practical considerations and clinical usefulness. Addiction 94:1279–1298, 1999

Wurst FM, Wiesbeck GA, Metzger JW, et al: On sensitivity, specificity, and the influence of various parameters on ethyl glucuronide levels in urine—results from the WHO/ISBRA study. Alcohol Clin Exp Res 28:1220–1228, 2004

Suggested Reading

Dupont RL, Brady LA: Drug Testing in Schools: Guidelines for Effective Use. Center City, MN, Hazelden, 2005

Relevant Websites

American Association of Medical Review Officers Registry: http://www.aamro.com

Institute for Behavior and Health: Guide to Responsible Family Drug Testing and Alcohol Testing and Smarter Student Drug Testing: http://www.ibhinc.org

State List of Certified Labs: http://workplace.samhsa.gov/DrugTesting/Level_1_Pages/CertifiedLabs.aspx

Placement Criteria and Treatment Planning for Adolescents With Substance Use Disorders

Marc Fishman, M.D.

Treatment planning for adolescents with substance use disorders (SUDs) begins with a comprehensive assessment and case formulation that informs the appropriate selection of treatment setting, objectives, and curriculum, including length of stay, intervention modalities, and intensity (i.e., dosage and fre-

Material in this chapter, notably Table 5–3, has been adapted with permission from Fishman M: "Treatment Planning, Matching, and Placement for Adolescents With Substance Use Disorders," in *Adolescent Substance Abuse: Psychiatric Comorbidity and High-Risk Behaviors*. Edited by Kaminer Y, Bukstein OG. New York, Routledge/Taylor & Francis, 2008.

quency) of the interventions provided. Placement should emerge from an individualized assessment. One size does not fit all (Fishman 2008). Placement decisions require consideration of the risk of progression, determination of treatment service needs, and then consideration of where and how those services should be effectively and safely delivered.

One of the productive trends moving the field of adolescent addiction treatment forward has been the development, refinement, and implementation of standardized treatment matching guidelines, with the goal of finding the optimal fit between patient needs and treatment available. *The American Society of Addiction Medicine Patient Placement Criteria*, 2nd Edition—Revised (ASAM PPC-2R) (Mee-Lee et al. 2001) has become the standard in the field. In addition to its function as an algorithm for level-of-care placement decisions, it is also a guideline for treatment matching and treatment planning in general. Its overall approach is to guide the clinician by organizing assessment data into six broad categories of assessment dimensions that serve to focus the assessment on key practical domains with central treatment implications. The six ASAM PPC-2R assessment dimensions are listed and described in Table 5–1.

The ASAM PPC-2R is also a consensus picture of the adolescent service delivery model. In its outline of various levels of care (see Table 5–2), as well as its descriptions of the broad range of service components that are expected in each of these individual levels of care, the ASAM PPC-2R is a prescription for the adolescent continuum of care. Of course, such a prescription should not be construed rigidly, because flexibility and innovation are encouraged. Furthermore, not all services or levels of care are available in all communities, particularly in rural communities. Also, every community has potential constraints on the availability of services (e.g., limitations of providers, reimbursement, treatment slots).

General Principles of Treatment Planning and Placement

An important general principle of treatment planning is the need for a longitudinal view, taking into account the need for continuity of care and coordination of treatment across episodes of care. Envisioning treatment matching as a black-box intervention at a particular level-of-care placement, from which

Table 5–1. ASAM PPC-2R assessment dimensions

Dimension	Description
1. Intoxication and withdrawal potential	Relating to the potential for acute and subacute intoxication and withdrawal and ensuing treatment needs
2. Biomedical conditions and complications	Relating to medical symptoms and comorbidity—preexisting, substance-induced, and substance-exacerbated conditions, and ensuing treatment needs
3. Emotional, behavioral, and cognitive conditions and complications	Relating to psychiatric symptoms and comorbidity—preexisting, substance-induced, and substance-exacerbated conditions, and ensuing treatment needs
4. Readiness to change	Relating to treatment engagement, motivation, resistance, and stages of change
5. Relapse and continued use potential	Relating to the likelihood of relapse, continuation of substance use and associated problems, along with potential consequences and ensuing treatment needs
6. Recovery environment	Relating to the family, peers, living situation, and home setting

Note. ASAM PPC-2R = *The American Society of Addiction Medicine Patient Placement Criteria*, 2nd Edition, Revised.
Source. Mee-Lee et al. 2001.

adolescents will emerge cured or fixed, is naive. Although many adolescents with mild to moderate severity do respond to time-limited, discrete interventions, many do not. Moreover, the higher the severity, the less likely this response is. Much more typical is a waxing-waning, remitting-relapsing course over a prolonged period of time and across several episodes of care at different levels of care, with different kinds of services and interventions.

The ideal is a treatment system in which patients can move fluidly and flexibly up (i.e., step-up) and down (step-down) levels of care as necessary to meet their contemporary needs. Treatment at higher levels of care should be followed by longer episodes of step-down continuing care or aftercare. Treatment at lower levels of care may need to be punctuated by periodic briefer episodes

Table 5–2.   ASAM PPC-2R levels of care

Level 0.5	Early intervention
Level I	Outpatient
Level II	Intensive outpatient and partial hospital
II.1	Intensive outpatient
II.5	Partial hospital/day program
Level III	Residential/inpatient
III.1	Clinically managed, low-intensity residential
III.5	Clinically managed, medium-intensity residential
III.7	Medically monitored, high-intensity residential/inpatient
Level IV	Hospital

Note.   ASAM PPC-2R = *The American Society of Addiction Medicine Patient Placement Criteria,* 2nd Edition, Revised.
Source.   Mee-Lee et al. 2001.

of treatment at higher levels of care in response to exacerbations. Repeated episodes of treatment are not so much an indicator of treatment failure as much as a marker of severity. Ongoing continuing care, extended monitoring phases, repeated booster doses, and in some cases indefinite maintenance should be the rule.

Another general principle of treatment planning and matching is that increased severity and impairment require increased intensity of services. This usually translates into increased level of care, because lower levels of care may not be as effective (Dasinger et al. 2004) or may not even be able to engage or "capture" (as in the case of a runaway who does not show up for a partial hospital program) the higher-severity adolescent. Increased intensity, however, can sometimes be counterproductive if it increases resistance by the youth or family. In these circumstances, it is useful to enhance motivation for change and increased engagement (see the discussion of Dimension 4 below).

Treatment planning needs to be realistic, and feasibility and acceptability need to be considered in terms of expectations of the youth and family and the availability of resources. Considerations include availability of services, financial costs of care, transportation, difficulties navigating complex agencies and systems, and so forth. Clinicians need to appreciate the burdens of treatment on both adolescents and families. Part of effective treatment planning is attempting to balance the prescription of what adolescents and families need with accommodating what they are willing and able to accomplish. One approach is to offer contingent and staged choices regarding intensity, modality, and level of care. This approach involves 1) starting engagement with a more convenient or more palatable choice, with the prospect of future intensification or modification if there are problems, or 2) asking the patient and family to try more at first, but with the offer of a recipe for stepping down as soon as things are going well.

Substance-involved adolescents generally need an array of services that are broader than "pure" substance abuse counseling alone for the multiple problems they face. Provision of services should be coordinated, taking into consideration that often even when services are available, they might be fragmented and/or only partially effective. Examples of frequently needed linkages include psychiatric, medical, family, social welfare, special education, school support, and juvenile justice. Case management, integration of services by a single provider, co-location within a single institution ("one-stop shopping"), interdisciplinary teams, cross-training and broadening of disciplinary focus, active coordination of service linkages among separate providers, and primary provider team leadership are all approaches that are attempted, but unfortunately integration is rare. Generally, the higher the severity of the adolescent's addiction, the higher the need for intensity, breadth, and integration of adjunctive services.

Dimensional Assessment and Treatment Planning Using the ASAM PPC-2R

In this section, clinical considerations are reviewed for treatment planning and matching by each of the six ASAM PPC-2R assessment dimensions.

Dimension 1: Intoxication and Withdrawal Potential

One of the critical considerations in Dimension 1 is the need for detoxification services when there is potential for physiological withdrawal. Intensive management of withdrawal is most frequently needed in adolescents with opioid dependence, the rates of which are increasing with the concurrent modern epidemics of heroin and diverted prescription opioids. The trend for treatment of severe opioid withdrawal in adolescents, as in adults, is the use of tapering doses of the partial agonist buprenorphine, which replaces or is added to more indirect symptom reduction agents such as clonidine (Marsch et al. 2005). Opioid dependence is generally an indicator of increased psychosocial impairment (Clemmey et al. 2004), with increased severity in all of the assessment dimensions. In particular, the presence of withdrawal symptoms of sufficient severity to require pharmacological intervention is considered a marker for very high risk of relapse, with resultant need for higher levels of monitoring and treatment intensity, including environmental control to decrease access to substances and to increase likelihood of initiation of the next phase of treatment and the induction of continuing care. Less frequently, this same principle applies to detoxification from alcohol, benzodiazepines, and other sedative-hypnotics. Unlike the trend for ambulatory detoxification in adults, detoxification in adolescents should be conducted with residential support (see Chapter 7, "Pharmacotherapy of Adolescent Substance Use Disorders").

Another Dimension 1 consideration is the persistence of subacute psychiatric intoxication and withdrawal symptoms and syndromes. These issues overlap considerably with the assessment for Dimension 3, and are especially salient because of potential direct links to the toxic effects of substances and the frequent confusion in diagnosis and treatment. In patients in whom substance toxicity has caused serious psychiatric morbidity (e.g., methamphetamine-induced or hallucinogen-induced psychosis, or inhalant-induced cognitive clouding), the emphasis should be on detoxification and the need to ensure abstinence, possibly by confinement if necessary. Where there are difficult diagnostic dilemmas in distinguishing substance-induced symptoms from autonomous syndromes (e.g., major depressive disorder vs. stimulant withdrawal depression), there is a need for increased intensity of monitoring, and often a period of short-term residential abstinence is required to clarify diagnosis and treatment.

Dimension 2: Biomedical Conditions and Complications

Important considerations in Dimension 2 include treatment services for the wide variety of medical conditions commonly associated with adolescent substance use. Furthermore, these medical complications tend to be a marker for overall severity and progression of SUDs. One important example is the need for assessment and treatment of the sexually transmitted infections associated with high-risk sexual behaviors in substance-involved adolescents, including chlamydial and gonococcal infections, human papillomavirus, syphilis, and so on. Both urethritis in boys and cervicitis in girls are relatively common but too often overlooked because they are frequently asymptomatic. Access to contraception and education regarding barrier methods for prevention of sexually transmitted infections are essential. Screening for HIV and hepatitis C virus is important in adolescents with injection drug use and high-risk sexual behaviors. When treatment services are being selected, the special needs and medical vulnerabilities of pregnant substance-using teenagers require particular care. Overall, the need for education, prevention, and treatment services related to sexual behaviors cannot be overemphasized.

The involvement of primary care medicine (pediatrics and family medicine) in substance abuse treatment can make a valuable contribution but unfortunately occurs infrequently. Primary care settings are often among the most important for delivering early intervention services. Primary care providers also have the advantage of providing longitudinal continuity and could serve as an essential hub for the coordination of episodes of specialty care across time. Increasing interest is being shown in staged models of care, organized along the lines of screening, brief intervention, referral, and treatment (SBIRT). Such models would be especially applicable in the general medical setting, where lower-severity cases might respond to briefer, time-limited interventions, whereas more complex or refractory cases would be linked to specialty care. The emergency department is another setting where screening and linkages to treatment are crucial, especially given the underrecognized association of medical trauma with intoxication.

Certain chronic medical conditions in adolescents can be profoundly exacerbated and complicated by SUDs. Examples include diabetes, reactive airway disease, chronic pain, and sickle cell disease. In these and other situations, the need for matching substance abuse treatment with coordinated medical capacity is important. Above and beyond the need for additional medical services, medical conditions and complications add complexity and potential morbidity, increasing the overall profile of severity, and generally increasing the need for intensity of treatment.

Dimension 3: Emotional, Behavioral, and Cognitive Conditions and Complications

As discussed throughout this volume, psychiatric comorbidity is the rule rather than the exception among adolescents with SUDs. Certainly, the first element of treatment matching is obtaining appropriate psychiatric evaluation as needed. Unfortunately, given the shortage of available psychiatric services in most adolescent addiction programs, especially in the public sector, the difficulty of obtaining appropriate evaluation is a major barrier to adequate treatment (Libby and Riggs 2008).

Even adolescents who have not been diagnosed with a psychiatric disorder—either because they have not yet had a formal psychiatric evaluation or because their symptoms are subsyndromal and do not meet the diagnostic criteria—often have problems in Dimension 3 that need to be considered in making treatment decisions. Examples include hyperactivity or distractibility without a diagnosis of attention-deficit/hyperactivity disorder, mood lability and explosive temper without a diagnosis of bipolar disorder, and dysphoric mood and loss of interests without a diagnosis of depression. Various nonspecific symptoms—such as problems with anger management or impulse control, poor frustration tolerance, and social withdrawal—also may be induced or exacerbated by substance use.

One aspect of the Dimension 3 assessment that features prominently in early triage for treatment matching is the assessment for dangerousness—that is, whether the adolescent needs placement or urgent services for suicidality, assaultiveness, risk of victimization, acute psychosis, or other issues related to safety of self or others. An important indicator of severity is the extent to which emotional or behavioral symptoms interfere with or distract from treatment and recovery efforts. Examples include difficulty attending to treatment sessions because of problems with attention and concentration, difficulty in completing recovery assignments or absorbing treatment material because of problems with memory or comprehension, inability to attend treatment sessions consistently because of running away, inability to participate in treatment because of disruptive behavior or poor peer relations, and distraction from treatment caused by preoccupying worries. Another useful metric is the impact of emotional or behavioral problems on social functioning and difficulties in meeting role responsibilities in the major arenas of family, school, work, and personal relationships. Examples include problems managing peer or family conflict, legal and conduct problems, problems with truancy or school performance, ungovernability at home, and narrowing of social repertoire and isolation. Another consideration is the extent to which ability for self-care or management of daily living activities has been affected. Examples include behaviors associated with patterns of victimization, high-risk or indiscriminate sexual behaviors, disorganization that interferes with emerging independent living skills, poor self-regulation (or poor cooperation with external regulation) of daily routine, and problems with hygiene or nutrition.

Another important concern related to adolescent treatment in Dimension 3 involves behavior and its management. The expectation of adult, or mature, behavior may be questionable in adult treatment settings, but it is certainly absurd in adolescent settings. The acquisition of self-regulation skills is an essential goal of treatment for substance users of all ages, but it also is a work in progress for all adolescents, including those without substance use problems. Treatment of adolescents must constantly seek a balance between an emphasis on limit setting and some degree of tolerance for chaos, as part of the necessary recognition that adolescents still are partly children. Moreover, the penchant for mischief among youngsters is not always an indicator of antisocial traits. Careful assessment of the broad range of adolescent misbehavior forms the basis of powerful treatment interventions that target improvements in family monitoring, supervision, and behavioral management. Disruptive behavior should be an expected feature of the profile of the drug-involved adolescent, and the capacity to manage behavior should be a focus of treatment, increasing with intensity of level of care. By inflexibly dismissing adolescents for nondangerous disruption, rule infractions, or noncooperation, payers or providers are dismissing an opportunity to improve that behavior and to intervene in a major source of interference with recovery efforts.

There is a great need for program development and cross-training of counselors and youth workers regarding psychiatric or dual-diagnosis disorders and treatments, in order to create treatment that is at least dual-diagnosis capable and preferably dual-diagnosis enhanced. This nomenclature refers not only to the intensity of available professional psychiatric services (psychiatry, nursing, therapy, etc.) but also to the ability of the nonlicensed staff and the overall milieu to tolerate (dual-diagnosis capable) or to provide meaningful interventions for (dual-diagnosis enhanced) potentially provocative or disruptive psychiatric symptoms and behaviors (e.g., aggression, oppositionality, suicidal thoughts, psychosis, self-induced vomiting, self-injurious behaviors such as cutting). Some programs, however, remain committed to the notion that all Dimension 3 problems should be exclusively addressed through abstinence and spiritual transformation, to the detriment of many youth with co-occurring disorders.

Dimension 4: Readiness to Change

The key considerations in Dimension 4 are motivation and engagement. Elements of motivation include motivation to change, motivation to attempt to change, motivation to contemplate change, and both internal and external motivation. Elements of engagement include ability and willingness to attend and participate in treatment, help-seeking stance, and the actual track record of treatment utilization. Assessments of and interventions for motivation and engagement are important both for the adolescent and for the adolescent's family or caregiver, and are often different.

On the whole, because of their developmental immaturity, adolescents tend to present at earlier stages of readiness to change than do adults. It is a mistake to assume that adolescents are "ready" for treatment at first presentation, and role induction is critical. Furthermore, although confrontation has a place in the repertoire of engagement techniques, it is not the place to start. When applied inflexibly, both confrontation and the traditional concept of "overcoming resistance" tend to reduce adolescents' engagement, rather than winning them over. In well-established techniques using the concepts of motivational interviewing and motivational enhancement therapy, an attempt is made to appreciate adolescents' own current sets of goals and motivations and to "meet them where they are" in order to gradually and incrementally enroll them into an evolving treatment agenda.

External pressures to seek treatment tend to be more effective for adolescents than adults (Deas et al. 2000). Common externally oriented goals and contingencies that tend to motivate adolescents include parental and other caregiver pressures and influences (e.g., approval, privileges, rewards, disciplinary consequences); legal mandates and sanctions; peer pressures, influences, and affiliations; and contingencies related to school (e.g., suspension, participation in athletic teams and other extracurricular activities). Manipulations of such external contingencies are often effective, even in the absence of subjective internal motivation. Emphasis on juvenile justice involvement, use of court mandates and monitoring, and application of legal contingencies can be extremely helpful. It is sometimes difficult, but nevertheless vital, to achieve effective cooperation and coordination between treatment providers and the juvenile justice system. Specific approaches that emphasize juvenile justice integration have been developed and may provide a good match for adolescents with low levels of treatment engagement in the context of delinquency and adjudication. One example is juvenile drug courts, which utilize a specified set of graduated sanctions and rewards, and which have staff whose training and goals cross between the justice and treatment systems.

An unrealistic expectation is that adolescents will achieve insight before they change, or even that some of them will ever have a subjective conversion experience. Self-recognition of problems and impairments does not come easily to most adolescents based on the normal course of maturation and development. Clinicians or parents should not be surprised that behavioral change often precedes cognitive change. One strategy is for the adults to use external pressures as the basis for treatment alliance, uniting with the adolescent in trying to respond to these pressures and hoping to link these efforts to a longer-term treatment goal in a staged approach. For example, in working with an adolescent who does not think that he or she has a drug problem, instead of starting with the potentially unrealistic goal of seeking abstinence, a counselor might instead propose the goal of joining forces to help the adolescent negotiate with the probation officer's demands and develop a treatment plan with realistic "milestone" gradual objectives. Only over time might the adolescent appreciate other benefits of the reduction or cessation of substance use that produced the negative urine screens that met the probation officer's initial goal.

A variety of other practical strategies may be effective in promoting engagement. These can include assertive outreach, such as social marketing, home visits, or telephone calls, for adolescents or families who are more difficult to engage. School-based services are an increasingly widespread method for improving engagement by co-locating treatment in convenient community settings. Also appropriate in some circumstances are strategies that target typical practical engagement barriers. These strategies could include providing transportation, assisting with public benefits (e.g., Medicaid), and developing advances and flexibility in reimbursement structures that increase access. For many adolescents, traditional treatment is not enticing enough to hold their attention; boredom may be a major barrier. Therefore, some treatment providers have adopted approaches that emphasize active rather than passive learning, using experiential activities that can be energetic and noisy while preserving serious therapeutic content. Another approach is to entice adolescents to serious treatment by alternating it with fun recreational activities.

Finally, treatment alliance is a powerful tool for engagement (Brown 2001). Treatment engagement is probably as much about the messenger as the message. Attention and expression of interest and concern are potent motivators for adolescents in general. Additionally, many substance-involved adolescents have had few connections with benevolent adults or few prosocial adult role models. Adolescents who are rewarded and engaged by a relationship with an adult and/or who have lacked positive adult supports may benefit from individual (rather than group) counseling or from mentoring over a longer duration. The subjective sense of a positive helping relationship with a provider (individual or even an institution) also often helps with reengagement following dropout or relapse. Engagement may also be enhanced by the adult's acknowledgment and even partial endorsement of adolescent culture, including its typical stance of nonconformity with adult and mainstream norms. Culturally and/or ethnically specific programming can also serve as an engagement tool.

Dimension 5: Relapse and Continued Use Potential

Important goals in Dimension 5 are to predict the risk of further substance use (either relapse or continuing use) and its potential dangerousness, and to choose appropriate interventions in response to risk. An adolescent's historical patterns of use and of change are often likely to predict future course of illness, including relapse potential. For example, some adolescents are more likely to have a rapid course of full reinstatement of substance dependence with severe impairment following a single lapse episode, whereas others are likely to have a more indolent course, with only gradual escalation of substance use. Knowledge of the individual's response to past treatment also may serve as a guide to placement. On the one hand, if a particular treatment intervention or modality, dose of treatment, or level of care led to a significant period of improvement for an adolescent in the past, then it may be appropriate to repeat that treatment following a relapse or exacerbation. Alternatively, the treatment may need modification to attempt to increase the persistence of the treatment effects. On the other hand, if a particular dose or placement was not effective in the past, this history may suggest the need for a different and/or more intensive intervention.

These recommendations apply not only to professional treatment but also to other interventions and circumstances, such as parental involvement and juvenile justice contingencies. This approach is one way of informing treatment and placement matching decisions on an individualized basis.

Although evidence is increasing for the enduring effectiveness of time-limited interventions (Dennis et al. 2004; Hser et al. 2001; Muck et al. 2003), many adolescents are refractory (at least initially) to treatment, and many adolescents have partial posttreatment improvements that are short of abstinence or "full" recovery. Furthermore, the course for many adolescents, especially those with higher severity, is characterized by remission and relapse, with multiple episodes of treatment over time. Dimension 5 assessment guides practitioners in planning longitudinal treatment that supports incremental improvements, accommodates shifting priorities, and responds to periodic relapse and/or exacerbation. It is sometimes difficult for parents, policy critics, and other stakeholders to accept and characterize partial improvements as successes; however, the substantial increases in psychosocial functioning that usually accompany partial decreases in substance use are an important measure of treatment effectiveness, and also a critical part of what shapes ongoing treatment planning in Dimension 5. The unrealistic expectation of "cure" also sometimes informs a cynical view of high-severity or refractory cases as "chronic" or hopeless and therefore not worthy of additional efforts or resources. This view is contrary to the more appropriate view of therapeutic optimism and problem management common to other health care arenas.

One area of particular recent interest related to Dimension 5 is that of continuing care. Ongoing treatment at less intensive levels of care (step-down, aftercare, or continuing care), with the intent of consolidating and sustaining gains initiated at more intensive levels of care, should be an expected feature of successful treatment across a continuum of care. Because enduring treatment effectiveness may be tempered by the attenuation of treatment effect over time, the need for ongoing reinforcement or periodic booster doses of treatment and/or monitoring checkups should be anticipated.

Rates of utilization of continuing care are alarmingly low following index episodes of residential (Fishman et al. 2005; Godley et al. 2007) and outpatient (Kaminer et al. 2008) treatment. Recent work focused on innovative strategies to enhance continuing care and overcome barriers to its utilization and effectiveness has been encouraging. One of the barriers to continuing care has been provider attitudes that place the burden of engagement on adolescents and families to make use of services if and when they are ready. Some of the newer approaches are more assertive, attempting in various ways to shift the burden and responsibility for engagement to the provider. In an assertive continuing care model used in a rural setting (Godley et al. 2003), continuing care following residential treatment was brought to adolescents and their families through home visits; this model demonstrated increases in continuing care utilization. This model suggests the possibility of a treatment-matching strategy that prescribes specialized (higher intensity or more assertive) continuing care based on particular assessment factors, such as high relapse potential in Dimension 5 and/or low treatment engagement in Dimension 4. Another assertive continuing care approach, in an urban setting in Baltimore, used small caseload case management and numerous telephone calls for treatment engagement "reminders" and brief telephone counseling following acute residential treatment (Fishman et al. 2005). Kaminer et al. (2008) also reported success with a protocol for telephone-based continuing care following episodes of outpatient treatment (Kaminer and Napolitano 2010).

The development of pharmacological strategies for management of relapse potential, involving the use of primary antiaddiction medications (sometimes referred to as anticraving agents, or medication-assisted recovery), holds exciting new promise, especially for patients with opioid dependence (see Chapter 7, "Pharmacotherapy of Adolescent Substance Use Disorders").

Dimension 6: Recovery Environment

In Dimension 6, the key is the home setting, including the influences of the parents and other caretakers, the home environment, peers, and the community. During assessment, families are necessary collateral informants. Adolescents themselves, once they are ready to provide confidential reports of their histories, often give richer detail of actual substance use than their parents can, but they may need some priming to get started. Furthermore, given the tendency of adolescents to minimize impairment, collateral informants usually present a more accurate account of psychosocial function. Adolescents' history should also be considered in a family system context. Despite their developmentally appropriate bravado of independence, adolescents continue to rely heavily on the supports and influences of adults. It is important to try to understand how the home environment, especially the family, shapes an adolescent's behavior. In turn, such an understanding can provide a basis for informing interventions and treatment.

A wide range of family-based intervention strategies have been introduced. These include family education, individual family counseling and therapy, multifamily groups, parenting interventions, enhancement of mutual family support, and others. Some interventions have the goal of improving parents' knowledge, because parents are often underinformed—about substances, substance use, access to substances, the course and treatment of SUDs, normative and deviant aspects of adolescent culture, access to treatment resources, and so forth. Some interventions have the goal of using the family's influence to enhance and support the adolescent's engagement and involvement in treatment.

Some interventions have the goal of helping the family to improve its approach to monitoring, supervision, and home interventions. These interventions are based on the concept that the adolescents themselves may not be the initial or most important locus of change. Rather, it may be more effective to expect that the family as the primary locus of change will in turn change the adolescent. Parents often need help with setting consistent limits, providing effective discipline, demonstrating credible concern, and modeling prosocial behaviors.

By the time of presentation to treatment, many parents are often stuck in an embattled and ineffective mode of monitoring and supervision that alternates unpredictably between overreactive, punitive responses and abdication of the parenting role. These families need encouragement and refereeing for both sides to find common ground for positive reengagement. Many parents need help with the unrealistic hope that their adolescents will somehow change through an internal epiphany and fundamental change in worldview, or with the nonsensical expectation that they will suddenly become more mature than they actually are or undergo a miraculous transformation of temperament. These parents are understandably weary of the unending battles, but are also overwhelmed by the amount of work required day in and day out to effectively shape—or more likely to *reshape*—behavior. Many parents need a road map or instruction manual for the use of behavioral contingencies, especially rewards, to reinforce desired behaviors. Families may be helped by instruction, guidance, and practice in how to conduct effective negotiations. Various skills-based interventions target communication skills, problem-solving skills, or home behavior management skills for adolescents or for caretakers or for both together. Although such family-based interventions may be used in a piecemeal fashion, arrayed with or added on to other treatment approaches, some approaches are committed to a primary role for family-based treatments.

Other Dimension 6 interventions may include efforts to attenuate toxic environmental influences. Examples of attempts to make the recovery environment safer include identification of and efforts to intervene in substance use, maltreatment, criminal behaviors, and antisocial attitudes in the home. Some adolescents have a social network composed primarily or even exclusively of family members or peers who are involved in substance use or criminal behaviors. This social context may portray deviance as normative. An adolescent may have no readily apparent role models for the rewards of abstinence. Some adolescents may have had no experience of living in an environment that fosters healthy prosocial development and functioning.

In severe situations, the best action may be temporary removal of adolescents from toxic home environments and placement in residential treatment to provide reprieve or counterbalancing interventions. Some preliminary work has suggested that adolescents with significant levels of acute traumatic stress may be more responsive to residential than to outpatient levels of care (Funk et al. 2003), based on their temporary removal from sources of stress. Longer-term residential treatments, such as modified therapeutic community programs, may be beneficial for adolescents whose home environments have been chronically unable to support recovery, and/or as an alternative to out-of-home juvenile justice detention placements, which are certainly not good recovery environments. For especially severe cases, efforts may be necessary to more definitively remove adolescents from toxic environments and find alternative living arrangements, such as placement with other family members or surrogate families (e.g., foster care), longer-term residential placements (e.g., group homes), and so forth.

Treatment Matching and Placement

Once treatment service needs and approaches have been determined, the next goal is to create the opportunity for their implementation through placement referral recommendations. Researchers and clinicians are just beginning to untangle the heterogeneity of the adolescent SUDs and to gain some broader understanding about staging and subgroups, as well as the treatment response patterns of those subgroups. As understanding develops, it will become more realistic to propose (and of course test) more specific and more operationalized treatment matching guidelines, which will eventually lead to specific practice guidelines that recommend specific treatment interventions, modalities, doses, lengths of treatment, and so on.

Table 5–3 both summarizes some of the material presented above and gives a speculative example in broad outline format of what a treatment matching grid based on the ASAM PPC-2R assessment dimensions might eventually look like as such specificity is developed in the future. The goals are to be able to perform treatment matching at the level of specific interventions and to use assessment profiles and individual patient characteristics to choose appropriately individualized treatment strategies. Although few empirical data are available to support such specific matching so far, there are some clinically driven strategies and emerging consensus approaches.

While work is ongoing to expand the underdeveloped continuum, practitioners have to adapt realistically to the resources at hand. Often, when a given level of care is not practicably available, a more intensive level of care that *is* available is the best substitute. Another approach that is sometimes successful is to creatively weave together a multidimensional array of services from a variety of sources that approximates the intensity of the unavailable level of care. An example of the former approach is the common practice in many communities of using inpatient psychiatric hospitalization as a setting for stabilization of substance-related crises when no medically monitored high-intensity residential program is available. Another example is the use of brief residential placement for daily support and monitoring when no Level II.5 partial hospitalization program (PHP)/day program is available. An example of the latter "patchwork" approach is substituting increased frequency of Level I outpatient sessions (say, two or three per week) for an unavailable Level II.1 intensive outpatient program. Another example might be combining a Level II.5 PHP/day program with an alternative, temporary living situation (e.g., with a relative) that is less problematic than the home environment as a substitution for an unavailable Level III.5 residential placement.

Table 5–3.   Speculative example of future treatment matching grid based on ASAM PPC-2R assessment dimensions

Assessment	Treatment services and placement
Dimension 1: Intoxication and withdrawal potential	
Physiological withdrawal	Aggressive pharmacological management for symptom reduction in opioid withdrawal, especially using partial agonists such as buprenorphine
	High-intensity services, environmental control in residential LOC because of high risk of dropout, focus on transition to and retention in ongoing treatment services
Prolonged subacute intoxication symptoms (e.g., substance-induced psychosis or severe mood disturbance, marijuana-induced amnestic syndrome, substance-induced cognitive impairment, hallucinogen-induced perceptual distortion syndrome)	Psychiatric assessment if persistent
	Explicit identification and tracking as a strategy to enhance problem self-recognition, treatment role induction, and engagement
	Consider increased intensity (e.g., residential treatment) if ongoing use produces significant impairment and/or prevents adequate assessment or treatment
Dimension 2: Biomedical conditions and complications	
High-risk sexual behaviors associated with substance use	Chlamydia/gonorrhea screening
	Explicit discussion of sexual risk behaviors
	Review of risk of sex-related danger associated with intoxication, especially for females
	Review of contraception possibilities
Presence of chronic health disorders, likelihood of exacerbation	Involvement in coordination with primary medical care providers
	Explicit identification of problem (e.g., marijuana-induced bronchospasm or general exercise intolerance) and tracking as a strategy to enhance problem self-recognition, treatment role induction, and engagement

Table 5–3. Speculative example of future treatment matching grid based on ASAM PPC-2R assessment dimensions (*continued*)

Assessment	Treatment services and placement
Dimension 3: Emotional, behavioral, and cognitive conditions and complications	
High levels of psychopathy, emerging antisocial personality disorder, and/or external locus of control	May not do as well with 12-step induction
High levels of social affiliation	May do well with 12-step induction
Cognitive impairment	May not do well with complex CBT, or alternatively may need modification of CBT materials
Specific comorbid psychiatric disorders	Specific pharmacotherapies Specific psychotherapies
Attention-deficit/hyperactivity disorder, executive function problems, cognitive impairment, or other factors that decrease capacity for attention and/or verbal learning	May benefit from experiential approaches, role-plays May need briefer sessions, more frequent repetition, etc.
Severe affective instability, not amenable to outpatient treatment	Psychiatric evaluation in a residential setting, with initiation or readjustment of pharmacotherapy once sufficient abstinence attained for diagnostic clarification

Table 5–3.   Speculative example of future treatment matching grid based on ASAM PPC-2R assessment dimensions *(continued)*

Assessment	Treatment services and placement
Dimension 4: Readiness to change	
Low degree of engagement/motivation	Utilization of strategies targeting motivation and engagement:
	Therapeutic alliance and relationship with a caring therapist or counselor
	Explicit identification of stage of change
	Contingency management, including specific use of experimental motivational incentive interventions, or more broadly, reward-consequence manipulations with increasingly specific, concrete, and frequent reinforcers as needed
	Strategies aimed at enhancing internal motivation, including motivational enhancement therapy, motivational interviewing, etc.
	Strategies for enhancing external motivation, including juvenile justice involvement, probationary monitoring, adjudicatory mandate, progressive sanctions, drug court, etc.
Low degree of service utilization	Strategies targeting increased service utilization:
	Assertive engagement techniques, including phone calls, home services, assertive stance, etc.
	Social marketing and outreach
	Transportation support
	Integration and/or co-location with other services
Dimension 5: Relapse and continued use potential	
High relapse potential	Increased frequency and/or intensity of monitoring
	Relapse prevention CBT, ACRA, etc.
	Assertive continuing care approaches
	Contingency "backup" planning
	Pharmacological treatments (antiaddiction/anticraving medications)

Table 5–3. Speculative example of future treatment matching grid based on ASAM PPC-2R assessment dimensions *(continued)*

Assessment	Treatment services and placement
Dimension 6: Recovery environment	
Drug-involved peer group	CBT relapse prevention interventions including cue avoidance and refusal skills
Maltreatment	Protection from abusive influences
	Residential LOC
Insufficient family supervision and/or	Family therapies
supports	Surrogate caregivers
	Incremental step-up in intensity and LOC
	Incremental step-down supervision intensity and LOC for community reintegration following residential treatment
Difficulties with effectiveness of parental involvement	Negotiate involvement of parents on as-needed basis, designate "alarm system" that supersedes desire for confidentiality
	Address struggles for autonomy in older adolescents
	Teach parents to "pick their battles"

Note. ACRA = Adolescent Community Reinforcement Approach; ASAM PPC-2R = *The American Society of Addiction Medicine Patient Placement Criteria*, 2nd Edition, Revised (Mee-Lee et al. 2001); CBT = cognitive-behavioral therapy; LOC = level of care.

Case Vignette

Tanya is a 16-year-old girl referred from detention for evaluation. Her substance use history is notable for onset of marijuana use at age 12, progressing to daily use by age 15; alcohol onset at age 13, with weekend binges to severe intoxication; and sporadic infrequent experimentation with nasal cocaine, hallucinogens, and prescription opioids. She was abstinent by confinement while in detention for the past 3 weeks. She had a few sessions of substance abuse counseling several months ago, but mostly was a no-show because her family couldn't "make her" attend.

Tanya lives with her grandmother. Her father is incarcerated, and Tanya was removed by the protective services agency from the care of her mother, who has a history of substance abuse and a "breakdown." There was an allegation of molestation by a neighbor at age 9. Tanya has been sexually active since age 13, with 10 lifetime partners, and currently engages in unprotected sex with older boys, often while intoxicated. Her educational history is notable for poor academic performance, having repeated third grade, being told she was a "slow learner," no special education services, multiple suspensions for disruptive behavior, and being assigned to tenth grade but truant most of the year. Most of her friends are involved with drugs and delinquent behaviors.

Tanya's medical history is notable for asthma, history of chlamydia, spontaneous abortion, and complaints of "stomachaches" that have been worse recently.

Tanya's legal history is notable for an arrest for possession of controlled dangerous substances on school grounds at age 14 (charges dropped); probation received at age 14 for assault; and house arrest at age 15 for intent to distribute controlled dangerous substances. Most recently she was detained with a violation of probation for theft and unauthorized use of a vehicle.

Tanya's psychiatric history is notable for inattention and hyperactivity since childhood, without treatment. She has had chronic emotional lability and dysphoric mood, tantrums, and explosive temper, which have been much worse since onset of substance use during the past few years. She has been progressively oppositional and ungovernable at home, she stays away from home habitually until late, and she ran away overnight once. She has chronic nighttime insomnia and sleeps late, with sleep-wake cycle disruption. She says marijuana helps her to "chill" and avoid fights with peers. She has had several attempts at family and school counseling, but never sustained. She has never had formal psychiatric evaluation. Her insomnia and irritability are worse since discontinuation of marijuana 3 weeks ago.

Table 5–4 illustrates treatment matching for this case example. For each of the ASAM PPC-2R dimensions, the table includes information related to assessment, ascertainment of treatment service needs, and determination of a suitable placement in which those service needs could be met. The table ends with an integration of those dimension-related placements into a single level-of-care placement recommendation using the ASAM PPC-2R decision rules.

Key Clinical Concepts

- The ASAM PPC-2R provides a standard approach and practical organization for treatment planning that includes three "steps": assessment of severity in each dimension; determination of treatment service needs in each assessment dimension; and selection of setting, program, and placement in an integrated treatment plan.

- The field is gradually accumulating knowledge about specific strategies for matching heterogeneous subtypes of adolescents with SUDs, based on their clinical assessment characteristics, to different treatment interventions, modalities, doses, and levels of care.

- The treatment service delivery system is being improved by broadening the continuum of care; utilizing that continuum more fully to include continuing care, longitudinal monitoring, and follow-up care; and coordinating between episodes of treatment at different levels of care.

References

Brown S: Facilitating change for adolescent alcohol problems: a multiple options approach, in Innovations in Adolescent Substance Abuse Interventions. Edited by Wagner E, Waldron H. Oxford, UK, Pergamon, 2001, pp 169–187

Clemmey P, Payne L, Fishman M: Clinical characteristics and treatment outcomes of adolescent heroin users. J Psychoactive Drugs 36:85–94, 2004

Dasinger L, Shane P, Martinovich Z: Assessing the effectiveness of community-based substance abuse treatment for adolescents. J Psychoactive Drugs 36:27–33, 2004

Deas D, Riggs P, Langenbucher J, et al: Adolescents are not adults: developmental considerations in alcohol users. Alcohol Clin Exp Res 24:232–237, 2000

Dennis M, Godley S, Diamond G, et al: The Cannabis Youth Treatment (CYT) study: main findings from two randomized trials. J Subst Abuse Treat 27:197–213, 2004

Table 5–4. Treatment matching for case vignette (assessment, treatment services, and placement)

Assessment	Treatment services	Placement
Dimension 1: Intoxication and withdrawal potential		
Abstinent for 3 weeks, some mild "subacute" persistent abstinence effects of insomnia and irritability	Needs education regarding sleep hygiene and insomnia as potential relapse trigger. Consider mild, non-habit-forming temporary sleep aid (e.g., diphenhydramine, low-dose trazodone).	Dimensional service needs met by Level I (outpatient) placement (and could be addressed in any level of care).
Dimension 2: Biomedical conditions and complications		
No acute problems. Exacerbation of chronic moderate-severity abdominal symptoms. At risk for sexually transmitted infections, given history. At risk for exacerbation of reactive airways disease from heavy marijuana use.	Needs nonurgent medical evaluation (differential diagnosis might include urinary tract infection, gastritis, cervicitis, somatic symptom of depression, etc.) and general health maintenance. Needs screening for sexually transmitted infections, contraception services, and sexual risk behavior counseling.	Dimensional service needs met by Level I (outpatient) placement (and could be addressed in any level of care).

Table 5–4. Treatment matching for case vignette (assessment, treatment services, and placement) *(continued)*

Assessment	Treatment services	Placement
Dimension 3: Emotional, behavioral, and cognitive conditions and complications		
Significant symptoms of affective disturbance but without evaluation or treatment. No imminent dangerousness. Social functioning significantly impaired in the school, legal, and family domains. Emotional and behavioral symptoms have caused severe interference with addiction recovery efforts through lack of cooperation with treatment, deviant peer group affiliation, and self-professed psychological benefits of substance use. Impaired ability for self-care characterized by ongoing sexual risk behaviors.	Needs psychiatric evaluation, including consideration of treatment for possible affective disorder, possible attention-deficit/hyperactivity disorder. Needs programmatic treatment setting for implementation and close monitoring of psychiatric treatment (pharmacological and/or psychotherapeutic). Needs at least moderately high-intensity daily structure and assessment of behavioral response.	Dimensional service needs probably met by Level II.5 (partial hospitalization/day program) placement, with psychiatric treatment either built into the substance abuse program or provided through coordinated psychiatric services. Consideration might reasonably be given to a Level III.5 (clinically managed, medium-intensity residential) placement, especially if additional details of assessment or lack of progress at Level II.5 suggest the need for higher intensity, including 24-hour structure and boundaries unavailable in the home environment to prevent further deterioration of social functioning.

Table 5–4. Treatment matching for case vignette (assessment, treatment services, and placement) *(continued)*

Assessment	Treatment services	Placement
Dimension 4: Readiness to change		
Currently in precontemplative stage of change. Patient sees self as having a probation officer problem, not a substance problem.	Needs significant treatment frequency, intensity, and programmatic milieu to support motivation and progression through stages of change. Needs motivational enhancement therapy techniques, including functional analysis of pros and cons of substance use, as well as juvenile justice leverage (e.g., probationary mandate) to improve treatment engagement.	Dimensional service needs met by Level II.5 placement for near-daily contact. Consideration might be given to Level II.1 (intensive outpatient) placement as motivation progresses or if patient becomes engaged in other prosocial structured activities.

Table 5–4. Treatment matching for case vignette (assessment, treatment services, and placement) *(continued)*

Assessment	Treatment services	Placement
Dimension 5: Relapse and continued use potential		
Despite brief abstinence during confinement, patient has had no appreciable acquisition of recovery skills and remains at very high risk of immediate continued use/relapse and functional deterioration. Patient has not been amenable to previous Level I treatment because would not attend.	Needs significant treatment intensity and structure to overcome pattern of habitual use, impulsive behaviors, and susceptibility to relapse triggers. Needs frequent monitoring with feedback and debriefing on temptations to use and/or anticipated actual use. Needs relapse prevention interventions, including relapse trigger identification and refusal skills rehearsal, guidance in support of alternative prosocial leisure activities and different peer group.	Dimensional service needs met by Level II.5 placement for near-daily monitoring.
Dimension 6: Recovery environment		
Grandmother is supportive but lacks the personal resources to effectively sustain treatment. Peer group is predominantly substance using.	Needs family intervention, including encouragement and training for grandmother on monitoring, home behavior negotiation and management, utilization of services and system (juvenile justice) leverage. Needs contact with peers beginning to succeed without substance use and fun social interactions without intoxication.	Dimensional service needs met by Level II.1 placement.

Table 5–4. Treatment matching for case vignette (assessment, treatment services, and placement) *(continued)*

Assessment	Treatment services	Placement
Dimensions 1–6: Integrated multidimensional placement		The PPC contains decision rules that combine the criteria and placement recommendations for each of the individual dimensions as above into an overall level-of-care recommendation. In this case, that recommendation would be for a Level II.5 placement (because patient meets criteria for II.5 in two of six dimensions).

Fishman M: Treatment planning, matching, and placement for adolescents with substance use disorders, in Adolescent Substance Abuse: Psychiatric Comorbidity and High-Risk Behaviors. Edited by Kaminer Y, Bukstein OG. New York, Routledge/Taylor & Francis, 2008, pp 87–110

Fishman M, Payne L, Clemmey P: Engagement in adolescent continuing care. Presentation at the Joint Meeting on Adolescent Treatment Effectiveness, Washington, DC, March 21, 2005

Funk RR, McDermeit M, Godley SH, et al: Maltreatment issues by level of adolescent substance abuse treatment: the extent of the problem at intake and relationship to early outcomes. Child Maltreat 8:36–45, 2003

Godley MD, Godley SH, Dennis MI: The effectiveness of assertive continuing care on continuing care linkage, adherence, and abstinence following residential treatment. Addiction 102:81–93, 2007

Godley S, Godley M, Karvinen T, et al: The assertive continuing care protocol: a case manager's manual for working with adolescents after residential treatment for alcohol and other substance use disorders. 2003. Available at: http://www.chestnut.org/LI/bookstore/Blurbs/Manuals/K107-Assertive_Continuing_Care.html. Accessed December 14, 2009.

Hser Y, Grella CE, Hubbard RL, et al: An evaluation of drug treatment for adolescents in 4 US cities. Arch Gen Psychiatry 58:689–695, 2001

Kaminer Y, Napolitano C: Telephone Continuing Care Therapy for Adolescents. Center City, MN, Hazelden, 2010

Kaminer Y, Burleson J, Burke R: Aftercare for adolescents with alcohol use disorders: a randomized controlled study. J Am Acad Child Adolesc Psychiatry 47:1405–1412, 2008

Libby AM, Riggs PD: Integrated substance use and mental health services for adolescents: challenges and opportunities, in Adolescent Substance Abuse: Psychiatric Comorbidity and High-Risk Behaviors. Edited by Kaminer Y, Bukstein OG. New York, Routledge/Taylor & Francis, 2008, pp 435–452

Marsch L, Bickel W, Badger G, et al: Comparison of pharmacological treatments for opioid-dependent adolescents: a randomized controlled trial. Arch Gen Psychiatry 62:1157–1164, 2005

Mee-Lee D, Shulman GD, Fishman M, et al (eds): ASAM Patient Placement Criteria for the Treatment of Substance-Related Disorders, 2nd Edition, Revised (ASAM PPC-2R). Chevy Chase, MD, American Society of Addiction Medicine, 2001

Muck R, Zempolich K, Titus J, et al: An overview of the effectiveness of adolescent substance abuse treatment models. Youth Soc 33:143–168, 2003

6

Adolescent Behavioral Change

Process and Outcomes

Ken C. Winters, Ph.D.
Yifrah Kaminer, M.D., M.B.A.

Substance use and abuse among youth are a significant public health concern. Adolescence represents a critical period for the potential initiation of substance use. Onset of substance use during the teenage years negatively impacts cognitive, physical, and psychosocial development; increases the likelihood for developing a substance use disorder (SUD); and for some youth, contributes to a progression to a longer-term addiction. Despite the high rates of use of nicotine, alcohol, and other drugs by young people, only a small segment (about 10%) of the adolescent subpopulation with SUDs, including those with high-severity SUDs (Waldron and Turner 2008), comorbid psychiatric disorders (Kaminer and Bukstein 2008), and legal problems (Dembo et al. 1997), end up in treatment (Substance Abuse and Mental Health Services Administration 2008).

We have three primary objectives in this chapter. First, we present an overview of adolescent substance abuse treatment outcome. Second, we address mechanisms of behavioral change in treatment. Third, we discuss aftercare and the emerging adaptive treatment concept and their role in providing continuity of care to maintain treatment gains, enhance treatment outcomes for poor responders, and prevent relapse in youth who have achieved partial or complete abstinence.

Advances in Youth Treatment Research

There are numerous controlled evaluations of drug treatments for adults (Miller and Wilbourne 2002). By comparison, only a modest number of controlled evaluations have been done of adolescent drug abuse treatments. The good news, however, is that great advances have been made since 1990 in the development and evaluation of treatments for adolescent drug abuse (Dennis and Kaminer 2006). These advances are reflected in the use of assessment tools that have been developed and validated on adolescent populations; treatment approaches that target multiple drugs, reflecting the fact that most clinical populations of teenagers abuse multiple substances; treatment manuals and specific protocols that permit treatment replication; and the increased rigor used in evaluating the effectiveness of these approaches.

This body of treatment-evaluation research reflects various interventions using different theory-related approaches. Family-based treatment, motivational enhancement, 12-step, therapeutic community, community reinforcement, cognitive-behavioral, and pharmacological approaches either have met standards of evidence-based treatments or have demonstrated modest empirical support (Williams and Chang 2000; Winters et al. 2009). Despite prominent differences in design and methodology, the most recent studies employing various treatment modalities in youth with SUDs in general have reported remarkably similar outcomes (Waldron and Kaminer 2004).

Brief interventions are receiving more attention for use in diverse settings, such as in emergency rooms, school-based clinics, and juvenile detention settings (O'Leary and Monti 2004). Nontraditional approaches to aftercare are also making inroads, including sober high schools (Moberg and Finch 2007) and technology-assisted aftercare via the computer and telephone (Kaminer and Napolitano 2004, 2010).

The Therapeutic Process

Clinicians typically focus on the single or repeated treatment episode at hand and determine that the treatment goal is abstinence. However, only a limited proportion of adolescents will achieve sobriety from alcohol or abstinence from substance abuse following a single episode of treatment. Some outpatient teens might be more appropriately considered as "continuing to use" rather than as having "relapsed," because in fact they did not abstain from alcohol or drugs while in treatment (Chung and Maisto 2006). Some research suggests an association between longer time in treatment and positive outcomes (Hser et al. 2001; Winters et al. 2000). Nevertheless, the majority of adolescents who "achieve" abstinence will relapse 3–6 months later (Deas and Thomas 2001; Winters et al. 2009).

Understanding the therapeutic process is not easy. Most evidence-based treatments are also "theory based," at least to some degree. However, tests of the mechanisms of action suggested by the theories on which the interventions are based often do not yield positive results (Apodaca and Longabaugh 2009; Morgenstern and Longabaugh 2000; Morgenstern and McKay 2007). Some theorists have argued that positive treatment effects are due primarily to what are referred to as "general" therapeutic factors, such as an empathic and caring therapist, and the structure and support provided by regularly scheduled treatment sessions over a prolonged period of time (Baskin et al. 2003; Wampold 2001). Increased motivation to change has often been cited as a predictor for positive outcome in both adult and youth literature. S. H. Godley et al. (2004) reported that motivated adolescents were three times more likely than nonmotivated youth to remain abstinent during aftercare and to show improved engagement.

L. C. Sobell et al. (2003) reported that some adults with problematic drinking stopped using alcohol by simply being exposed to an advertisement of a clinical trial. Others responded to advice by a clinician to stop smoking (Russell et al. 1979) or drinking (Edwards et al. 1977; Fleming et al. 2002) because it might be harmful to their health. The report by Russell et al. (1979) indicated that more participants quit smoking in the month immediately preceding the research assessment interview than had quit in the month following the brief intervention. According to the classic study by Edwards et al. (1977), two groups of "alcoholics" received either one counseling session or several months of inpatient and outpatient treatment. One year later, the two groups demonstrated no significant differences in outcome.

How to Differentiate Youth From Adults in Preparation for Treatment

Treated teens who use substances differ from their adult counterparts in length and severity of substance use, typical patterns and context of use, type of substance-related problems most often experienced, and source of referral to treatment (Chung and Maisto 2006; see also Chapter 1, "Prevalence and Clinical Course of Adolescent Substance Use and Substance Use Disorders"). Adolescent substance use and abuse should be evaluated from a developmental perspective. Some subgroups of adolescents have not yet started drinking or have not yet reached the peak of the trajectory characterizing their drinking pattern. Therefore, any effort to reduce or eliminate drinking amounts to "swimming against the tide or current." Furthermore, youth are also less motivated than adults to change substance use and often enter treatment because of external pressures (Battjes et al. 2003). This happens either as a suggested referral by a concerned parent, mental health clinician, or school staff, or as a mandated referral initiated by the legal system. Consequently, it appears unlikely that youth will respond to advice only. However, McCambridge et al. (2008) reported that advice may be an effective brief intervention with older adolescent cannabis users; moreover, when fidelity to the motivational interviewing treatment provided to those randomized to the experimental condition was not high (as is commonly the case), it was not more effective than advice.

In the search to identify the effective ingredients of successful psychotherapy, one therapist characteristic in particular, "accurate empathy," as defined by Carl Rogers (1957), has been shown to be a predictor of therapeutic success. Within the addiction field, the search for conditions that are necessary and sufficient to induce change led Miller and Sanchez (1994) to identify six critical elements, which some refer to as mechanisms of behavioral change. These six active ingredients of effective brief interventions are represented best by the acronym FRAMES:

1. Feedback regarding personal risk or impairment
2. Emphasis on personal Responsibility for change

3. Clear Advice to change
4. A Menu of alternative change options
5. Therapist Empathy
6. Facilitation of participant optimism about the potential to change and Self-efficacy

Therapeutic interventions containing some or all of these elements have been effective in initiating change and reducing alcohol use.

Assessment Reactivity

Participants in treatment outcome studies undergo extensive assessment protocols to assess their eligibility and to provide information before beginning therapy sessions. Participants might be exposed, therefore, to a professional who does not necessarily function as a therapist, such as a research assistant in a clinical trial or a nurse in an outpatient clinic setting. Such interactions containing some or all of the components or active ingredients of FRAMES might be effective in initiating change and reducing substance use, even though they were not intended to be therapeutic. This change is defined as assessment reactivity (Epstein et al. 2005). In this case, *assessment reactivity* refers to a change of substance use status from positive at baseline to negative at the time of initiation of the first therapy session. Assessment reactivity has also been reported in association with posttreatment follow-up assessments in adults (Clifford et al. 2000, 2007), as well as with adolescents in an assessment-only condition (McCambridge and Strang 2005).

Kaminer et al. (2008) conducted a study 1) to examine if a change from positive to negative alcohol use from baseline assessment to the onset of the first session (i.e., pretreatment phase)—that is, baseline assessment reactivity (BAR)—occurs in adolescents and 2) to compare what mediators differentiate BAR-positive and BAR-negative youths. Participants were 177 adolescents with alcohol use disorders attending nine weekly group sessions of cognitive-behavioral therapy. Self-report for alcohol use and urinalysis for drug use in the last 30 days before baseline assessment and immediately before the first session of treatment were obtained to determine BAR. The findings were highly significant: 51.4% of the adolescents reported abstinence for alcohol use at the first session, and 29% of those who were positive for other drugs at baseline assessment tested negative for drugs at the first session. The authors also reported that variables such as age, gender, criminal justice involvement, or waiting duration from baseline assessment to first session were not associated with BAR. The likelihood of manifesting BAR was significantly correlated with the level of readiness to change and with three of eight subscales measuring self-efficacy. It is noteworthy that in Kaminer et al.'s (2008) study, participants continued to improve from first to last session; that is, treatment outcome was not solely attributed to BAR.

The Kaminer et al. (2008) study is the only one to date that has reported on BAR in adolescents enrolled in treatment for an alcohol use disorder. Participants showed a highly significant shift to nonuse of alcohol from baseline assessment to first session. These findings support the validity of BAR as a construct relevant to youth waiting for the initiation of treatment for alcohol and other SUDs. Regarding the second objective of the study (i.e., determining what mediators differentiate BAR-positive and BAR-negative youths), it is worth considering the comments of Epstein et al. (2005), who found that alcohol assessment is therapeutic in adults. These authors provided three possible explanations for observed changes in adults' drinking prior to initiating treatment that may apply to adolescents' behavior as well:

> 1) decision making about changing drinking that is prompted by seeing an advertisement, 2) telling someone in the social network about a decision to seek help, resulting in a change in others' responses to drinking and abstinence, and 3) initiation of a therapeutic change process as a result of the assessment itself; for instance, realizing the extent and severity of one's drinking problems in the course of verbalizing them to another person. This possible explanation can be considered "Assessment Reactivity." (p. 369)

As in the study by Epstein et al. (2005), an assessment may have supported motivation to change in Kaminer et al.'s (2008) study. It is not known whether these youth would have changed their alcohol and substance use patterns based on sheer insight without the assessment, as might happen with adults (L. C. Sobell et al. 2003). Based on our clinical experience, this type of change is unlikely to happen with youth. Nonetheless, assessment reactivity needs to be identified and separated from treatment effects, because

> if change is indeed occurring prior to treatment proper and this initial change is not taken into account in interpreting outcome data, then positive findings

may be misattributed to the experimental treatment rather than to the processes of change that began prior to treatment. (Epstein et al. 2005, p. 377)

Heterogeneity of Response to Adolescent Treatment

Despite prominent differences in design and methodology, the most recent studies employing various treatment modalities in youth with SUDs have reported remarkably similar outcomes (Waldron and Turner 2008). The similarity of outcomes might suggest that similar mechanisms of behavioral change are the active ingredients of various treatment modalities that appear different in the way they are administered. Nevertheless, no data are available to support or negate the possibility that varied treatments might share active ingredients of mechanisms of behavioral change. Increasing efforts are being invested in studying mechanisms of behavioral change in adolescent substance abuse treatment. Potential mediator variables include readiness to change (O'Leary and Monti 2004), self-efficacy (Burleson and Kaminer 2005), and perceived family support (Liddle et al. 2001).

The traditional experimental designs for studies of youth SUDs have emphasized the comparison of standardized, fixed interventions as the primary method for evaluating treatment efficacy. Despite considerable variation in patient response, most treatments in the addictions strive to deliver essentially the same intervention to all patients, regardless of how the patient is responding. Indeed, treatment planning based on this approach has overlooked the most urgent challenges facing the field: the heterogeneity of adolescent response to treatment, the problem of poor response to treatment, and the difficulty of preventing relapse (Waldron and Turner 2008).

Data from numerous treatment studies indicate that there are large individual differences in patients' responsivity, even to effective treatments that have been standardized and with therapists who show high adherence to treatment manuals (Dennis et al. 2004; Waldron et al. 2001). Although a considerable percentage of the patients complete treatment and achieve abstinence, others attend most sessions but continue to drink or use drugs, and a sizable number of patients drop out during treatment (S. H. Godley et al. 2004).

There are usually two types of poor responders to substance abuse treatment: 1) those who are noncompleters of treatment (i.e., through dropout and administrative discharge) and 2) those who are retained in treatment and continue to use drugs, as evidenced by positive drug urinalysis. Rates of youth who are treatment noncompleters in clinical settings range from 30% to 50% (Kaminer and Bukstein 2008). Rates of positive drug urinalysis among treatment completers are even higher than noncompletion rates. For example, available unpublished data from the Cannabis Youth Treatment study indicate the following rates of positive urinalysis per study condition at the end of treatment: 57% for motivational enhancement therapy (MET)/CBT-5 (two individual motivational enhancement sessions followed by three cognitive-behavioral therapy [CBT] sessions), 55% for MET/CBT-12 (two individual motivational enhancement sessions followed by 10 CBT sessions), 50% for the adolescent community reinforcement approach, and 60% for multidimensional family therapy (M.L. Dennis and R. Funk, personal communication, May 19, 2009). The literature provides little guidance regarding what to do with poor responders to treatment. A review by M.D. Godley and Godley (2009) indicates that few programs clearly specify what types of efforts (if any) will be made for linking program completers to continuing care, and even fewer indicate what to do about treatment noncompleters.

Several studies published in a book focusing on treatment models for adolescent SUDs imply that to get services for the maintenance of treatment gains, an adolescent has to graduate or complete the treatment program (Stevens and Morral 2003). This popular approach is raising a public health concern because noncompleters are at higher risk for continued, exacerbated, or renewed substance use, as well as substance use–related consequences that affect the users, their family, and the community (Kaminer et al. 2008). Consequently, noncompleters have greater and perhaps more costly needs than treatment completers. M.D. Godley et al. (2007) posited that because several episodes of treatment and therefore several potential reentries are the rule rather than the exception for youth with SUDs, a noncompleter status does not necessarily indicate that the adolescent may fail to benefit from continued care. Although arranging the first session of the assigned adaptive treatment condition may be difficult due to the abrupt or unexpected departure of the adolescent from the initial treatment program, engaging dropouts has not been as difficult as might commonly be perceived when an effective tracking system has been in place (Scott and Dennis 1998; Scott et al. 2005).

Aftercare or Continued Care

Addiction treatment programs have traditionally provided fixed amounts or durations of intervention and evaluated their effects several months after treatment completion. The results provide an answer to the question, "How long do positive changes last following discharge?" (McLellan et al. 2005). However, the immediate goal of reducing substance use is necessary but rarely sufficient for the achievement of long-term abstinence. Consensus maintains that SUD is a chronic disorder (McKay 2005) with a relapsing-remitting course (McLellan et al. 2000). Very little has been done, however, to link and engage patients with aftercare programs and services (McKay 2005). Often, no coordinated effort is made to provide a system of continuing care. The lack of posttreatment support and monitoring of clients leaves them vulnerable to frequent relapse. Also, substantial within- and between-program variability exists in terms of the success in achieving goals for continued care. The most common approach to reducing recurrence of psychiatric disorders has been continued care by the addition of "booster" sessions, typically at a reduced frequency, after the end of more intensive acute treatments.

A common growing view of addiction treatment is that it is a process that requires a continuum of care, including management and monitoring similar to that for chronic disease (McKay 2005; Scott et al. 2005). The American Society of Addiction Medicine defined *continuing care* as

> the provision of a treatment plan and organizational structure that will ensure that a patient receives whatever kind of care he or she needs at the time. The treatment program thus is flexible and tailored to the shifting needs of the patient and his or her level of readiness to change. This term is preferred to the term "aftercare." (American Society of Addiction Medicine 2001, p. 361)

The vast majority of the research on continued care has been conducted with adults. The results of only two studies on youths receiving continued care have been published to date (M. D. Godley et al. 2007; Kaminer et al. 2008).

Reports on the importance of self-efficacy (Burleson and Kaminer 2005), coping skills (Waldron and Kaminer 2004), and readiness to change (O'Leary and Monti 2004) as mechanisms for treatment outcome are common in the literature on treatment for youth with SUDs. A possible mechanism that accounts for the relationship between aftercare and ultimate outcomes is the maintenance of during-treatment proximal outcome gains afforded by continuing care (e.g., increased self-efficacy, improved readiness to change). An important point is that alcohol and substance use increases in youth until they reach their early 20s, at which time young adults manifest moderation or cessation of use. The trajectory of increased substance use, therefore, compromises the likelihood of favorable response to treatment and increases the odds for relapse during the posttreatment phase. Furthermore, in contrast to adults, a considerable proportion of youth in treatment may be better considered "continuing users" who are not sufficiently motivated to abstain during and following the treatment phase (Chung and Maisto 2006).

One of the crucial goals of aftercare should be to prepare patients to cope effectively with high-risk situations for relapse in the future. Indeed, McKay (2009) suggested that an individualized relapse prevention program might be helpful for patients to facilitate maintenance of abstinence or to initiate abstinence for those who failed to achieve it during treatment.

Many communities lack aftercare services for adolescents with SUDs. Even if referrals are being made, many adolescents do not link to or only participate minimally in aftercare interventions. M.D. Godley et al. (2007) found that only 36% of adolescents discharged from residential treatment attended one or more aftercare sessions at community clinics. Among those who link to continued care, many attend only a few sessions.

As noted in the previous section, M.D. Godley et al. (2007) posited that because several episodes of treatment, and therefore several potential reentries, are the rule rather than the exception for youth with SUDs, a noncompleter status does not necessarily indicate that the adolescent may fail to benefit from continued care. According to M.D. Godley et al. (2007), unplanned discharges are treated essentially the same except that the case manager providing continuing care usually works harder to get the first session arranged due to the abrupt or unexpected departure of the adolescent from the program. M.D. Godley and Godley (in press) advocated that to inform their linkage practice, providers should, at a minimum, track linkage rates by type of discharge and whether or not the adolescent is referred to their own organization or another service provider.

Only one empirical study has been published examining the efficacy of aftercare interventions in adolescents with SUDs discharged from residential treatment programs. S.H. Godley et al. (2007) used an assertive aftercare model addressing outreach strategies for clients with mental health problems who were often reluctant or unable to attend office-based services. Assertive approaches transfer the responsibility for linkage and retention from the patient to the clinician (M. D. Godley et al. 2007). Adolescents referred to residential treatment have been characterized by high severity of SUDs and are at high risk for both relapse and poor linkage to aftercare programs. In this study, adolescents referred from residential treatment were assigned to one of two conditions: 1) assertive continuing care services, which included case management, home visits, and the adolescent community reinforcement approach, or 2) usual continuing care, which included outpatient treatment services and encouragement to attend self-help groups. Those who were assigned to assertive continuing care were significantly more likely to initiate and receive more continuing care services, to be abstinent from marijuana at 3 months postdischarge, and to have reduced days of alcohol use at 3 months postdischarge. S. H. Godley et al. (2007) also found that motivated adolescents were three times more likely than nonmotivated youth to remain abstinent during aftercare and to show improved engagement. Based on these findings, it appears that adolescents who are reentering the community after a treatment episode (whether completed or not completed) require coordinated case management that will ensure linkage and retention, and ultimately improve outcomes.

Kaminer et al. (2008) studied aftercare for youth with alcohol use disorders in an outpatient program for the following reasons: 1) adolescents have high posttreatment rates of continued use and of relapse; 2) the literature provides little guidance for the implementation of continued care programs for youth after a treatment episode in an outpatient clinic; and 3) very little research has been done to investigate the relationship among self-efficacy, readiness to change, social support, and engagement as it pertains to outcomes of continued care for adolescents with SUDs. The study was developed to test the relative efficacy of three randomized aftercare conditions for treatment completers during the 3-month period following treatment: 1) individualized 50-minute integrated motivational enhancement and cognitive-behavioral therapies; 2) individualized integrated motivational enhancement and cognitive-behavioral therapies via 15-minute therapeutic phone contacts only; and 3) no-intervention control condition. Ninety percent of treatment completers finished the assigned aftercare conditions. The phone intervention was found to be feasible and acceptable to both adolescents and therapists (Burleson and Kaminer

2007). A significant reduction occurred for number of drinking occasions, heavy drinking occasions, and drinks per occasion, as well as highest number of drinks per occasion, as a function of combined active aftercare conditions versus the no-intervention condition.

More than 80% of the cohort in Kaminer et al.'s (2008) study also met criteria for cannabis use disorders. The study also found a significant change in readiness for change in marijuana use, such that youth in the active aftercare conditions collectively showed significantly more readiness to change than youth in the no-intervention control condition. Similar to the findings regarding alcohol use disorders, a significant reduction in cannabis-positive urinalysis occurred as a function of combined active aftercare conditions versus the no active aftercare condition. No significant difference was found between the two active interventions regarding alcohol use disorders or cannabis use disorders (Kaminer et al. 2008). These results were maintained at 12 months following aftercare completion (Burleson and Kaminer 2009). Suicidal ideation decreased significantly following the individualized aftercare condition and showed a trend in the same direction following the phone intervention, compared with the no-intervention control condition (Kaminer et al. 2006).

Adaptive Treatment for Youth

Research in adaptive treatment for adult substance abusers has been ongoing during the last decade to address the heterogeneity in both clinical severity and treatment response (Collins et al. 2004; Murphy et al. 2007; M.B. Sobell and Sobell 2000). Adaptive treatment is a promising performance-based procedure in which individuals who respond poorly to an initial level of evidence-based efficacious treatment are then provided a different or a more enhanced version of the same treatment (McKay 2009). The definitions of nonresponse or poor response and the timing of change are pivotal decision rules in an adaptive treatment protocol, which includes an intervention options algorithm.

Although adaptive treatment studies are a relatively new development in addictions treatment research, a total of 15 adult studies were identified and reviewed by McKay (2009). Most of these studies yielded favorable results in which adaptive procedures 1) led to better substance use outcomes, 2) led to equivalent outcomes yet were associated with other advantages (e.g., lower cost, lower patient burden, greater safety), or 3) produced algorithms that specified which patients would benefit most from what continuation treatments. These results are highly encouraging with regard to the potential acceptability and effectiveness of adaptive interventions for SUDs.

One of the key questions in treatment is what to do with patients who do not respond to an initial treatment. The important consideration is whether the patients' initial treatment should be switched to something else, and if so, to what treatment, or whether they should receive another treatment to augment their current treatment (McKay 2009). In accordance with the stepped care approach, patients are started at the lowest appropriate level of care, and then "stepped up" to more intensive treatment if warranted by poor initial response. This approach has the potential to increase rates of participation, because it may be more palatable to patients due to the fact that it places a lower burden on them at the beginning of treatment. Stepped care may also increase cost-effectiveness and cost-benefit, because lower-intensity treatments are often less costly (McKay 2009). Adaptive or stepped care treatment algorithms have been developed and evaluated for a number of disorders, including depression and anxiety (Fava et al. 2006; Otto et al. 2000; Scogin et al. 2003). Although practicing child and adolescent psychiatrists have developed their own algorithms to address the issue of nonresponse (e.g., the Texas algorithm for depression; Hughes et al. 2007), the field of adolescent substance abuse treatment, which relies mostly on psychosocial interventions, has not generated an empirically supported set of tailoring variables and decision rules specifying the intervention that is most likely to be effective in the face of initial nonresponse.

Adolescent substance abuse treatment consists of repeated, isolated episodes of acute care. The perspective that addiction is a long-term problem that requires multiple treatment episodes before abstinence might be achieved is another argument for pursuing evidence-based adaptive treatments for youth. Based on the extant adult SUD-oriented literature and the youth psychopharmacological algorithm literature, there is reason to believe that this approach should be expanded to youth substance abuse treatment outcome research in order to overcome the limitations of traditional interventions and to advance the field.

Future Directions

Perhaps the most important future research priority in the field of adolescent substance abuse treatment is to address the question of what to do with poor responders to treatment. Little research attention has been directed toward enhancing treatment engagement strategies (Winters et al. 2009), and only a few programs clearly specify what types of efforts (if any) will be made for linking adolescent clients to continuing care (M.D. Godley and Godley 2009). Because research has started to identify some factors that influence recovery— aftercare involvement, coexisting disorders, coping skills, peer drug use, parental support, and motivational factors—a high priority for research is to identify ways to tailor treatment approaches in order to promote engagement and the recovery process.

Future research should also explore in more depth factors that affect extended recovery. The field has identified general principles of recovery, but little is known about the recovery process for various types of teenagers, such as those who have attention-deficit/hyperactivity disorder versus those who have depression. Also, technology-based aftercare services seem to be a promising approach, given the ease of administrating these services, the comfort level for youth using electronic communication, and the applicability regardless of the location of the client.

Key Clinical Concepts

- The six active ingredients of effective brief interventions are represented best by the acronym FRAMES: Feedback, Responsibility, Advice, Menu, Empathy, and Self-efficacy.
- Baseline assessment reactivity should be considered when evaluating treatment outcomes.
- Regardless of varying treatment modalities, treatment outcomes across conditions have been similar due in part to high levels of motivation.
- Standardized treatment manuals and specific protocols that permit treatment replication are available for a variety of interventions.
- Aftercare is needed to maintain treatment gains and prevent relapse.

References

American Society of Addiction Medicine: Patient Placement Criteria for Treatment of Substance-Related Disorders, 2nd Edition, Revised. Chevy Chase, MD, American Society of Addiction Medicine, 2001

Apodaca TR, Longabaugh R: Mechanisms of change in motivational interviewing: a review and preliminary evaluation of the evidence. Addiction 104:705–715, 2009

Baskin TW, Tierney SC, Minami T, et al: Establishing specificity in psychotherapy: a meta-analysis of structural equivalence of placebo controls. J Consult Clin Psychol 71:973–979, 2003

Battjes RJ, Gordon MS, O'Grady KE, et al: Factors that predict adolescent motivation for substance abuse treatment. J Subst Abuse Treat 24:221–232, 2003

Burleson J, Kaminer Y: Adolescent substance use disorders: self-efficacy as a predictor of relapse. Addict Behav 20:751–764, 2005

Burleson JA, Kaminer Y: Aftercare for adolescent alcohol use disorder: feasibility and acceptability of a phone intervention. Am J Addict 16:202–205, 2007

Burleson J, Kaminer Y: Outcomes at nine-month follow-up of aftercare for adolescents with alcohol use disorders. Paper presented at the annual meeting of the Research Society on Alcoholism, San Diego, CA, June 2009

Chung T, Maisto SA: Review and reconsideration of relapse as a change point in clinical course in treated adolescents. Clin Psychol Rev 26:149–161, 2006

Clifford PR, Maisto SA, Franzke LH, et al: Alcohol treatment research follow-up interviews and drinking behaviors. J Stud Alcohol 61:736–743, 2000

Clifford PR, Maisto SA, Davis CM: Alcohol treatment research assessment exposure subject reactivity effects, part I: alcohol use and related consequences. J Stud Alcohol Drugs 68:519–528, 2007

Collins LM, Murphy SA, Bierman KL: A conceptual framework for adaptive preventive interventions. Prev Sci 5:185–196, 2004

Deas D, Thomas SE: An overview of controlled studies of adolescent substance abuse treatment. Am J Addict 10:178–189, 2001

Dembo R, Pacheco K, Schmeidler J, et al: Drug use and delinquent behavior among high risk youths. J Child Adolesc Subst Abuse 6:1–25, 1997

Dennis ML, Kaminer Y: Introduction to special issue on advances in the assessment and treatment of adolescent substance use disorders. Am J Addict 15 (suppl 1):1–3, 2006

Dennis ML, Godley SH, Diamond G, et al: The Cannabis Youth Treatment (CYT) study: main findings from two randomized trials. J Subst Abuse Treat 27:197–213, 2004

Edwards G, Orford J, Egert S, et al: Alcoholism: a controlled trial of treatment and advice. J Stud Alcohol 38:1004–1031, 1977

Epstein EE, Drapkin ML, Yusko DA, et al: Is alcohol assessment therapeutic? Pretreatment change in drinking among alcohol-dependent women. J Stud Alcohol 66:369–378, 2005

Fava M, Rush AJ, Wisniewski SR, et al; STAR*D Study Team: A comparison of mirtazapine and nortriptyline following two consecutive failed medication treatments for depressed outpatients: a STAR*D report. Am J Psychiatry 163:1161–1172, 2006

Fleming MF, Mundt MP, French MT, et al: Brief physician advice for problem drinkers: long-term efficacy and benefit-cost analysis. Alcohol Clin Exp Res 26:36–43, 2002

Godley MD, Godley SH: Continuing care following residential treatment: history, current practice, critical issues, and emergency approaches, in Understanding and Treating Adolescent Substance Use Disorders. Edited by Jainchill N. Kingston, NJ, Civic Research Institute (in press)

Godley MD, Godley SH, Dennis ML, et al: The effect of assertive continuing care on continuing care linkage, adherence and abstinence following residential treatment for adolescents with substance use. Addiction 102:81–93, 2007

Godley SH, Dennis ML, Godley MD, et al: Thirty-month relapse trajectory cluster groups among adolescents discharged from out-patient treatment. Addiction 99 (suppl 2):129–139, 2004

Hser YI, Grella CE, Hubbard RL, et al: An evaluation of drug treatments for adolescents in 4 U.S. cities. Arch Gen Psychiatry 58:689–695, 2001

Hughes CW, Emslie GJ, Crismon ML, et al: Texas Children's Medication Algorithm Project: update from Texas Consensus Conference Panel on Medication Treatment of Childhood Major Depressive Disorder. J Am Acad Child Adolesc Psychiatry 46:667–686, 2007

Kaminer Y, Bukstein OG (eds): Adolescent Substance Abuse: Psychiatric Comorbidity and High-Risk Behaviors. New York, Routledge/Taylor & Francis, 2008

Kaminer Y, Napolitano C: Dial for therapy: aftercare for adolescent substance use disorders. J Am Acad Child Adolesc Psychiatry 43:171–174, 2004

Kaminer Y, Napolitano C: Dial for Therapy: Manual for the Aftercare of Adolescents With Alcohol and Other Substance Use Disorders. Minneapolis, MN, Hazelden, 2010

Kaminer Y, Litt MD, Burke RH, et al: An interactive voice response (IVR) system for adolescents with alcohol use disorders: a pilot study. Am J Addict 15:122–125, 2006

Kaminer Y, Burleson JA, Burke RH: Efficacy of outpatient aftercare for adolescents with alcohol use disorders: a randomized controlled study. J Am Acad Child Adolesc Psychiatry 47:1405–1412, 2008

Liddle HA, Dakof GA, Diamond G: Multidimensional family therapy for adolescent substance abuse: results of a randomized clinical trial. Am J Drug Alcohol Abuse 27:651–687, 2001

McCambridge J, Strang J: Deterioration over time in effect of motivational interviewing in reducing drug consumption and related risk among young people. Addiction 100:470–478, 2005

McCambridge J, Slym RL, Strang J: Randomized controlled trial of motivational interviewing compared with drug information and advice for early intervention among young cannabis users. Addiction 103:1809–1818, 2008

McKay JR: Is there a case for extended interventions for alcohol and drug use disorders? Addiction 100:1594–1610, 2005

McKay JR: Continuing care research: what we have learned and where we are going. J Subst Abuse Treat 36:131–145, 2009

McLellan AT, Lewis DC, O'Brien CP, et al: Drug dependence, a chronic mental illness: implications for treatment, insurance, and outcomes evaluation. JAMA 284:1689–1695, 2000

McLellan AT, McKay JR, Forman R, et al: Reconsidering the evaluation of addiction treatment: from retrospective follow-up to concurrent recovery monitoring. Addiction 100:447–458, 2005

Miller WR, Sanchez V: Motivating young adults for treatment and lifestyle change, in Issues in Alcohol Use and Misuse by Young Adults. Edited by Howard G, Nathan P. Notre Dame, IN, University of Notre Dame Press, 1994, pp 51–81

Miller WR, Wilbourne PL: Mesa Grande: a methodological analysis of clinical trials of treatment for alcohol use disorders. Addiction 97:265–277, 2002

Moberg DP, Finch A: Recovery high schools: a descriptive study of school programs and students. J Groups Addict Recover 2:128–161, 2007

Morgenstern J, Longabaugh R: Cognitive-behavioral treatment for alcohol dependence: a review of evidence for its hypothesized mechanisms of action. Addiction 95:1475–1490, 2000

Morgenstern J, McKay JR: Rethinking the paradigms that inform behavioral treatment research for substance use disorders. Addiction 102:1377–1389, 2007

Murphy SA, Lynch KG, Oslin D, et al: Developing adaptive treatment strategies in substance abuse research. Drug Alcohol Depend 88:S24–S30, 2007

O'Leary TT, Monti PM: Motivational enhancement and other brief interventions for adolescent substance abuse: foundations, applications and evaluations. Addiction 99 (suppl 2):63–75, 2004

Otto MW, Pollack MH, Maki KM: Empirically supported treatments for panic disorder: costs, benefits, and stepped care. J Consult Clin Psychol 68:556–563, 2000

Rogers CR: The necessary and sufficient conditions for therapeutic personality change. J Consult Psychol 21:95–103, 1957

Russell MA, Wilson C, Taylor C, et al: Effect of general practitioners' advice against smoking. Br Med J 2:231–235, 1979

Scogin FR, Hanson A, Welsh D: Self-administered treatment in stepped-care models of depression treatment. J Clin Psychol 59:341–349, 2003

Scott CK, Dennis ML: Illinois Health Survey Laboratory Adolescent Follow-Up Manual. Chicago, IL, Chestnut Health Systems, 1998

Scott CK, Foss MA, Dennis ML: Utilizing recovery management checkups to shorten the cycle of relapse, treatment reentry, and recovery. Drug Alcohol Depend 78:325–338, 2005

Sobell LC, Agrawal S, Sobell MB, et al: Responding to an advertisement: a critical event in promoting self-change of drinking behavior. Poster presented at the 37th annual meeting of the Association for the Advancement of Behavior Therapy, Boston, MA, November 2003

Sobell MB, Sobell LC: Stepped care as a heuristic approach to the treatment of alcohol problems. J Consult Clin Psychol 68:573–579, 2000

Stevens SJ, Morral AR (eds): Adolescent Substance Abuse Treatment in the United States: Exemplary Models From a National Evaluation Study. Binghampton, NY, Haworth Press, 2003

Substance Abuse and Mental Health Services Administration, Office of Applied Studies: Results from the 2007 National Survey on Drug Use and Health: national findings (NSDUH Series H-34, DHHS Publ No SMA-08-4343). Rockville, MD, Substance Abuse and Mental Health Services Administration, 2008

Waldron H, Kaminer Y: On the learning curve: cognitive behavioral therapies for adolescent substance abuse. Addiction 99 (suppl 2):93–105, 2004

Waldron HB, Turner CW: Evidence-based psychosocial treatments for adolescent substance abuse. J Clin Child Adolesc Psychol 37:238–261, 2008

Waldron HB, Slesnick N, Brody JL, et al: Treatment outcomes for adolescent substance abuse at 4- and 7-month assessments. J Consult Clin Psychol 69:802–813, 2001

Wampold BE: The Great Psychotherapy Debate: Models, Methods, and Findings. Mahwah, NJ, Erlbaum, 2001

Williams RJ, Chang SY: A comprehensive and comparative review of adolescent substance abuse treatment outcome. Clinical Psychology: Science and Practice 7:138–166, 2000

Winters KC, Stinchfield RD, Opland E, et al: The effectiveness of the Minnesota Model approach in the treatment of adolescent drug abusers. Addiction 95:601–612, 2000

Winters KC, Botzet AM, Fahnhorst T, et al: Adolescent substance abuse treatment: a review of evidence-based research, in Handbook on the Prevention and Treatment of Substance Abuse in Adolescence. Edited by Leukefeld C, Gullotta T, Staton Tindall M. New York, Springer, 2009, pp 73–96

Suggested Reading

Kaminer Y, Bukstein OG (eds): Adolescent Substance Abuse: Psychiatric Comorbidity and High-Risk Behaviors. New York, Routledge/Taylor & Francis Group, 2008

7

Pharmacotherapy of Adolescent Substance Use Disorders

Yifrah Kaminer, M.D., M.B.A.

Lisa A. Marsch, Ph.D.

The majority of research on the pharmacotherapy of adolescent alcohol and other substance use disorders (AOSUDs) has been lagging behind both the adult AOSUD pharmacological research and the research evaluating the efficacy of psychosocial interventions for youth. The emerging consensus among treatment researchers is that a biopsychosocial, multidimensional, problem-oriented approach is necessary to meet the needs of adolescents with AOSUDs. The objectives of this chapter are twofold: 1) to clarify the reasons behind the relative scarcity of research and publications on pharmacological interventions for youth with AOSUDs and 2) to review the present knowledge concerning pharmacotherapy for adolescents with AOSUDs. We conclude by addressing future directions.

Challenges in the Development of Pharmacotherapy for Adolescents With AOSUDs

Despite increased acceptance of pharmacotherapy for adults with AOSUDs, little systematic research has been done evaluating the safety and efficacy of psychotropic medications in the treatment of adolescents with AOSUDs (Waxmonsky and Wilens 2005). The potential risks versus benefits of psychopharmacotherapy for youth have been continuously debated over the last two decades (Biederman 1992; Gibbons and Mann 2009; Vitiello et al. 1999). The deliberation has been complicated by the recent controversy regarding the alleged potential increase in suicidal behavior by youth treated with selective serotonin reuptake inhibitors (Gibbons and Mann 2009). It is not surprising that these debates contribute to the unfavorable public perceptions of pediatric psychopharmacology, which are compounded by the outdated belief that medications represent "chemical restraints." Many parents, therefore, face the question of whether their belief in their offspring's potential to outgrow early-onset psychiatric disorders without pharmacological intervention is a realistic expectation or merely a form of denial and rationalization that may have profound negative consequences if a potentially treatable disorder is left untreated.

Psychopharmacological approaches may be inconsistent with some perspectives on recovery from AOSUD. For example, Hoffmann et al. (1987) noted that 12-step self-help groups, such as Alcoholics Anonymous, do not acknowledge the importance of accurate medical and psychiatric diagnoses, which are a necessary component of psychopharmacotherapy. Furthermore, given the 12-step perspective's general orientation toward abstinence from alcohol and other drugs, 12-step sponsors of dually diagnosed adolescents participating in self-help groups may have a strong objection to any medication, even those such as lithium and neuroleptics that have no known abuse potential. This perspective can have the negative consequence of exposing the dually diagnosed adolescent to increased risk for relapse to substance use and/or other disorders (Kaminer and Bukstein 2008).

Additionally, there is substantial evidence regarding the common phenomenon of diversion of psychotropic medications, such as stimulants by adolescents with attention-deficit/hyperactivity disorder (ADHD) (Wilens et al. 2006). The diversion might be for pleasure or for the drugs' stimulating effects (e.g., to help a student stay awake and study before an examination). Lack of knowledge and training of pediatricians and child and adolescent psychiatrists regarding how to identify and prevent diversion and abuse of stimulants may lead to physicians' poor management of this phenomenon and may further promote negative perceptions of pediatric psychopharmacology (Winters and Kaminer 2008).

Drug-Specific Pharmacotherapy

In a review of the pharmacological treatment of adolescent AOSUDs, Kaminer (1995) referred to four drug-specific pharmacological strategies that are commonly used for the treatment of AOSUDs:

1. Make psychoactive substance administration aversive (e.g., by giving disulfiram to patients with alcohol dependence).
2. Substitute for the psychoactive substance an agonist medication that has a similar mechanism of action as the abused drug or involves administration of a key component of the abused drug via a different route (e.g., methadone or buprenorphine for heroin dependence; nicotine replacement therapy for nicotine dependence) (many agonist medications are longer acting than the abused drug, stabilize an individual who is drug dependent, reduce symptoms of withdrawal, are generally well tolerated, and may attenuate the reinforcing effects of the abused substance in the case of relapse)
3. Block the reinforcing effects of the psychoactive substance by the use of a receptor antagonist (e.g., naltrexone for opioid abuse).
4. Relieve craving and withdrawal (e.g., acamprosate for alcohol; clonidine for heroin dependence).

In this section, we review pharmacotherapy for the abuse and dependence of nicotine, alcohol, opioids, cocaine, and cannabis for youth. Other drugs of abuse (e.g., hallucinogens, inhalants, anabolic steroids) are not discussed in this review due to lack of empirical data on their pharmacotherapy. Also, no scientific information is currently available on the pharmacotherapy of polysubstance abuse in adolescents, or on potential interactions between psychoactive drugs and psychotropic medications (Kaminer et al. 2010).

Detoxification

To reduce or prevent withdrawal symptoms, detoxification from opioids, alcohol, barbiturates, benzodiazepines, and other psychoactive agents needs to follow rigorous procedures in a timely fashion. Few empirical studies are available on detoxification of adolescents with AOSUDs (e.g., Marsch et al. 2005); however, clinical experience suggests that detoxification of adolescents should not be much different from that of adults with AOSUDs. Legal assent is necessary before treating the adolescent.

The majority of adolescents may undergo detoxification in an outpatient setting if they meet the following indications: mild to moderate withdrawal symptoms, no medical or neurological illness, no infection, psychiatric stability, no history of seizures or delirium tremens, reliable support person (for care and transportation), and need to reassess in a period that is not shorter than 24 hours (Myrick and Wright 2008).

Nicotine

Cigarette smoking among youth continues to be a major public health concern. Cigarette smoking during adolescence is associated with immediate health effects, compromised fitness and endurance (Colby and Gwaltney 2007), and poorer mental health, including substance abuse, depression, conduct disorder, and increased suicidality (Alvarado and Breslau 2005). Smoking prevalence varies widely among different racial and ethnic groups of youth (Centers for Disease Control and Prevention 2006). The highest smoking prevalence among adolescents is among Native Americans and Alaskans (23%), followed by non-Hispanic whites (15%), Hispanics (9%), non-Hispanic blacks (6.5%), and Asians (4.3%), among whom the lowest prevalence is among Vietnamese Americans.

Adolescent smokers frequently consider and attempt quitting smoking, yet they seldom succeed on their own. Therefore, they may benefit from a smoking cessation intervention to enhance abstinence. Adolescent developmental issues are a critical consideration when designing teen-specific interventions. The role of peers in teen smoking must be understood within the context of developing social identity (e.g., cigarette use in relation to self-perception, perception of others, and perception of self as viewed by others) rather than exclusively as "peer pressure" (Myers et al. 2000). Therefore, addressing cigarette-related social perceptions and attitudes, particularly among teens who abuse alcohol and other drugs, will be important in effecting behavior change. In addition, evidence for the influence of parental smoking and the perception by youth that smoking is normative indicates a need for providing psychoeducation and involving parents when intervening with adolescent smoking.

Cessation interventions typically incorporate components focused on 1) reducing dependence on nicotine, 2) behavioral habit control strategies, and 3) strategies to assist in the maintenance of cessation. The relevance of these strategies to adolescent smokers is supported by several studies in youth (Myers and Brown 2005).

Based on two large reviews of studies of teen cigarette smoking cessation, Sussman et al. (2006) concluded that teen smoking cessation programming shows promise for the short term. This is especially true for those programs incorporating elements sensitive to "stage of change," or adolescents' level of motivation to change their smoking behavior (Grimshaw and Stanton 2006). Relatively higher quit rates were associated with programs consisting of at least five sessions that included a motivation-enhancement component, cognitive-behavioral techniques, and social-influence approaches. Also, adolescent social factors related to smoking may be more salient and effectively addressed in a group, rather than in individual sessions (Myers and Brown 2005). Nevertheless, further studies are necessary to develop better and more enduring clinically desirable outcomes.

Pharmacotherapy for Nicotine Dependence

The few published randomized, placebo-controlled studies of pharmacotherapy for adolescent smoking cessation have involved nicotine replacement therapy (Hanson et al. 2003; Moolchan et al. 2005), bupropion, or both. Although not approved by the U.S. Food and Drug Administration (FDA) for individuals younger than age 18 years, nicotine replacement therapy and bupropion slow release (SR) have been studied in this population.

Nicotine replacement therapy. The primary pharmacotherapy for nicotine dependence involves the strategy of developing nicotine replacement therapy—that is, a substitute therapy resulting in the reduction of nicotine withdrawal symptoms during smoking cessation. The agents available include nicotine gum, transdermal patch, inhaler, lozenge, and nasal spray. The introduction of these agents in the 1990s doubled smoking cessation success rates

of treatment programs for adults from about 15% (validated long-term abstinence) to about 30% (West 1992). Furthermore, the success of nicotine replacement therapies in treating nicotine dependence and promoting smoking
cessation improved even more when these therapies were integrated with behavioral or cognitive therapy (Lichtenstein and Glasgow 1992).

Some of the nicotine replacement therapy agents have negative side effects.
For example, nicotine gum tastes bad and can cause sore mouth and jaws, because it is hard to chew. The patch may increase nicotine's toxic effects, such as
rapid heart rate and nausea, particularly if the person continues to smoke. It
can irritate the user's skin locally and disrupt sleep if left on for 24 hours. The
nicotine spray can cause irritation to the user's mucous membranes. Moreover,
some people find it difficult to wean themselves off these nicotine replacement
therapies (Lichtenstein and Glasgow 1992). None of these therapies should be
used by active smokers.

Bupropion (Zyban, Wellbutrin).   Bupropion is a dopamine and norepinephrine reuptake inhibitor and nicotine receptor antagonist. Adverse effects include a small risk of seizure, weight loss, and insomnia. One study conducted
with adolescent smokers demonstrated no difference between bupropion SR
and placebo (Killen et al. 2004), and in two other studies there was a short-
lived response rate in smoking cessation of between 5% and 30% (Muramoto
et al. 2007; Upadhyaya et al. 2004). In recent reviews of pharmacotherapy for
adolescent smoking cessation, authors concluded that the evidence for nicotine
replacement therapy for youth is insufficient and that bupropion studies with
and without a combination of nicotine replacement therapy have not demonstrated effectiveness (Colby and Gwaltney 2007; Grimshaw and Stanton 2006);
these authors also explain the limitations of these studies and encourage well-
designed, adequately powered randomized controlled trials with a rigorous
definition of smoking cessation. Colby and Gwaltney (2007) provided practical guidelines for the clinician:

> Referral to appropriate psychosocial intervention is the most appropriate ini-
> tial treatment for adolescent smokers. Although these interventions produce
> relatively low quit rates, they increase the odds of quitting over no treatment.
> While pharmacotherapies may be considered, they should be prescribed only
> after careful consideration of the patient's intention to quit and under close
> monitoring. (p. 2184)

Verduin and Upadhyaya (2007) suggested that teens who are nicotine dependent should be encouraged to reduce tobacco use by one cigarette per day over the 2 weeks before their quit date to minimize withdrawal symptoms. They also recommended the following dosing guidelines if pharmacotherapy is used: When using bupropion SR for adolescents weighing under 90 pounds, the maximum dosage is 150 mg in the morning if tolerated. Patients over 90 pounds can take 150 mg once in the morning for 3–6 days, then 150 mg twice a day for 12 weeks. When using transdermal nicotine replacement therapy for an adolescent who smokes fewer than 10 cigarettes per day, the recommendation is 14 mg/day for 6 weeks, then 7 mg/day for 2 weeks, then discontinue. For youth who smoke 10 or more cigarettes per day, the recommendation is 21 mg/day for 6 weeks, then 14 mg/day for 2 weeks, then 7 mg/day for 2 weeks, then discontinue.

Varenicline (Chantix, Champix). Varenicline is a nicotine receptor partial agonist that acts both as an agonist (i.e., maintaining moderate levels of dopamine to counteract withdrawal symptoms) and as an antagonist (i.e., reducing smoking satisfaction). It has been reported to be more effective than placebo or bupropion in the treatment of smoking dependence (Cahill et al. 2008). Varenicline is available in Canada; however, its side-effect profile, which includes depressed mood, irritability and suicidal thoughts, is under review by the FDA. The use of this agent has not yet been reported in youth smokers.

Combined Behavioral and Pharmacological Treatment

A noteworthy finding is that youth who received motivational interviewing for smoking cessation during psychiatric hospitalization also manifested improvement of substance use outcomes during the 6 months posttreatment (Brown et al. 2009). Therefore, combining integrative treatment for both smoking cessation and substance abuse should be considered.

Alcohol

According to the U.S. school-based Monitoring the Future (2008) study, over 72% of twelfth graders reported ever having used alcohol, and about 55% reported ever having been drunk. Alcohol use, abuse, and dependence continue to be a public health concern. Alcohol is significantly associated with mortality from automobile accidents, homicide, suicide, and drowning. It has also been implicated with other high-risk behaviors, such as physical and sexual violence and unprotected sex (e.g., Sindelar et al. 2004).

Disulfiram, naltrexone, and acamprosate are approved by the FDA for relapse prevention in adults with alcohol use disorders.

Disulfiram (Antabuse)

Disulfiram is an antidipsotropic agent that produces a reaction with ethanol by inhibiting the liver enzyme aldehyde dehydrogenase, which catalyzes the oxidation of aldehyde (the major metabolic product of ethanol to acetate). The resulting accumulation of acetaldehyde is responsible for the aversive symptoms (e.g., nausea, vomiting, flushing of the skin). With experience, these aversive symptoms become paired with ethanol consumption, and thus decrease the likelihood that alcohol will be consumed. The success of this controversial pharmacotherapy has been mediocre at best (Alterman et al. 1991). Voluntary self-administration of disulfiram has been shown to help reduce drinking frequency in a very limited number of controlled clinical trials in adults (American College of Physicians 1989; Schuckit 1985).

Aversive therapy in children and adolescents has always been controversial. It appears unlikely that wide use of aversive pharmacotherapy for adolescents with alcohol dependence will be accepted. A report of two adolescent males with alcohol dependence who were prescribed disulfiram showed a limited short-term benefit with one person only (Myers et al. 1994). A small placebo-controlled double-blind trial with alcohol-dependent adolescents resulted in a significantly superior longer duration of abstinence and higher rates of sustained abstinence from alcohol among the disulfiram users (Niederhofer and Staffen 2003a). Although compliance rates were not reported, gastrointestinal adverse effects were more common with the medication than with the placebo.

Disulfiram should be considered for youth only after a thorough consideration of previous treatment attempts. There are two potential concerns with disulfiram use with adolescents: 1) the unpleasant aversive reactions and 2) the uncommon yet problematic self-abusive behavior of combining disulfiram with alcohol consumption. Therefore, determining eligibility for the use of disulfiram should include establishing a patient's physical-medical status, intellectual competency, insightfulness, and high motivation for recovery. Finally, adolescents should be closely monitored when prescribed disulfiram.

Naltrexone (Revia) and Nalmefene (Revex)

Research regarding pharmacotherapy for alcoholism generated interest in the impact of alcohol consumption on opioid receptors and the potential utility of an opioid antagonist such as naltrexone for blocking the reinforcing properties of alcohol. A large meta-analysis of randomized controlled studies revealed that naltrexone is safe and effective in reducing drinking frequency, rates of relapse, levels of craving, and number of drinks, both as a stand-alone treatment (Srisurapanont and Jarusuraisin 2005) and with adjunctive psychotherapy in the COMBINE trial (which evaluated medication and behavioral therapies for the treatment of alcohol dependence; Anton et al. 2006). Not all studies of naltrexone have revealed positive results, suggesting there may be subtypes of individuals who are more likely to respond to naltrexone. The drug may be preferred by those whose reward craving can be blocked by exogenous opioids, thereby diminishing the pleasant effects of alcohol consumption (Myrick and Wright 2008). In a case report, Wold and Kaminer (1997) reported on the successful short-term treatment of an alcohol-dependent adolescent with oral naltrexone 50 mg/day. A small open-label trial of naltrexone in adolescents found that it was well tolerated and reduced craving and drinking among adolescents who were dependent on alcohol (Deas et al. 2005).

Nalmefene is an opioid antagonist that is structurally similar to naltrexone but with a number of potential pharmacological advantages, including its longer half-life and greater oral bioavailability. To our knowledge, nalmefene has not been systematically studied in the treatment of alcohol use disorders among adolescents.

Acamprosate (Campral)

Acamprosate is a compound that is structurally similar to gamma-aminobutyric acid (GABA), an inhibitory neurotransmitter in the central nervous system, with a diversity of actions in several neurotransmitter systems affected by chronic ethanol intake. Acamprosate has been shown to interfere with transmission of excitatory amino acids, primarily glutamate, and to positively modulate GABA transport in different brain areas. Two meta-analyses of placebo-controlled studies showed statistically significant differences in cumulative abstinence in alcohol-dependent individuals who had stopped drinking for patients who received acamprosate versus those receiving placebo (Bouza et al. 2004; Mann et al. 2004). The COMBINE study did not show a superior effect of naltrexone and acamprosate over naltrexone alone (Anton et al. 2006). Niederhofer and Staffen (2003b) reported that acamprosate was associated with a significantly longer duration of abstinence compared with placebo in adolescents with alcohol dependence.

Benzodiazepines

The treatment of choice for alcohol withdrawal symptoms is benzodiazepines. (See Mayo-Smith 1997 for evidence-based guidelines and a meta-analysis.) Similar guidelines apply for youth.

Opioids

In the United States in 2008, about 1.3% of surveyed twelfth graders reported having used heroin in their lifetime. Perhaps most alarming, the nonmedical use of prescription opioids among adolescents has increased markedly in recent years. About 5% of twelfth-graders reported nonmedical use of OxyContin, and about 10% of this age group reported nonmedical use of Vicodin (Monitoring the Future 2008). Opioid use among adolescents has been associated with high rates of academic problems (e.g., skipping school, being expelled or suspended) and high rates of other substance use. Additionally, opioid abuse can lead to serious health complications, including emergency department visits and death, especially when opioids are consumed with other central nervous system depressants, such as alcohol and benzodiazepines.

Four maintenance pharmacotherapies are currently used in the United States for treatment of opioid abuse: methadone, naltrexone, L-α-acetylmethadol (LAAM), and buprenorphine. LAAM and buprenorphine address some limitations of methadone and naltrexone, including illicit diversion of take-home methadone doses, difficulties with detoxification from methadone maintenance to a drug-free state, and poor compliance of patients taking naltrexone (Kosten and McCance 1996).

Methadone

Methadone maintenance is a common form of opioid substitution therapy and is usually reserved for the treatment of adult heroin addicts. The desired response from methadone maintenance is threefold: 1) to prevent the onset of opioid abstinence syndrome, 2) to eliminate drug hunger or craving, and 3) to block the euphoric effects of any illicitly self-administered opioids. As a general rule, patients who have not been dependent on opioids for at least 1 year or who have not previously made any attempt at withdrawal are not appropriate candidates for prolonged opioid maintenance (Jaffe 1986).

Methadone maintenance should not rely on methadone administration alone, even in adequate daily dosage, as a "magic bullet" for curing heroin addiction. McLellan et al. (1993) reported that patients in a methadone maintenance program who also received a psychosocial services package fared better than two other groups of patients who received either counseling in addition to methadone maintenance or only methadone maintenance, underscoring the importance of combined pharmacological and psychosocial treatment.

No person under age 18 years may be admitted to a methadone maintenance treatment program in the United States unless an authorized adult signs an official consent form (FDA Form 2635). To be eligible for methadone maintenance, patients under age 18 are required to have two documented attempts at short-term detoxification or drug-free treatment. A 1-week waiting list period is required after a detoxification attempt. However, before an attempt is repeated, the program physician has to document in the minor's record that the patient continues to be or is again physiologically dependent on narcotic drugs (Parrino 1992). Methadone maintenance, and not opioid detoxification, is the treatment of choice for pregnant adolescents who abuse heroin. This daily pharmacotherapy decreases the possibility of contracting HIV infection from a contaminated needle, due to reduced injection drug use. It also ensures a relatively stable plasma level of methadone, which reduces the fetus's risk of developing intrauterine distress, as compared to heroin, which has a short half-life and causes abrupt changes in plasma level (Finnegan and Kandall 1992).

Few research studies have examined the effectiveness and safety of methadone with opioid-dependent adolescents. An early study by Sells and Simpson (1979) examined outcomes from four treatment modalities for youth 19 years and younger who used heroin and other opioids, as part of the Drug Abuse Reporting Program, a database of patients in a variety of U.S. substance abuse treatment programs. The four treatment modalities to which youth were not randomly assigned were methadone maintenance, outpatient drug-free treatment, therapeutic communities, and medication-assisted withdrawal (termed "detoxification"). Results indicated that youth who used opiates daily had significantly greater retention in methadone maintenance treatment. Additionally, all treatment modalities were associated with a reduction in opiate use, and time in treatment was the strongest significant positive predictor of reduced opiate use, despite treatment modality. If patients who were not receiving methadone maintenance remained in treatment at least 6 months, their outcomes were comparable to those of patients who received methadone maintenance treatment.

DeAngelis and Lehmann (1973) reported an 18-month abstinence rate of 35% for subjects ages 15–24 following methadone detoxification with dosages of 10–60 mg/day.

Crome et al. (1998) evaluated outcomes for heroin-dependent adolescents who entered methadone maintenance treatment at a community-based treatment program in the United Kingdom during a 2-year period. Patients were provided with mean methadone dosages of 28.3 mg/day (range=15–50) and weekly counseling and urinary drug tests. Limited results are available; however, retention in treatment was reported to be 80%. Also, by the end of the evaluation window, approximately 50% were reportedly either drug free or in methadone reduction programs, 30% had shown no improvement, and about 20% were lost to contact.

Finally, Kellogg and colleagues (2006) reported 48% retention rates at 1 year among opioid-dependent adolescents and young adults (ages 15–23 years) who were admitted to a community-based methadone maintenance treatment program and significant reductions in opioid use among those retained for a 1-year period.

Levo-alpha-acetylmethadol

LAAM is quite similar to methadone in its pharmacological actions, and it has been approved by the FDA for treatment of opioid dependence. It is converted into active metabolites that have longer biological half-lives than methadone. Opioid withdrawal symptoms are not experienced for 72–96 hours after the last oral dose; therefore, LAAM needs to be given only three times per week. LAAM has been shown to have equivalent effects to methadone in terms of suppressing illicit opioid abuse and encouraging a more productive lifestyle (Jaffe 1986). LAAM has been withdrawn from the U.S. market by its manufacturer, largely in light of a postmarketing surveillance report of its association with a prolonged QT interval, as measured by electrocardiogram readings, and several reports of torsades de pointes, a life-threatening heart ventricular arrhythmia (Kreek and Vocci 2002).

Buprenorphine (Subutex) and Buprenorphine-Naloxone (Suboxone)
Currently, no effective standard of care exists for the treatment of opioid-
dependent adolescents; however, research and clinical experience have highlighted the importance of providing pharmacotherapy as part of substance
abuse treatment to this population. Agonist (methadone) or partial agonist
(sublingual buprenorphine) medications have been shown to produce the best
treatment outcomes, and buprenorphine may be especially appealing for treating this young population due to its safety profile. Buprenorphine is a partial
opioid agonist-antagonist, and also is used as an analgesic due to its ability to
produce morphine-like effects at low dosages. This agent relieves opiate withdrawal, diminishes craving, and does not produce euphoria in opioid-dependent
individuals. It is more difficult to overdose on buprenorphine than on methadone because of the former's opioid antagonist effects in high dosages (Rosen
and Kosten 1991).

Additionally, certified physicians more readily provide buprenorphine than
methadone treatment to eligible youth in the United States (those age 16 years
or older), because youth under age 18 years may only be placed in maintenance
treatment with methadone after they have two unsuccessful attempts at short-
term detoxification or drug-free treatment (Department of Health and Human
Services 2001). Additionally, although clonidine (an α_2-adrenergic agonist) appears to be safe in the medication-assisted withdrawal of opioid-dependent
adolescents, it has been shown to be less efficacious relative to opioid pharmacotherapy in promoting treatment retention and opioid abstinence, and in managing opioid withdrawal (Kellogg et al. 2006; Marsch et al. 2005; Woody et al.
2008).

To date, both clinical and research experience providing buprenorphine to
opioid-dependent youth suggest that slower medication-assisted withdrawal
(>30 days) may produce better outcomes than faster withdrawal regimens
(Minozzi et al. 2009a, 2009b; Woody et al. 2008), although the conditions under which buprenorphine maintenance treatment for youth (as opposed to a
taper) is warranted remain unclear. As in the treatment of opioid-dependent
adults, initial doses of buprenorphine provided to opioid-dependent youth
have been provided, in research to date, when youth are in early stages of withdrawal (a minimum of 6–12 hours after their last consumption of a short-acting
opioid). Initial doses have generally been between 2 and 8 mg, with additional

medication provided as clinically warranted depending on the extent to which withdrawal symptoms are controlled. For example, in one study with opioid-dependent adolescents and young adults, an initial 2-mg dose of buprenorphine (Suboxone, a 4:1 combination of buprenorphine and naloxone) was provided on the day of buprenorphine induction, with an additional dose of 2–6 mg provided 1.5–2 hours later as appropriate (based on standardized observed and self-reported withdrawal measures) (Woody et al. 2008). In a controlled trial with opioid-dependent adolescents, day 1 starting dosages of 6 or 8 mg of buprenorphine (Subutex) were provided to youth (Marsch et al. 2005). To our knowledge, a maximum daily dosage of 24 mg of buprenorphine has been provided to opioid-dependent youth during buprenorphine treatment (Woody et al. 2008), but low-moderate daily dosages (e.g., 8–16 mg) appear efficacious for many opioid-dependent youth, especially for youth with lower levels of dependence (Marsch and Solhkhah 2008; Marsch et al. 2005).

Optimal treatment outcomes for opioid-dependent youth are generally achieved when pharmacotherapy is provided along with psychosocial treatment. Importantly, combined behavioral and buprenorphine treatment appears safe and efficacious for both adolescents dependent on heroin and youth dependent on prescription opioids (Motamed et al. 2008). Additionally, both male and female youth have been shown to experience positive treatment outcomes from buprenorphine treatment (Solhkhah et al. 2007). Moreover, the opioid agonist naltrexone may play a useful role in preventing relapse to opioid use after a medication-assisted withdrawal (Marsch et al. 2005) and in preventing opioid overdose after an adolescent is no longer dependent (Hulse and Tait 2003).

As with all types of substance abuse treatment for youth, providing evidence-based treatment to opioid-dependent adolescents early in their drug involvement may hold great promise for reducing their likelihood of continued and escalating substance involvement. Future research needs include more systematic evaluations of optimal durations and medication dosing regimens for opioid-dependent youth and models of care for delivering such treatment.

Finally, some heroin-dependent individuals also abuse cocaine, which "speeds" the rush from heroin injected alone (i.e., a speed ball). Methadone maintenance treatment has not been shown to reduce cocaine abuse for many patients. Some limited evidence suggests that buprenorphine may reduce cocaine use in opiate-dependent individuals (Kosten et al. 1989).

Cocaine

Over 7% of twelfth graders in the United States reported having used cocaine, and about 3% reported having used crack (Monitoring the Future 2008). Research has implicated the neurotransmitter dopamine as the leading catecholamine responsible for the specific reinforcing effects of cocaine and the craving/withdrawal symptoms among cocaine users (Kosten 1990). Neuroleptics were hypothesized to block the cocaine-induced euphoria initiated by mesolimbic and mesocortical neuroanatomical reward pathways, leading to attenuation of cocaine self-administration by animals (Gawin et al. 1989). However, neuroleptics are known to produce anhedonia and considerable neurological and metabolic side effects, and compliance has been problematic.

The pharmacological treatment strategy for cocaine abuse has been focused mainly on the reduction or elimination of cocaine abstinence–related craving. This effort is essential to improve relapse prevention rates by reducing attrition from treatment and to enable the introduction of additional therapeutic interventions.

Based on the theory that chronic stimulant use results in depletion of dopamine and reduction in dopaminergic activity, it has been hypothesized that craving for cocaine would be reduced by increasing dopaminergic stimulation (Meyer 1992). Sparse evidence is available to support the depletion theory. However, the following direct and indirect dopaminergic agents have shown some efficacy in open trials in adults: levodopa, carbidopa, bromocriptine, amantadine, methylphenidate, and mazindol (Kosten et al. 2008).

Another theory that appears to have neurobiological support suggests that craving is mediated by supersensitivity of presynaptic inhibiting dopaminergic autoreceptors. The tricyclic antidepressant desipramine was found to desensitize these receptors and facilitate cocaine abstinence by attenuating craving for 7–14 days from the onset of therapy. Kosten et al. (1992) presented 6-month follow-up data on 43 of the original 72 patients. They reported that self-reported cocaine abstinence during the 6-month period was significantly greater in patients treated with desipramine (44%) than in those treated with lithium (19%) or placebo (27%).

Only one detailed case study has supported the use of desipramine for treatment of cocaine use by an adolescent (Kaminer 1992). A 6-month follow-up confirmed continued abstinence. In this case, desipramine treatment (200 mg/

day, plasma level stabilized around 130 µg/L) was instituted for the treatment of three psychiatric disorders simultaneously (i.e., cocaine dependence, major depressive disorder, and ADHD), thus preventing polypharmacy.

Other research has found that the intensity of cocaine craving is independent of depression during the first week of abstinence among newly abstinent chronic cocaine abusers (Ho et al. 1991). This finding suggests that withdrawal-related dysphoria during the first week of abstinence will not respond to the antidepressant properties of desipramine, and may be alleviated earlier than the depressive symptomatology of a patient diagnosed with cocaine dependence and major depressive disorder. This may also differentiate a cocaine-dependent adolescent from a dually diagnosed one. The results from a single case study, however, should be viewed with caution until such findings are replicated in other studies. Two other cases in which cocaine-dependent adolescents were treated with desipramine had less positive outcomes (Kaminer 1994). One adolescent's clinical symptoms responded favorably to desipramine for about 30 days, at which time the patient dropped out of treatment. The second adolescent, who had abused amitriptyline prior to treatment, developed postural hypotension following the introduction of desipramine. As a result, the medication was discontinued.

Dopamine system dysregulation is probably not the only mechanism underlying cocaine addiction. The serotonin system has been implicated as well, although small open-label studies of serotonergic agents showed conflicting results in the treatment of cocaine abuse (Kosten and McCance 1996).

Another development in the pharmacological treatment of cocaine dependence is the use of carbamazepine. The theoretical rationale for this intervention is that the agent blocks cocaine-induced kindling and increases dopamine concentration. However, double-blind trials using carbamazepine have not supported this theory.

Stimulants have proven useful for the treatment of children and adolescents diagnosed with ADHD. The pharmacokinetic similarities between an illegal stimulant such as cocaine and therapeutic stimulants such as methylphenidate, magnesium pemoline, and dextroamphetamine have led to the assumption that they might be useful for the treatment of cocaine abuse. Modafinil, a novel stimulant, provided a significant reduction in cocaine use in a double-blind, placebo-controlled study (Dackis et al. 2005).

Various medications and compounds with different pharmaceutical mechanisms (e.g., GABAergic agents, disulfiram, cocaine antagonists, opiate antagonists) have been examined in research studies for cocaine dependence, with varying success. These findings are beyond the scope of this review, because studies involving adolescents have not been reported. For a comprehensive review, readers are referred to Kosten et al. (2008). No pharmacotherapies have yet been approved by the FDA for the treatment of stimulant dependence in the United States.

Marijuana

About 42% of twelfth graders reported having tried marijuana (Monitoring the Future 2008). Cannabis withdrawal syndrome is not included in the *Diagnostic and Statistical Manual of Mental Disorders*, 4th Edition, Text Revision (DSM-IV-TR; American Psychiatric Association 2000); however, strong consideration for its inclusion in the next revision of DSM is justified due to growing evidence that cannabis withdrawal syndrome is a valid syndrome that appears similar to tobacco withdrawal in magnitude and severity (Budney et al. 2004). Cannabis withdrawal syndrome has also been described in youth (Milin et al. 2008).

Quitting marijuana use for individuals who are dependent is no easier than trying to stop using other substances. Outcomes of treatment using psychosocial interventions indicate that achieving abstinence is difficult and relapse is common. Recently, investigators have started to study the neurobiological properties of cannabis in an effort to examine potential pharmacotherapy. According to reviews of recent and ongoing pharmacotherapy studies, the focus of research is on medications that alleviate symptoms of cannabis withdrawal or those that directly affect endogenous cannabinoid receptor function (Vandrey and Hanes 2009). Oral medications (tetrahydrocannabinol [THC]) that target the cannabinoid B1 receptor may hold promise for treating cannabis dependence, reducing drug seeking, and attenuating withdrawal symptoms. A recent double-blind study in a small cohort of older adolescents (ages 16–21) indicated that oral THC was well tolerated (Gray et al. 2008). However, controlled clinical trials are needed to support clinical use of these medications.

Future Directions and Conclusion

Providing pharmacotherapy to youth with AOSUDs has historically been controversial, and limited research has been conducted to date evaluating the safety and effectiveness of pharmacotherapy for AOSUD. Additional research is undoubtedly needed to provide clinical guidance on the safe and effective use of medications with youth who have AOSUDs.

Eichelman (1988) described four important principles for the pharmacological treatment of adults: 1) treat the primary illness, 2) use the most benign interventions when treating empirically, 3) have some quantifiable means of assessing efficacy, and 4) institute drug trials systematically. These principles are arguably even more important with younger patients. Ethical principles must govern clinical research and treatment in adolescent AOSUDs and comorbid psychiatric disorders (Munir and Earls 1992). Improved communication with and education of the public, parents, and patients regarding the nature of AOSUD and the efficacy of pharmacotherapy are necessary. Implementation of and training in AOSUD screening, and treatment curricula for physicians who work primarily with youth, are crucial (Winters and Kaminer 2008).

Future research must include the systematic study of new therapeutic agents. For example, recent immunological research has focused on the development of vaccines to treat abuse of drugs such as cocaine, nicotine, phencyclidine (PCP), and methamphetamine (Volkow 2008). Those vaccines stimulate the immune system to produce antibodies that will attach to drug molecules, forming a compound molecule that is too big to cross the blood-brain barrier easily. By slowing drugs' entry into the brain, and preventing or reducing binding to receptors in the brain, the vaccines reduce or prevent the euphoria that promotes addiction.

The continued development of pharmacotherapy for the treatment of adolescents with AOSUDs is warranted, and may ultimately improve treatment options and outcomes for substance-abusing teens. However, pharmacotherapy alone cannot deal with polysubstance abuse and the associated problems in various life domains experienced by the adolescent with AOSUD during the recovery process. Indeed, McLellan et al. (1993) confirmed an additive effect of integrated pharmacotherapy and psychosocial interventions. Additionally, Carroll (1997) advocated for the concomitant provision of some form of psychosocial treatment with pharmacotherapy in the treatment of AOSUDs.

She argued that this approach will foster replicability of findings and address several common problems in clinical trials (e.g., attrition, medication noncompliance, reduction of error variance, ethical issues associated with placebo controls). "Careful selection and standardization of the psychosocial context in which medications are delivered will improve the validity, precision, and power of pharmacotherapy efficacy research" (Carroll 1997, p. 923). Increasing understanding of how to optimize treatment outcomes with youth using combinations of behavioral and pharmacological treatments is a clinically important endeavor.

Key Clinical Concepts

- The main drug-specific pharmacological strategies commonly used for the treatment of adolescent alcohol and other substance use disorders are using drug substitution, blocking reinforcing effects, relieving craving and withdrawal, and making drug administration aversive.

- Technically, detoxification for adolescents is similar to that of adults. However, legal assent is necessary.

- Treatment of cigarette smoking improves the likelihood of achieving positive outcome while treating a concomitant AOSOD.

- Both methadone and buprenorphine have been shown to have clinical utility for opioid-dependent youth. However, buprenorphine has a greater safety profile and less restrictive treatment regulations.

- Interactions between psychotropic medications and drugs have not been found to result in adverse effects.

References

Alterman AI, O'Brien CP, McLellan AT: Differential therapeutics for substance abuse, in Clinical Textbook of Addictive Disorders. Edited by Frances RJ, Miller SI. New York, Guilford, 1991, pp 369–390

Alvarado GF, Breslau N: Smoking and young people's mental health. Curr Opin Psychiatry 18:397–400, 2005

American College of Physicians: Disulfiram treatment of alcoholism. Ann Intern Med 111:943–945, 1989

American Psychiatric Association: Diagnostic and Statistical Manual of Mental Disorders, 4th Edition, Text Revision. Washington, DC, American Psychiatric Association, 2000

Anton RF, O'Malley SS, Ciraulo DA, et al: Combined pharmacotherapies and behavioral interventions for alcohol dependence: the COMBINE study: a randomized controlled trial. JAMA 295:2003–2017, 2006

Biederman J: New developments in pediatric psychopharmacology. J Am Acad Child Adolesc Psychiatry 31:14–15, 1992

Bouza C, Angeles M, Munoz A, et al: Efficacy and safety of naltrexone and acamprosate in the treatment of alcohol dependence: a systematic review. Addiction 99:811–828, 2004

Brown RA, Strong DR, Abrantes AM, et al: Effects on substance use outcomes in adolescents receiving motivational interviewing for smoking cessation during psychiatric hospitalization. Addict Behav 34:887–891, 2009

Budney AJ, Hughes JR, Moore BA, et al: Review of the validity and significance of cannabis withdrawal syndrome. Am J Psychiatry 161:1967–1977, 2004

Cahill K, Stead LF, Lancaster T: Nicotine receptor partial agonists for smoking cessation. Cochrane Database Syst Rev CD006103, 2008

Carroll KM: Manual-guided psychosocial treatment: a new virtual requirement for pharmacotherapy trials? Arch Gen Psychiatry 54:923–928, 1997

Centers for Disease Control and Prevention: Racial/ethnic differences among youths in cigarette smoking and susceptibility to start smoking—United States, 2002–2004. MMWR Morb Mortal Wkly Rep 55:1275–1277, 2006

Colby SM, Gwaltney CJ: Pharmacotherapy for adolescent smoking cessation. JAMA 298:2182–2184, 2007

Crome IB, Christian J, Green C: Tip of the national iceberg? Profile of adolescent patients prescribed methadone in an innovative community drug service. Drugs: Education, Prevention and Policy 5:195–197, 1998

Dackis C, Lynch K, Yu E: Modafinil and cocaine: a double-blind placebo-controlled drug interaction study. Drug Alcohol Depend 30:205–211, 2005

DeAngelis GG, Lehmann WX: Adolescents and short term, low dose methadone maintenance. Int J Addict 8:853–863, 1973

Deas D, May MP, Randall C, et al: Naltrexone treatment of adolescent alcoholics: an open-label pilot study. J Child Adolesc Psychopharmacol 15:723–728, 2005

Department of Health and Human Services, Substance Abuse and Mental Health Services Administration: Part II: Opioid Drugs in Maintenance and Detoxification Treatment of Opiate Addiction: Final Rule. 21 CFR Part 291 and 42 CFR Part 8. Federal Register, Vol 66, No 11, January 17, 2009. Available at: http://www.dpt.samhsa.gov/pdf/regs.pdf. Accessed June 14, 2010.

Eichelman B: Toward a rational pharmacotherapy for aggressive and violent behavior. Hosp Community Psychiatry 39:31–39, 1988

Finnegan LP, Kandall SR: Maternal and neonatal effects of alcohol and drugs, in Substance Abuse: A Comprehensive Textbook. Edited by Lowinson JH, Ruiz P, Millman RB, et al. Baltimore, MD, Williams & Wilkins, 1992, pp 628–656

Gawin FH, Allen D, Humblestone B: Outpatient treatment of "crack" cocaine smoking with flupenthixol decanoate: a preliminary report. Arch Gen Psychiatry 46:322–325, 1989

Gibbons R, Mann JJ: Proper studies of selective serotonin reuptake inhibitors are needed for youth with depression. CMAJ 180:270–271, 2009

Gray KM, Hart CL, Christie DK, et al: Tolerability and effects of oral delta 9-tetrahydrocannabinol in older adolescents with marijuana use disorders. Pharmacol Biochem Behav 91:67–70, 2008

Grimshaw GM, Stanton A: Tobacco cessation interventions for young people. Cochrane Database Syst Rev CD003289, 2006

Hanson K, Allen S, Jensen S, et al: Treatment of adolescent smokers with the nicotine patch. Nicotine Tob Res 5:515–526, 2003

Ho A, Cambor R, Bodner G: Intensity of craving is independent of depression in newly abstinent chronic cocaine abusers. Presented at the annual scientific meeting of the Committee on Problems of Drug Dependence, Palm Beach, FL, 1991

Hoffmann NG, Sonis WA, Halikas JA: Issues in the evaluation of chemical dependency treatment programs for adolescents. Pediatr Clin North Am 34:449–459, 1987

Hulse GK, Tait RJ: A pilot study to assess the impact of naltrexone implant on accidental opiate overdose in "high-risk" adolescent heroin users. Addict Biol 8:337–342, 2003

Jaffe JH: Opioids, in Psychiatry Update: The American Psychiatric Association Annual Review, Vol 5. Edited by Frances AJ, Hales RE. Washington, DC, American Psychiatric Press, 1986, pp 137–159

Kaminer Y: Desipramine facilitation of cocaine abstinence in an adolescent. J Am Acad Child Adolesc Psychiatry 31:312–317, 1992

Kaminer Y: Tricyclic antidepressants: therapeutic use for cocaine craving and potential for abuse (letter). J Am Acad Child Adolesc Psychiatry 33:592, 1994

Kaminer Y: Issues in the pharmacological treatment of adolescent substance abuse. J Child Adolesc Psychopharmacol 5:93–106, 1995

Kaminer Y, Bukstein O (eds): Adolescent Substance Abuse: Psychiatric Comorbidity and High-Risk Behaviors. New York, Routledge/Taylor & Francis, 2008

Kaminer Y, Goldberg P, Connor D: Psychotropic medications and substances of abuse interactions in youth. Subst Abus 31:53–57, 2010

Kellogg S, Melia D, Khuri E, et al: Adolescent and young adult heroin patients: drug use and success in methadone maintenance treatment. J Addict Dis 25:15–25, 2006

Killen JD, Robinson TN, Ammerman S, et al: Randomized clinical trial of the efficacy of bupropion combined with nicotine patch in the treatment of adolescent smokers. J Consult Clin Psychol 72:729–735, 2004

Kosten TR: Neurobiology of abused drugs: opioids and stimulants. J Nerv Ment Dis 178:217–227, 1990

Kosten TR, McCance E: A review of pharmacotherapies for substance abuse. Am J Addict 5:58–65, 1996

Kosten TR, Kleber HD, Morgan C: Treatment of cocaine abuse with buprenorphine. Biol Psychiatry 26:637–639, 1989

Kosten TR, Gawin FH, Kosten TA, et al: Six-month follow-up of short-term pharmacotherapy for cocaine dependence. Am J Addict 1:40–49, 1992

Kosten TR, Sofuoglu M, Gardner TJ: Clinical management: cocaine, in The American Psychiatric Publishing Textbook of Substance Abuse Treatment, 4th Edition. Edited by Galanter M, Kleber HD. Washington, DC, American Psychiatric Publishing, 2008, pp 157–168

Kreek MJ, Vocci FJ: History and current status of opioid maintenance treatments: blending conference session. J Subst Abuse Treat 23:93–105, 2002

Lichtenstein E, Glasgow RE: Smoking cessation: what have we learned over the past decade? J Consult Clin Psychol 60:518–527, 1992

Mann K, Lehert P, Morgan MY: The efficacy of acamprosate in the maintenance of abstinence in alcohol-dependent individuals: results of a meta-analysis. Alcohol Clin Exp Res 28:51–63, 2004

Marsch LA, Solhkhah R: Evidence-based behavioral and pharmacological treatment for opioid-dependent adolescents. Paper presented at the annual meeting of the American Psychiatric Association, Washington, DC, May 3–8, 2008

Marsch LA, Bickel WK, Badger GJ, et al: Comparison of pharmacological treatments for opioid-dependent adolescents: a randomized controlled trial. Arch Gen Psychiatry 62:1157–1164, 2005

Mayo-Smith MF: Pharmacological management of alcohol withdrawal: a meta-analysis and evidence-based practice guideline. American Society of Addiction Medicine Working Group on Pharmacological Management of Alcohol Withdrawal. JAMA 278:144–151, 1997

McLellan AT, Arndt IO, Metzger DS, et al: The effects of psychosocial services in substance abuse treatment. JAMA 269:1953–1959, 1993

Meyer RE: New pharmacotherapies for cocaine dependence...revisited. Arch Gen Psychiatry 49:900–904, 1992

Milin R, Manion I, Dare G, et al: Prospective assessment of cannabis withdrawal in adolescents with cannabis dependence: a pilot study. J Am Acad Child Adolesc Psychiatry 47:174–178, 2008

Minozzi S, Amato L, Davoli M: Detoxification treatments for opiate dependent adolescents. Cochrane Database Syst Rev CD006749, 2009a

Minozzi S, Amato L, Davoli M: Maintenance treatments for opiate dependent adolescents. Cochrane Database Syst Rev CD007210, 2009b

Monitoring the Future, 2008 survey results: Available online at: http://www.monitoringthefuture.org, 2008

Moolchan ET, Robinson ML, Ernst M, et al: Safety and efficacy of the nicotine patch and gum for the treatment of adolescent tobacco addiction. Pediatrics 115:407–414, 2005

Motamed M, Marsch LA, Solhkhah R, et al: Differences in treatment outcomes between prescription opioid–dependent and heroin-dependent adolescents. J Addict Med 2:158–164, 2008

Munir K, Earls F: Ethical principles governing research in child and adolescent psychiatry. J Am Acad Child Adolesc Psychiatry 31:408–414, 1992

Muramoto ML, Leischow SJ, Sherrill D, et al: Randomized, double-blind, placebo-controlled trial of 2 dosages of sustained-release bupropion for adolescent smoking cessation. Arch Pediatr Adolesc Med 161:1068–1074, 2007

Myers MG, Brown SA: A controlled study of a cigarette smoking cessation intervention for adolescents in substance abuse treatment. Psychol Addict Behav 19:230–233, 2005

Myers MG, Brown SA, Kelly JF: A smoking intervention for substance abusing adolescents: outcomes, predictors of cessation attempts, and post-treatment substance use. J Child Adolesc Subst Abuse 9:77–91, 2000

Myers WC, Donahue JE, Goldstein MR: Disulfiram for alcohol use disorders in adolescents. J Am Acad Child Adolesc Psychiatry 33:484–489, 1994

Myrick H, Wright T: Clinical management of alcohol abuse and dependence, in The American Psychiatric Publishing Textbook of Substance Abuse Treatment, 4th Edition. Edited by Galanter M, Kleber HD. Washington, DC, American Psychiatric Publishing, 2008, pp 129–142

Niederhofer H, Staffen W: Acamprosate and its efficacy in treating alcohol dependent adolescents. Eur Child Adolesc Psychiatry 12:144–148, 2003a

Niederhofer H, Staffen W: Comparison of disulfiram and placebo in treatment of alcohol dependence of adolescents. Drug Alcohol Rev 22:295–297, 2003b

Parrino MW: State Methadone Maintenance Treatment Guidelines. Rockville, MD, U.S. Department of Health and Human Services, 1992

Rosen MI, Kosten TR: Buprenorphine: beyond methadone? Hosp Community Psychiatry 42:347–349, 1991

Schuckit MA: A one-year follow-up of men alcoholics given disulfiram. J Stud Alcohol 46:191–195, 1985

Sells SB, Simpson DD: Evaluation of treatment outcome for youths in the Drug Abuse Reporting Program (DARP): a follow-up study, in Youth Drug Abuse: Problems, Issues and Treatment. Edited by Beschner GM, Friedman AS. Lanham, MD, Lexington Books, 1979, pp 571–622

Sindelar HA, Barnett NP, Spirito A: Adolescent alcohol use and injury: a summary and critical review of the literature. Minerva Pediatr 56:291–309, 2004

Solhkhah R, Marsch LA, Waldbaum M, et al: Gender differences in treatment outcome among opioid-dependent adolescents. Poster presented at the third annual Joint Meeting on Adolescent Treatment Effectiveness. Washington, DC, 2007

Srisurapanont M, Jarusuraisin N: Opioid antagonists for alcohol dependence. Cochrane Database Syst Rev CD001867, 2005

Sussman S, Sun P, Dent CW: A meta-analysis of teen cigarette smoking cessation. Health Psychol 25:549–557, 2006

Upadhyaya HP, Brady KT, Wang W: Bupropion SR in adolescents with comorbid ADHD and nicotine dependence: a pilot study. J Am Acad Child Adolesc Psychiatry 43:199–205, 2004

Vandrey R, Hanes M: Pharmacotherapy for cannabis dependence: how close are we? CNS Drugs 23:543–553, 2009

Verduin M, Upadhyaya H: Beating nicotine: medication algorithm helps teens quit. Curr Psychiatry Rep 7:65–74, 2007

Vitiello B, Bhatara VS, Jensen PS: Current knowledge and unmet needs in pediatric psychopharmacology. J Am Acad Child Adolesc Psychiatry 38:501–502, 1999

Volkow ND: New vaccines are being developed against addiction and relapse. NIDA Notes, September 2008, p 2

Waxmonsky JG, Wilens TE: Pharmacotherapy of adolescent substance use disorders: a review of the literature. J Child Adolesc Psychopharmacol 15:810–825, 2005

West R: The 'nicotine replacement paradox' in smoking cessation: how does nicotine gum really work? Br J Addict 87:165–167, 1992

Wilens TE, Gignac M, Swezey A, et al: Characteristics of adolescents and young adults with ADHD who divert or misuse their prescribed medications. J Am Acad Child Adolesc Psychiatry 45:408–414, 2006

Winters KC, Kaminer Y: Screening and assessing adolescent substance use disorders in clinical populations. J Am Acad Child Adolesc Psychiatry 47:740–744, 2008

Wold M, Kaminer Y: Naltrexone for alcohol abuse. J Am Acad Child Adolesc Psychiatry 36:6–7, 1997

Woody GE, Poole SA, Subramaniam G, et al: Extended vs. short-term buprenorphine-naloxone for treatment of opioid-addicted youth: a randomized trial. JAMA 300:2003–2011, 2008

Club Drug, Prescription Drug, and Over-the-Counter Medication Abuse

Description, Diagnosis, and Intervention

Christian Hopfer, M.D.

Abuse of club drugs, prescription medicines, and over-the-counter (OTC) medications is a growing problem among adolescents and young adults. The use of so-called club drugs became popular during the 1990s. The latest trend in drug abuse by adolescents is "pharming"—that is, the nonmedical use of prescription and OTC cough and cold medicines. The steady growth in pharming since 2002 (Johnston et al. 2008) contrasts with the decline seen in the rate of

Support from the national Institute on Drug Abuse to develop the manuscript of this chapter was received from NIDA grants 5R01DA021913 abd 5P60DA011015.

use of any illicit drug. Currently, only alcohol, tobacco, and cannabis have higher rates of use by adolescents than prescription drugs (Schepis and Krishnan-Sarin 2009). Pharming is associated with an increased risk of polysubstance abuse with alcohol and other drugs, which can cause additional morbidity and potential substance use disorders (Levine 2007).

In this chapter I address the abuse of club drugs, prescription medications, and OTC medications. The following drugs and associated treatment-related issues are reviewed: MDMA (3,4-methylenedioxymethamphetamine), commonly known as "ecstasy"; GHB (gamma-hydroxybutyrate); ketamine; methamphetamine; LSD (lysergic acid diethylamide); opiates such as hydrocodone; benzodiazepines; and dextromethorphan (*d*-3-methoxy-*N*-methylmorphinan), which is an active ingredient in cough suppressants and cold medicines.

Club Drugs

Overview

During the 1990s, epidemiological surveys detected the increased use of a group of drugs that were commonly associated with all-night dance parties called "raves," which were frequented by older adolescents and young adults. The moniker "club drugs" was coined as an umbrella term referring to substances commonly consumed at raves or at other dance clubs. This category of drugs is quite broad and includes MDMA, LSD, GHB, ketamine, and methamphetamine (Tellier 2002). These substances, with the exception of GHB, have hallucinogenic properties that "enhance" the experience of dancing to electronic music and/or facilitate the ability to participate in all-night dances by increasing energy or depressing the need for food or sleep. Although initially associated with all-night dance parties and dance clubs, these substances are now consumed by adolescents and young adults outside of this particular milieu (Hopfer et al. 2006).

MDMA

Brief History

MDMA was initially synthesized in 1891 as an appetite suppressant (Haber 1891); however, it was not widely used until the 1970s. Some psychotherapists reported that its use facilitated introspective states and closeness with the therapist. It gradually became more popular as an illicit substance and became most commonly known as "ecstasy" in its street form. MDMA use was first reported to be part of a youth subculture in the early 1980s, with reports initially surfacing in Europe and later appearing in North America in the early 1990s. It was declared a Schedule I substance in 1985 due to concerns about its abuse potential and potential neurotoxicity (Cottler et al. 2001; Freese et al. 2002; Scheier et al. 2008).

Chemical Name and Mechanisms of Action

MDMA is a semisynthetic substance that can produce both stimulant and psychedelic effects. As indicated by its chemical name, 3,4-methylenedioxymethylamphetamine, MDMA is a member of the amphetamine class. However, it also shares chemical similarities to the hallucinogen mescaline (Koesters et al. 2002). It functions as an indirect sympathomimetic, acting at dopaminergic and adrenergic receptors, but also inhibiting the reuptake of serotonin (which is thought to be related to its hallucinogenic properties).

Street Names and Typical Doses

MDMA is most commonly known as "ecstasy" or "X." Other names include "E," "the love drug," "the hug drug," "Adam," and "Stacey" (Cottler et al. 2001). Studies of actual street MDMA tablets report that typically doses range from 75 to 150 mg. Also of clinical note, street MDMA tablets or capsules sold as "ecstasy" often contain additional psychoactive drugs. Tests of these tablets have revealed that the active substances in the tablet or capsule vary considerably and may include methamphetamine, phencyclidine (PCP), ketamine, MDA (3,4-methylenedioxyamphetamine), and MDEA (N-ethyl-3,4-methylenedioxyamphetamine), as well as OTC substances such as caffeine, ephedrine, aspirin, acetaminophen, and dextromethorphan (National Institute on Drug Abuse 2006a).

Route of Administration

MDMA is taken orally in a tablet or a capsule form.

Physical and Psychological Effects

MDMA typically has an onset of action of 20–40 minutes, with a peak effect at 60–90 minutes, and the effects last about 3–6 hours. The reported desired effects of MDMA include elevated mood; a sense of intimacy, sensuality, and a desire to be touched (ergo the names "love drug" and "hug drug"); altered visual, sensual, or emotional feelings; and increased energy and self-confidence. Adverse effects may include increases in both heart rate and blood pressure. Because it is often used in raves with extended dancing, MDMA may cause dangerous increases in body temperature and dehydration, which might lead to medical complications and death (Grob 1998). Other possible adverse effects include derealization and depersonalization, jaw clenching, gait disturbances, and hyponatremia (Koesters et al. 2002).

Epidemiology

In the 2007 Monitoring the Future survey, 6.5% of twelfth graders, 5.2% of tenth graders, and 2.3% of eighth graders reported having ever using MDMA. Annual prevalence of use was 4.5%, 3.5%, and 1.5%, respectively. Past 30-day prevalence was 1.6%, 1.2%, and 0.6%, respectively (Johnston et al. 2008).

Patterns of Use and Risk of Abuse and Dependence

Studies of MDMA users have demonstrated that although MDMA is currently classified as a hallucinogen and withdrawal is not recognized in the *Diagnostic and Statistical Manual of Mental Disorders*, 4th Edition, Text Revision (American Psychiatric Association 2000), there is evidence that withdrawal symptoms are associated with MDMA abstinence. Symptoms may include generalized fatigue, trouble concentrating, anxiety, depression, and insomnia and may last 1–3 days (Curran and Travill 1997). Furthermore, MDMA users have a significantly higher risk of developing dependence than do LSD users (Leung and Cottler 2008), and they report varied patterns of psychological and behavioral impairment that may not fall into an abuse or dependence category. Of MDMA users, 20% report a "severe-dependent" cluster of behavioral and psychological symptoms, underscoring the risk of developing severe dependence on MDMA (Scheier et al. 2008). Other findings of note are that MDMA use typically co-occurs with use and abuse of and dependence on other drugs (Wu et al. 2006), including other club drugs.

Specific Treatment Issues

The typical length of time that MDMA is detectable through urine toxicology is 1–2 days; thus, a frequent program of random urine monitoring is necessary to detect MDMA use. MDMA is not always detected in standard urinalyses, although it may cross-react with and be detected as amphetamines. Thus, it is important to clarify that the laboratory one is using detects MDMA.

Two particular clinical issues deserve additional attention: concerns about neurotoxicity stemming from chronic MDMA abuse, and the medical management of MDMA overdoses. One of the major concerns about MDMA use is whether, in addition to developing abuse or dependence, users may experience chronic neurotoxic effects. Animal studies demonstrate that MDMA use results in substantial loss of serotonergic neurons. Human studies are all complicated by the fact that MDMA users tend to use other substances, so it is difficult to isolate the effects of MDMA. However, substantial evidence exists for one to suspect that chronic MDMA use is associated with a range of psychiatric problems, including sleep disturbances, neuropsychological impairment, and mood and anxiety disorders (Montoya et al. 2002). Acute MDMA toxicity may include hyperthermia, seizures, cardiac arrhythmias, and hyponatremia. Management, which typically involves supportive therapy, is reviewed by Koesters et al. (2002).

Case Vignette

Brian is a 19-year-old white male who presented for treatment for alcohol and MDMA dependence. He reported that he had used alcohol extensively since age 14, often consuming more than a six-pack every day of the weekend. In the last 2 years, he developed increased tolerance, episodes of blackouts, and a range of negative academic and psychosocial consequences. In addition, he reported use of 5–6 tablets of MDMA daily for 3–4 years starting his junior year in high school. He initially used these as part of the club scene, but eventually became dependent on taking the tablets daily.

Brian participated in an outpatient drug and alcohol treatment program consisting of weekly individual counseling and group counseling, as well as random urinalyses, and achieved abstinence from use after about 3 months of treatment. He was referred for a psychiatric consultation due to ongoing complaints of difficulty with memory, learning, and attention that persisted even after 2 months of continuous abstinence. He had completed high school and reported good grades; however, on presentation he noted that he was enrolled in community college and he found learning new material increasingly difficult. He also reported some mild depressive symptoms. The patient reported no previous history of learning disorders or attention-deficit/hyperactivity disorder (ADHD).

Case Discussion

As is typical of many chronic MDMA users, Brian reported a concurrent use of other substances, in this case alcohol. His complaints of neuropsychological impairment are more severe than those attributed to his alcohol use disorder and may be associated with his heavy use of MDMA for several years (Halpern et al. 2004). Currently, it is still unknown to what extent users who complain of neuropsychological difficulties recover function after achieving sustained abstinence. Treatment should include continued emphasis on maintaining sobriety by psychosocial interventions as well as periodic neuropsychological testing.

GHB

Brief History

GHB's history dates back to its development in the 1960s as a possible analogue for gamma-aminobutyric acid (GABA) and as an anesthetic. It later was found to be an endogenous product of the human brain, with GHB-specific receptors being identified (Okun et al. 2001). It was legally available in the early 1990s and was marketed for its effects as an anabolic agent and also sold in health food stores as a possible treatment for narcolepsy and alcohol dependence and withdrawal. Because of numerous reports of adverse effects, including comas and seizures, it was banned by the Drug Enforcement Administration in the late 1990s. GHB has been used as a treatment for alcoholism and is approved as a treatment for narcolepsy in Europe.

Chemical Name and Mechanisms of Action

GHB, which stands for gamma-hydroxybutyrate, is chemically similar to the inhibitory neurotransmitter GABA and has some limited activity at the GABA receptor. The brain has specific GHB receptors, and GHB's mechanism of action is thought to be mediated through these specific GHB receptors as well as through $GABA_B$ receptors and through inhibitory actions on the dopaminergic receptors (Okun et al. 2001).

Street Names and Typical Doses

The most common street names of GHB are "GHB" and "liquid ecstasy." Other names for GHB include "easy lay," "soap," "Georgia homeboy," "liquid X," "renutrient," "scoop," "salty water," and "grievous bodily harm." It is typically sold as a clear, salty liquid and is taken in teaspoons or capsules. The concentrations can vary markedly, ranging from 500 mg to 5 g per dose, which may account for cases of overdose.

Route of Administration

GHB is available in a liquid, a capsule, or a powder form and is orally administered.

Physical and Psychological Effects

GHB is rapidly absorbed and has a rapid onset of action, often within 15 minutes. It reaches peak concentrations in 20–60 minutes and is metabolized rapidly, with a half-life of 30 minutes. The duration of effect is usually 2–6 hours. Substantial individual variation occurs in response to GHB, and effects can include sedation or coma. The desired effects are described as similar to alcohol intoxication; however, the effects are typically more unpredictable. Users report enhanced social activity or improved sleep. Side effects can include drowsiness, vomiting, nystagmus, and ataxia, with possible death resulting from high doses (Freese et al. 2002). GHB is also considered a "date rape" drug, because it can easily be added to drinks and render the victim disinhibited or unconscious, and thus vulnerable to rape.

Epidemiology

GHB use is fairly uncommon among adolescents. In the 2007 Monitoring the Future study, the annual reported rates of GHB use were 0.9% among twelfth graders, 0.6% among tenth graders, and 0.7% among eighth graders (Johnston et al. 2008).

Patterns of Use and Risk of Abuse and Dependence

Knowledge about typical patterns of GHB use is very scarce. Most use occurs in the context of polysubstance use, and daily users may develop withdrawal syndromes (Degenhardt et al. 2002; Miotto et al. 2001). Case reports indicate that users can develop severe dependence, which may be characterized by very heavy use. There are reports of "round-the-clock" users who take GHB every 2–4 hours (Freese et al. 2002). If patients take GHB to be able to sleep, the rapid elimination of GHB often results in a rebound insomnia after 2–3 hours, and users might take additional doses to return to sleep. Because physical tolerance can develop to GHB and dependent users might escalate their intake, dependent users might take 25–100 g/day of GHB (Freese et al. 2002). Withdrawal also can occur in dependent users and can be severe because the withdrawal syndrome is similar to benzodiazepine or alcohol withdrawal. Onset may begin 1–6 hours after last use, and early symptoms include anxiety, insomnia, tremors, nausea, and vomiting. Autonomic instability can develop, and diaphoresis, hypertension, tremor, and tachycardia may be present. Severe cases of withdrawal may present as similar to delirium tremens (van Noorden et al. 2009). Longer term, a protracted withdrawal state may last for 3–6 months, characterized by dysphoria, memory problems, anxiety, and insomnia.

Specific Treatment Issues

Because of the rapid elimination of GHB, urine detection is possible only within an 8-hour time frame; therefore, frequent random urinalysis is required to detect GHB abuse. Treatment of GHB-induced coma is generally conservative, focusing on aspiration precautions and observing pulse oximetry. Gastric lavage is not indicated for GHB overdose due to its rapid absorption. Neither naloxone nor flumazenil has been shown to reverse GHB-induced coma. Recovery usually occurs rapidly within 4–6 hours. Physostigmine, 2 mg intravenously, may be used to reverse the effects of GHB if necessary, but its routine use is not recommended (Okun et al. 2001).

Ketamine

Brief History

Ketamine was initially developed in 1962 and used as an anesthetic agent in adult surgical patients; however, after reports emerged of severe adverse reactions, its use rapidly diminished (Wolff and Winstock 2006). Because of its hallucinogenic properties, ketamine came into use as a street drug. It first gained popularity in the 1980s, when large doses were found to cause dreamlike states similar to those associated with PCP use.

Chemical Name and Mechanisms of Action

Ketamine (2-[2-chlorophenyl]-2-[methylamino]cyclohexanone) is a derivative of phencyclidine (l-[l-phenylcyclohexyl]piperidine). Ketamine is classified as an antagonist of the N-methyl-D-aspartate (NMDA) receptor; however, it also has activity at the opiate, serotonin, and acetylcholine receptors (Wolff and Winstock 2006).

Street Names and Availability

Ketamine, known as "K," "special K," "kat food," and "vitamin K," is an anesthetic approved for both human and animal use, although about 90% of the ketamine sold today is intended for veterinary use only. Street preparations typically include powder forms for intranasal use of approximately 100–400 mg, and liquid, capsule, and powder forms for ingestion in doses of about 300–500 mg.

Route of Administration

Ketamine can be administered orally, intravenously, intranasally, and subcutaneously.

Physical and Psychological Effects

Ketamine has a short half-life, and effects typically last 1–3 hours. Onset of action is typically rapid, within 30 minutes. Desired effects of ketamine include mood elevation and some perceptual changes, including visual hallucinations and experiences of derealization or depersonalization. Low doses also may result in impaired attention, learning ability, and memory. At high doses, ketamine can cause delirium, amnesia, impaired motor function, high blood pressure, depression, vomiting, slurred speech, and potentially fatal respiratory problems. High-dose users report intense dissociative experiences, including out-of-body and near-death experiences. Visual disturbances can occur weeks after use (Wolff and Winstock 2006).

Epidemiology

Ketamine use is relatively rare among adolescents. Based on the 2007 Monitoring the Future survey, annual prevalence rates among twelfth, tenth, and eighth graders were reported to be 1.3%, 0.8%, and 1.0%, respectively (Johnston et al. 2008).

Patterns of Use and Risk of Abuse and Dependence

Studies of ketamine users are limited. Many users also appear to be users of other club drugs (Dillon et al. 2003). No studies specifically target adolescent ketamine users; however, ketamine use is likely to occur within a context of polysubstance use. In case studies, dependent users have reported loss of control over use, as well as other cognitive and behavioral changes associated with a dependence syndrome (e.g., Hurt and Ritchie 1994).

Specific Treatment Issues

Users of ketamine may report persistent perceptual problems similar to those that occur with use of LSD. Management of acute toxicity is typically supportive. Haloperidol has limited effects on the psychosis associated with ketamine (Wolff and Winstock 2006), and benzodiazepines may be useful to combat agitation. Long-term users may experience persistent cognitive difficulties. Pharmacological management may include medications that improve attention and focus.

Methamphetamine

Brief History

Methamphetamine was initially synthesized from ephedrine in 1887 but was not widely used until World War II, when it was used by soldiers to maintain alertness. Its use as an illicit substance became more widespread in the 1970s, and its use continues to be a growing problem. Methamphetamine can be fairly easily synthesized by a reduction reaction from precursor compounds ephedrine or pseudoephedrine, a fact that has led to laws regulating the distribution of these agents.

Chemical Name and Mechanisms of Action

Methamphetamine ([2S]-*N*-methyl-1-phenylpropan-2-amine) has two isomers: a levorotatory (r-form) isomer, which is used as a nasal decongestant, and a dextrorotatory (s-form) isomer, which is the active ingredient in the illicit substance of abuse. Methamphetamine is structurally similar to amphetamine, but the methyl group both increases its ability to cross the blood-brain barrier and makes it more resistant to degradation by monoamine oxygenase. Methamphetamine is a stimulant and acts by stimulating the release of dopamine, norepinephrine, and serotonin. At higher doses, it also inhibits the reuptake of these neurotransmitters (Cook et al. 1992, 1993).

Street Names and Typical Doses

Methamphetamine is known by a variety of street names, including "speed," "ice," "crystal," "glass," and "crank." Typical street doses vary but range from 100 to 250 mg.

Route of Administration

Methamphetamine can be smoked or can be administered intranasally, intravenously, or subcutaneously.

Physical and Psychological Effects

Methamphetamine has a rapid onset of action and a half-life of 9–15 hours; effects can last up to 30 hours. Desired effects of methamphetamine include increased energy, sense of well-being, libido, alertness, and activity; excitement; and decreased appetite. Physical effects include elevated blood pressure, body temperature, and respiration. Adverse effects include medical problems associated with excess doses and may include seizures or strokes, as well as hypertensive crises. Psychological effects may include the development of paranoia and hallucinations, psychosis, and suicidal or homicidal ideation, as well as cognitive impairments. Insomnia is a common effect of methamphetamine use, resulting in patterns of staying awake for days and then "crashing." Withdrawal depression is common. Methamphetamine use has also been linked with engaging in high-risk sexual behaviors.

Epidemiology

Reported lifetime prevalence rates of methamphetamine use by twelfth, tenth, and eighth graders, respectively, were 3.0%, 2.8%, and 1.8% in 2007. The 2007 annual prevalence rates were 1.7%, 1.6%, and 1.1%. The 30-day prevalence rates were 0.6%, 0.4%, and 0.6% (Johnston et al. 2008).

Patterns of Use and Risk of Abuse and Dependence

Methamphetamine is a highly addictive substance, and there is a strong likelihood of users becoming dependent (National Institute on Drug Abuse 2006b). A review of studies of adolescent methamphetamine users concluded that its use was associated with other drug use and engaging in risky behaviors (Russell et al. 2008). Gonzales et al. (2008) reported that compared with a sample of marijuana-abusing youth, methamphetamine-abusing youth were older, were more likely to be white and female, were more likely to have had prior treatment episodes, and had poorer treatment retention. Of particular clinical note is that girls who use methamphetamine may do so for reasons such as weight control, and particular attention should be given to this concern during treatment.

Specific Treatment Issues

Methamphetamine is detectable for 2–3 days by urinalysis; thus, a program of one or two weekly random urine drug screens should detect most dependent users. Typical approaches to treatment include contingency management approaches, 12-step group facilitation, and cognitive-behavioral approaches. Ling et al. (2006) provided an excellent review of behavioral treatment approaches and of promising pharmacotherapies, which include bupropion, modafinil, and baclofen as adjunct agents. A practical clinical issue is what to do if users complain about problems with attention after desisting from use (Kalechstein et al. 2003). There are numerous reports of methamphetamine use being associated with subsequent neuropsychological impairment, and many users may have preexisting problems with ADHD. Laboratories can discriminate between amphetamines prescribed for ADHD and methamphetamines; however, a discussion should be held with the laboratory to confirm their procedures for making this differentiation. Essentially, because methamphetamines are metabolized to amphetamines, if amphetamines are prescribed, urinalysis should reveal only amphetamines, not methamphetamine. Clinically, it is important to be clear with patients in advance how testing will be conducted and what consequences may occur if methamphetamines are detected in the urine (i.e., it would be considered a relapse).

In general, treatment for ADHD in patients with a history of methamphetamine use should focus on treatment with nonabusable medications. If a determination is made that stimulants would be the best treatment option, the clinician should clarify whether the lab can with confidence detect the difference between methamphetamine use and use of prescription stimulants.

LSD

Brief History

Although LSD was first synthesized in 1938, its psychedelic properties were not recognized until 5 years later. Initial tests by researchers at the Swiss company Sandoz Laboratories resulted in reports that even very small doses (measured in micrograms) produced hallucinogenic effects (National Institute on Drug Abuse 2001). LSD was available legally in the United States as an experimental psychiatric agent until 1966, when it was declared a Schedule I drug. It has been manufactured and sold illegally since the 1960s in the United States.

LSD use has waxed and waned in popularity, with its use rising in the 1960s, declining in the 1970s and 1980s, and experiencing a resurgence in the 1990s (Johnston 2008). In the 2000s, rates of use have trended down from their high rates in the 1990s.

Chemical Name and Mechanisms of Action

LSD (lysergic acid diethylamide) is synthesized from lysergic acid, an ergot. It affects a large number of G protein–coupled receptors, including dopamine and serotonergic receptors. Its mechanism of action is complex and not completely understood, but its psychotropic effects appear to be due in part to agonism of the serotonin 5-HT$_{2A}$ receptors (Freese et al. 2002).

Street Names and Typical Doses

The most common street name for LSD is "acid," although other names include "yellow sunshine" and "boomers." LSD doses are much smaller than most pharmacologically active substances, having effects at the microgram level. Minimal doses that have some psychotropic effects are between 20 and 25 μg, with typical doses being between 100 and 500 μg.

Route of Administration

LSD typically is sold as a liquid (often packaged in small bottles designed to hold breath freshener drops) or applied to blotter paper, sugar cubes, gelatin squares, or tablets. It is orally ingested.

Physical and Psychological Effects

As a hallucinogen, LSD produces abnormalities in sensory perception. Its effects are unpredictable depending on dose, surroundings, and the user's mood and personality. Typically taking the drug by mouth in tablet or blotter paper form, an LSD user begins to feel effects within 30–90 minutes. These effects include dilated pupils, increased body temperature, increased heart rate and blood pressure, sweating, dry mouth, and tremors. Long-term problems associated with LSD include persistent psychosis and hallucinogen persisting perception disorder (i.e., flashbacks) (Abraham et al. 1996; Halpern and Pope 2003). A rare yet serious effect reported in adults and youth is LSD-induced chronic visual disturbance (Kaminer and Hrecznyj 1991).

Epidemiology

Lifetime prevalence rates of LSD use reported in 2007 by twelfth, tenth, and eighth graders were 3.4%, 3.0%, and 1.6%, respectively. The 2007 annual prevalence rates were 1.7%, 1.7%, and 0.9%, respectively. The 30-day prevalence rates were 0.7%, 0.5%, and 0.5%, respectively (Johnston et al. 2008).

Patterns of Use and Risk of Abuse and Dependence

LSD use is typically not characterized by the development of a dependence syndrome, although heavy users might ingest LSD daily (Abraham et al. 1996).

Specific Treatment Issues

Detection of LSD use requires special laboratory procedures, and clinicians must specifically request testing because the drug is not normally detected by standard urine toxicology tests. Due to its low concentrations, LSD typically is not tested for using standard procedures, and detection is difficult. LSD is detectable for up to 7–10 days with special procedures. Management of LSD-related persistent perceptual disorders may include selective serotonin reuptake inhibitors (SSRIs), antipsychotic agents, or benzodiazepines (Halpern and Pope 2003).

Prescription and Over-the-Counter Medications

Overview

The abuse of prescription and OTC medications is common among youth for several reasons: these medications are readily available at home and in the pharmacy, are inexpensive, may be easily purchased on the Internet, are legal, and are erroneously perceived as harmless (Levine 2007). Abuse of medications prescribed for medical or psychiatric conditions has surged during the past decade and has become a major area of concern. Approximately 6.9 million individuals age 12 years and older were past-month nonmedical users of prescription psychotherapeutic drugs in 2007 (National Drug Intelligence Center 2009). In particular, recent reports that adolescents and young adults experimented with opiates more frequently than with illicit drugs, except marijuana, raised attention that this is a growing national problem (Compton and Volkow 2006a,

2006b; National Institute on Drug Abuse 2005). On the basis of a survey of 37,000 adolescents, Schepis and Krishnan-Sarin (2009) reported that the most common medication source was friends or family, for free; other sources include physicians and pharmacies (purchased medications).

According to the National Prescription Drug Threat Assessment (National Drug Intelligence Center 2009), along with the rise in the misuse of prescription substances, there has been a marked yearly increase in deaths attributable to prescription drugs, primarily opiates. In 2001, prescription opiates were cited as the cause of death in 3,994 cases; by 2005, this number had increased by 114% to 8,541. Furthermore, prescription opioid abuse might be fueling heroin abuse rates in some areas of the United States.

In addition, abuse of OTC medications, primarily dextromethorphan, which is an active ingredient in cough suppressants, has received increased attention due to reports of the increasing incidence of abuse of dextromethorphan (Bryner et al. 2006). In the following subsections, I focus on prescription opiate and benzodiazepine dependence, as well as abuse of dextromethorphan.

Opiates

Brief History

Opiates have long been used by humans to induce euphoria and manage pain. Illicit opiate use in the United States involves primarily heroin and is rare among adolescents; however, a growing concern is the misuse and abuse of prescription opiates by adolescents, with morbid and lethal consequences. Most recently, the U.S. Food and Drug Administration expressed concerns regarding safety of a common opioid pain-relieving product and has required the manufacturers of propoxyphene-containing products (e.g., Darvon, Darvocet) to strengthen the label's boxed warning to address the risk of overdose. In the following subsections, I focus on the most common prescription opiates abused by adolescents. These include hydrocodone, most commonly in the form of Vicodin, and oxycodone, most commonly marketed as OxyContin.

Chemical Name and Mechanisms of Action

The chemical name of OxyContin (oxycodone) is 4,5-epoxy-14-hydroxy-3-methoxy-17-methylmorphinan-6-one. The drug is marketed in a sustained-release preparation typically used for moderate to severe pain control (see http://www.drugbank.ca/drugs/DB00497). Vicodin consists of a combination of hydrocodone, which is a synthetic narcotic also typically used for pain control, and acetaminophen. Both agents act on the mu, kappa, and delta opioid receptors (see http://www.drugbank.ca/drugs/DB00956).

Street Names and Typical Doses

OxyContin is most frequently known on the street as "OC," "OX," "oxy," "oxycotton," "Hillbilly heroin," and "kicker." Typical OxyContin doses are between 10 and 80 mg.

Vicodin is known as "vike" and "Watson 387" (this refers to the imprint on the pill). Vicodin tablets typically contain 5 mg of hydrocodone and 500 mg of acetaminophen.

Route of Administration

Typically, both OxyContin and Vicodin are administered orally, although they can be injected.

Physical and Psychological Effects

The use of opioids results in the relief of pain and the induction of euphoria. Opiates typically cause respiratory depression and reduced gastrointestinal motility, along with drowsiness. Constricted pupils are a hallmark of opiate use. Regular use induces substantial tolerance, and withdrawal states may occur upon discontinuation. Withdrawal may be characterized by diarrhea, muscle pain, nausea, piloerection, and dilated pupils. Withdrawal may last 3–7 days (Jasinski 1981).

Epidemiology

Use of OxyContin has been increasing since the drug first became available in 1995. Various studies have documented a dramatic surge in the use of prescription opiates, starting in the late 1990s and reaching epidemic proportions around 2000 (Sung et al. 2005). In 2007, annual prevalence of OxyContin use by twelfth, tenth, and eighth graders was 5.2%, 3.9%, and 1.8%, respectively. The rate for Vicodin was 9.6%, 7.2%, and 2.7%, respectively. Of clinical note, adolescents and young adults frequently obtain prescription medications from peers or family members (McCabe and Boyd 2005), and inquiring about the sources of these medications should be a routine part of the clinical assessment.

Patterns of Use and Risk of Abuse and Dependence

Oxycodone has a high potential for abuse and the development of dependence and is a Schedule II medication. The risk for Vicodin is somewhat lower, as a Schedule III medication. A population-based study of adolescents found that of those who misused prescription medications (primarily opiates), approximately 17% reported symptoms of either substance abuse or dependence (Schepis and Krishnan-Sarin 2008).

Specific Treatment Issues

Studies of the characteristics of treatment-seeking adolescents reported that compared with users of cannabis and alcohol, opioid users were more likely to be white and to have dropped out of school. They also had greater substance use severity, with a higher proportion of current sedative and multiple substance use disorders (Subramaniam et al. 2009). Another comparison was made between treatment-seeking prescription opiate abusers and heroin-using adolescents with opioid use disorder (Subramaniam and Stitzer 2009). Both groups were older (mean = 17 years), predominantly suburban white youth, with high rates of psychiatric comorbidity (83%). The heroin-using group was more likely to drop out of school, be dependent on opioids, and inject drugs. The prescription opioid–using youth were more likely to meet criteria for multiple substance use disorders (including prescription sedatives and psychostimulants) and current ADHD, as well as to report selling drugs. These differences may have implications for the design of treatment programs, specifically indicating the need for more psychiatric services in these populations to address comorbidity.

For most patients, detoxification from opiates should be attempted, usually by utilizing other agonist therapies, such as buprenorphine or methadone. Methadone treatment can be administered only by a clinic licensed to treat opioid dependence (Hopfer et al. 2003). (See Chapter 7, "Pharmacotherapy of Adolescent Substance Use Disorders," for more information on the pharmacological treatment of heroin dependence.) It is noteworthy that patients need to be educated that if they detoxify, they will not be as tolerant to opiates as they were when they were using, and that should they relapse, they are at risk for overdosing. Another clinical issue of substantial importance is distinguishing legitimate use of prescription medications from misuse, abuse, or dependence. As discussed by Hertz and Knight (2006), symptoms of misuse, abuse, or dependence include diversion of medications, nonadherence behaviors, losing prescriptions, and demonstrating signs of declining functioning. Any pharmacological treatment should be integrated with other evidence-based psychosocial treatment approaches to managing substance use disorders (see chapters in this manual discussing the specific approaches for more details).

Benzodiazepines

Brief History

Benzodiazepines were developed in the 1950s and became more widespread as therapeutic agents in the 1960s. The growing recognition that this class of medications has abuse and dependence potential led to their being declared controlled substances. Most benzodiazepines are classified as Schedule IV controlled substances in the United States.

Misuse of prescription benzodiazepines is the second most common form of misuse of prescription medications, after misuse of prescription opiates. Additionally, the benzodiazepine flunitrazepam (Rohypnol), which is not available as a prescription benzodiazepine in the United States, is considered a club drug (Wu et al. 2006).

Chemical Name and Mechanisms of Action

A large number of benzodiazepines have been developed, all with different half-lives and different degrees of sedative or hypnotic properties. All act by modulation of the GABA receptors. Duration of effect varies depending on half-life. A commonly abused benzodiazepine is alprazolam, which typically has a duration of action of 2–6 hours (Erowid 2009).

Street Names and Typical Doses

Most street names of benzodiazepines are similar to the brand name of the benzodiazepine. Doses are similar to those used therapeutically.

Route of Administration

The typical route of administration of benzodiazepines is oral; however, these medications can also be injected.

Physical and Psychological Effects

Benzodiazepines reduce anxiety and can cause sedation at higher doses. In combination with other central nervous system depressants, there is a risk of respiratory depression. Tolerance will develop if benzodiazepines are used regularly, and withdrawal can result in seizures.

Epidemiology

Abuse or misuse of prescription benzodiazepines has remained fairly steady among adolescents over the past decade. In 2007, the reported annual prevalence rate of nonmedical use of "tranquilizers" among twelfth, tenth, and eighth graders was 6.2%, 5.3%, and 2.4%, respectively, indicating that misuse of these medications is fairly common among adolescents (Johnston et al. 2008).

Patterns of Use and Risk of Abuse and Dependence

The rate at which adolescents progress from misuse of benzodiazepines to abuse or dependence is not known. Clinically, dependence on benzodiazepines is characterized by the DSM-IV-TR constellation of symptoms that constitute dependence.

Specific Treatment Issues

A practical concern for clinicians treating adolescents is how to recognize whether an adolescent being treated for an anxiety disorder is developing abuse of or dependence on benzodiazepines. Requests for more medications do not by themselves indicate dependence. Signs to look for are evidence of engaging in antisocial or manipulative behaviors around benzodiazepine use, as well as evidence of intoxication on benzodiazepines or problems fulfilling role obligations. If patients are determined to be dependent on benzodiazepines, generally it is advisable to taper them off benzodiazepines and engage them in substance abuse treatment. A difficult issue is the management of complaints of anxiety, which may worsen when a patient is tapering off benzodiazepine use. SSRIs and buspirone may be helpful, as may cognitive-behavioral therapies that focus on managing anxiety (Martin and Volkmar 2007).

Over-the-Counter Medications: Dextromethorphan

Brief History

Although a number of OTC medications have abuse potential, abuse of dextromethorphan is clinically most concerning. Dextromethorphan has been used for many years as a cough suppressant in many OTC cold or cough preparations, such as Coricidin.

Chemical Name and Mechanisms of Action

Dextromethorphan (d-3-methoxy-N-methylmorphinan) is a morphine derivative and acts on the sigma opioid receptor, and therefore is thought to not have abuse potential. However, high doses are metabolized to dextrorphan, which acts on the NMDA receptor. Thus, high doses result in a similar pharmacology as PCP and ketamine. Typically, dextromethorphan takes about 30–60 minutes to have effects, and effects usually last about 6 hours.

Street Names and Typical Doses

Street names include most commonly "DXM," and also "CCC," "triple C," "Dex," "poor man's PCP," "Robo," and "Skittles."

Route of Administration

Dextromethorphan is taken orally as a capsule or syrup.

Physical and Psychological Effects

Dextromethorphan is primarily an antitussive agent. In high doses, such as greater than 180 mg, however, it has dissociative hallucinogenic properties.

Epidemiology

Abuse of dextromethorphan has grown in popularity among adolescents. Abuse cases reported to the California Poison Control System increased 10-fold between 1999 and 2004 (Bryner et al. 2006).

Patterns of Use and Risk of Abuse and Dependence

Most users of dextromethorphan do not abuse it, and the risk of developing abuse or dependence is unknown. Cases of abuse have been reported since the 1960s (Williams and Kokotailo 2006). The most extreme case of abuse reported in the literature was a 23-year-old man who reported using 36–48 oz of Robitussin DM daily for over 5 years (Wolfe and Caravatti 1995).

Specific Treatment Issues

Treatment of dextromethorphan abuse or dependence involves the usual strategies to address substance abuse disorders. High doses, particularly when combined with alcohol, may result in death. Typically, management of dextromethorphan overdoses is supportive. Case reports have indicated that naltrexone assists with reducing cravings for dextromethorphan (Williams and Kokotailo 2006).

Case Vignette

Ted is an 18-year-old male who reported that he began abusing Coricidin at age 12. He discovered that by taking 20–30 tablets at a time, he could induce a dissociative state, in which he would hallucinate for a couple of hours. He engaged in this behavior on a daily basis and was hospitalized a number of times when discovered by his family in a state of intoxication. He reported relatively little other substance use, although he abused alcohol on occasion. His peak consumption involved taking 40 tablets at a time. Ted reported that standard urinalysis tests did not reveal that he had been using Coricidin, and that his behavior was usually discovered because he admitted to it or he was observed to be intoxicated. Ted participated in a number of substance abuse treatment programs, ranging from residential treatment to outpatient treatment that involved multisystemic therapy. His clinical course was characterized by periods of remission and relapse.

Case Discussion

Ted found the dissociative state induced by high doses of dextromethorphan to be highly reinforcing and repetitively engaged in taking high doses. Obtaining the substance was relatively easy because it could be purchased at most drugstores. He clearly met criteria for dependence because he repeatedly used it, despite adverse social and medical consequences, and he spent a substantial amount of time using or recovering from use. His use was medically dangerous, particularly when he combined dextromethorphan with alcohol, and resulted in multiple hospitalizations. A substantial element of his treatment involved working with his family to provide appropriate supervision and monitoring of his behaviors, as well as trying to reinforce non-substance-using behaviors.

Conclusion

In this chapter, I have reviewed a broad range of substances of abuse, with varying pharmacological properties as well as different profiles of potential to develop abuse or dependence. It is important to note that for the substances reviewed in this chapter, general principles of substance abuse treatment apply, as reviewed in Chapter 7, "Pharmacotherapy of Adolescent Substance Use Disorders." However, a few practical issues bear noting. The first is that opiate dependence, whether in adolescents or in adults, is one of the few substance dependence syndromes for which pharmacotherapy, typically with agonists such as methadone or buprenorphine, may be indicated. Although clinicians may be unfamiliar with this treatment or consider it inappropriate for adolescents, careful consideration must be given to the risk of death from continued opiate use and the risk of progressing from prescription opiate dependence to heroin dependence, which is associated with substantial morbidity and mortality. Agonist therapy may help stabilize the patient and allow him or her to engage in psychosocial treatments.

Another practical issue is how to manage comorbid psychiatric or medical problems, such as anxiety, in the presence of benzodiazepine dependence, pain in the management of opiate dependence, or ADHD, when patients are abusing or have a history of MDMA or methamphetamine dependence. Clinically, it is highly advisable to avoid controlled substances when treating these comorbid conditions, and if they are used, to consider how abuse or dependence could be detected and be differentiated from appropriate use. This may require consultation with a laboratory that conducts urinalysis to confirm that the specific medications being prescribed are detectable, as well as substances that are abused, and clarification about what metabolites may be detected (e.g., whether methamphetamine can be distinguished from prescription stimulants).

Key Clinical Concepts

- Physicians need to be aware of the risk of diversion and abuse of prescription medications, such as painkillers and stimulants. This is particularly important in families in which substance abuse has been diagnosed.

- Clinicians should provide education to parents and adolescents regarding the peril of abusing prescription and OTC medications.

- Prescription medications should be stored in a place that cannot be accessed by adolescents. Pills should be frequently counted, and any discrepancy should be reported immediately to the prescribing physician.

References

Abraham HD, Aldridge AM, Gogia P: The psychopharmacology of hallucinogens. Neuropsychopharmacology 14:285–298, 1996

American Psychiatric Association: Diagnostic and Statistical Manual of Mental Disorders, 4th Edition, Text Revision. Washington, DC, American Psychiatric Association, 2000

Bryner JK, Wang UK, Hui JW, et al: Dextromethorphan abuse in adolescence: an increasing trend: 1999–2004. Arch Pediatr Adolesc Med 160:1217–1222, 2006

Compton WM, Volkow ND: Abuse of prescription drugs and the risk of addiction. Drug Alcohol Depend 83:S4–S7, 2006a

Compton WM, Volkow ND: Major increases in opioid analgesic abuse in the United States: concerns and strategies. Drug Alcohol Depend 81:103–107, 2006b

Cook CE, Jeffcoat AR, Sadler BM, et al: Pharmacokinetics of oral methamphetamine and effects of repeated daily dosing in humans. Drug Metab Dispos 20:856–862, 1992

Cook CE, Jeffcoat AR, Hill JM, et al: Pharmacokinetics of methamphetamine self-administered to human subjects by smoking S-(+)-methamphetamine hydrochloride. Drug Metab Dispos 21:717–723, 1993

Cottler LB, Womack SB, Compton WM, et al: Ecstasy abuse and dependence among adolescents and young adults: applicability and reliability of DSM-IV criteria. Hum Psychopharmacol 16:599–606, 2001

Curran HV, Travill RA: Mood and cognitive effects of +/− 3,4-methylenedioxymethamphetamine (MDMA, "ecstasy"): week-end "high" followed by mid-week low. Addiction 92:821–831, 1997

Degenhardt L, Darke S, Dillon P: GHB use among Australians: characteristics, use patterns and associated harm. Drug Alcohol Depend 67:89–94, 2002

Dillon P, Copeland J, Jansen K: Patterns of use and harms associated with non-medical ketamine use. Drug Alcohol Depend 69:23–28, 2003

Erowid: Alprazolam. September 2009. Available at http://www.erowid.org/pharms/alprazolam/alprazolam.shtml. Accessed January 2, 2010.

Freese TE, Miotto K, Reback CJ: The effects and consequences of selected club drugs. J Subst Abuse Treat 23:151–156, 2002

Gonzales R, Ang A, McCann MJ, et al: An emerging problem: methamphetamine abuse among treatment seeking youth. Subst Abus 29:71–80, 2008

Grob C: MDMA research: preliminary investigations with human subjects. Int J Drug Policy 9:119–124, 1998

Haber F: Ueber einige Derivate des Piperonals. Berichte der Deutschen Chemischen Gesellschaft 24:617–626, 1891

Halpern JH, Pope HG Jr: Hallucinogen persisting perception disorder: what do we know after 50 years? Drug Alcohol Depend 69:109–119, 2003

Halpern JH, Pope HG Jr, Sherwood AR, et al: Residual neuropsychological effects of illicit 3,4-methylenedioxymethamphetamine (MDMA) in individuals with minimal exposure to other drugs. Drug Alcohol Depend 75:135–147, 2004

Hertz JA, Knight JR: Prescription drug misuse: a growing national problem. Adolesc Med Clin 17:751–769; abstract xiii, 2006

Hopfer C, Khuri E, Crowley T, et al: Treating adolescent heroin use. J Am Acad Child Adolesc Psychiatry 42:609–611, 2003

Hopfer C, Mendelson B, Van Leeuwen JM, et al: Club drug use among youths in treatment for substance abuse. Am J Addict 15:94–99, 2006

Hurt PH, Ritchie EC: A case of ketamine dependence (letter). Am J Psychiatry 151:779, 1994

Jasinski DR: Opiate withdrawal syndrome: acute and protracted aspects. Ann NY Acad Sci 362:183–186, 1981

Johnston LD, O'Malley PM, Bachman JG, et al: Monitoring the Future National Survey Results on Drug Use, 1975–2007, Volume I: Secondary School Students (NIH Publ No 08-6418A). Bethesda, MD, National Institute on Drug Abuse, 2008

Kalechstein AD, Newton TF, Green M: Methamphetamine dependence is associated with neurocognitive impairment in the initial phases of abstinence. J Neuropsychiatry Clin Neurosci 15:215–220, 2003

Kaminer Y, Hrecznyj B: LSD induced chronic visual disturbances in an adolescent. J Nerv Ment Dis 179:173–174, 1991

Koesters SC, Rogers PD, Rajasingham CR: MDMA ("ecstasy") and other "club drugs." The new epidemic. Pediatr Clin North Am 49:415–433, 2002

Leung KS, Cottler LB: Ecstasy and other club drugs: a review of recent epidemiologic studies. Curr Opin Psychiatry 21:234–241, 2008

Levine DA: "Pharming": the abuse of prescription and over-the-counter drugs in teens. Curr Opin Pediatr 19:270–274, 2007

Ling W, Rawson R, Shoptow S, et al: Management of methamphetamine abuse and dependence. Curr Psychiatry Rep 8:345–354, 2006

Martin A, Volkmar FR: Lewis's Child and Adolescent Psychiatry: A Comprehensive Textbook, 4th Edition. Baltimore, MD, Lippincott Williams & Wilkins, 2007

McCabe SE, Boyd CJ: Sources of prescription drugs for illicit use. Addict Behav 30:1342–1350, 2005

Miotto K, Darakjian J, Basch J, et al: Gamma-hydroxybutyric acid: patterns of use, effects and withdrawal. Am J Addict 10:232–241, 2001

Montoya AG, Sorrentino R, Lukas SE, et al: Long-term neuropsychiatric consequences of "ecstasy" (MDMA): a review. Harv Rev Psychiatry 10:212–220, 2002

National Drug Intelligence Center: National prescription drug threat assessment 2009. April 2009. Available at: http://www.justice.gov/ndic/pubs33/33775/ index.htm. Accessed January 2, 2010.

National Institute on Drug Abuse: NIDA Research Report Series: Hallucinogens and dissociative drugs, including LSD, PCP, ketamine, and dextromethorphan (NIH Publ No 01-4209). March 2001. Available at: http://www.nida.nih.gov/PDF/ RRHalluc.pdf. Accessed January 2, 2010.

National Institute on Drug Abuse: NIDA Research Report Series: Prescription drugs: abuse and addiction (NIH Publ No 05-4881). August 2005. Available at: http:/ /www.nida.nih.gov/PDF/RRPrescription.pdf. Accessed January 2, 2010.

National Institute on Drug Abuse: NIDA Research Report Series: MDMA (ecstasy) abuse (NIH Publ No 06-4728). March 2006a. Available at: http://www.drugabuse. gov/PDF/RRmdma.pdf. Accessed January 2, 2010.

National Institute on Drug Abuse: NIDA Research Report Series: Methamphetamine: abuse and addiction (NIH Publ No 06-4210). September 2006b. Available at: http://www.nida.nih.gov/PDF/RRMetham.pdf. Accessed January 2, 2010.

Okun MS, Boothby LA, Bartfield RB, et al: GHB: an important pharmacologic and clinical update. J Pharm Pharm Sci 4:167–175, 2001

Russell K, Dryden DM, Liang Y, et al: Risk factors for methamphetamine use in youth: a systematic review. BMC Pediatr 8:48, 2008

Scheier LM, Ben-Abdallah A, Inciardi JA, et al: Tri-city study of ecstasy use problems: a latent class analysis. Drug Alcohol Depend 98:249–263, 2008

Schepis TS, Krishnan-Sarin S: Characterizing adolescent prescription misusers: a population-based study. J Am Acad Child Adolesc Psychiatry 47:745–754, 2008

Schepis TS, Krishnan-Sarin S: Sources of prescriptions for misuse by adolescents: differences in sex, ethnicity, and severity of misuse in a population-based study. J Am Acad Child Adolesc Psychiatry 48:828–836, 2009

Subramaniam GA, Stitzer MA: Clinical characteristics of treatment-seeking prescription opioid vs. heroin-using adolescents with opioid use disorder. Drug Alcohol Depend 101:13–19, 2009

Subramaniam GA, Stitzer MA, Woody G, et al: Clinical characteristics of treatment-seeking adolescents with opioid versus cannabis/alcohol use disorders. Drug Alcohol Depend 99:141–149, 2009

Sung HE, Richter L, Vaughan R, et al: Nonmedical use of prescription opioids among teenagers in the United States: trends and correlates. J Adolesc Health 37:44–51, 2005

Tellier PP: Club drugs: is it all ecstasy? Pediatr Ann 31:550–556, 2002 van Noorden MS, van Dongen LC, Zitman FG, et al: Gamma-hydroxybutyrate withdrawal syndrome: dangerous but not well known. Gen Hosp Psychiatry 31:394–396, 2009

Williams JF, Kokotailo PK: Abuse of proprietary (over-the-counter) drugs. Adolesc Med Clin 17:733–750; abstract xiii, 2006

Wolfe TR, Caravati EM: Massive dextromethorphan ingestion and abuse. Am J Emerg Med 13:174–176, 1995

Wolff K, Winstock AR: Ketamine: from medicine to misuse. CNS Drugs 20:199–218, 2006

Wu LT, Schlenger WE, Galvin DM: Concurrent use of methamphetamine, MDMA, LSD, ketamine, GHB, and flunitrazepam among American youths. Drug Alcohol Depend 84:102–113, 2006

Relevant Websites

National Institute on Drug Abuse (NIDA): http://www.nida.nih.gov. Contains research reports that can be accessed online, including the following:

NIDA Research Report Series: MDMA (ecstasy) abuse (NIH Publ No 06-4728). March 2006. Available at: http://www.drugabuse.gov/PDF/RRmdma.pdf. Accessed January 24, 2010.

NIDA Research Report Series: Prescription drugs: abuse and addiction (NIH Publ No 05-4881). August 2005. Available at: http://www.nida.nih.gov/PDF/RRPrescription.pdf. Accessed January 24, 2010.

NIDA Research Report Series: Methamphetamine: abuse and addiction (NIH Publ No 06-4210). September 2006. Available at: http://www.nida.nih.gov/PDF/RRMetham.pdf. Accessed January 24, 2010.

NIDA Research Report Series: Hallucinogens and dissociative drugs, including LSD, PCP, ketamine, and dextromethorphan (NIH Publ No 01-4209). March 2001. Available at: http://www.nida.nih.gov/PDF/RRHalluc.pdf. Accessed January 24, 2010.

Substance Abuse and Mental Health Services Administration: http://www.samhsa.gov. Contains links to treatment locators and updates on reports on drugs of abuse.

Brief Motivational Interventions, Cognitive-Behavioral Therapy, and Contingency Management for Youth Substance Use Disorders

Yifrah Kaminer, M.D., M.B.A.

Anthony Spirito, Ph.D., A.B.P.P.

William Lewander, M.D.

Research has shown that early onset of substance use problems can predict continuing substance abuse problems in adulthood (Hill et al. 2000). Individuals who seek help at earlier stages of drug dependence often experience more favorable outcomes, highlighting the importance of working with adolescents who are beginning their involvement with drugs (McLellan et al. 1983). Several approaches to treating adolescent substance abuse have been evaluated in the literature, but the majority of these approaches have little support for use with adolescents. Also, although therapy appears to help, little evidence is available to suggest that one therapy is more effective than another therapy (Waldron and Turner 2008). Even less is known about what therapy works for various populations, including ethnic or cultural groups (Gil et al. 2004) and adolescents with comorbid diagnoses (Kaminer and Bukstein 2008).

Waldron and Turner (2008) provided a meta-analysis based on a review of 17 studies of controlled evaluations for adolescent substance abuse treatment since 1998. The sample included 2,307 adolescents in 7 individual cognitive-behavioral therapy (CBT), 13 group CBT, 17 family therapy, and 9 minimal-treatment control conditions. The total sample was composed of 75% males, 45% white, 25% Hispanic, and 25% African American. The authors concluded that multidimensional family therapy (Liddle 2002), functional family therapy (Waldron et al. 2001), and group CBT (Kaminer et al. 2002) received the highest levels of empirical support. However, a number of other models are probably efficacious (Dennis et al. 2004), and none of the treatment approaches appeared to be clearly superior to any others in terms of treatment effectiveness.

Most of the treatment research on adolescent substance abuse is at the efficacy level, which establishes the value of an intervention in a well-controlled population, and little research is available from which to draw conclusions regarding the effectiveness of interventions in less controlled conditions of real-world populations (Bukstein and Winters 2004). Treatments with strong efficacy might not be effective in community practice. Therefore, attention to treatment fidelity, supervision, and practitioner training will be important foci of future research.

In this chapter, we review outpatient brief motivational interventions (BMIs), CBT, and the contingency management reinforcement approach for youth with alcohol and/or substance use disorders.

Brief Motivational Interventions

The theoretical basis of BMIs is grounded in client-centered therapy (Rogers 1957), social learning theory (Bandura 1977), CBT (Marlatt and Gordon 1985), and the transtheoretical paradigm of change (Prochaska et al. 1992).

This approach, in turn, resulted in the gradual shift from viewing motivation as a "trait" to a "state" (Maisto et al. 1999).

In the search to identify the effective ingredients of successful psychotherapy, one therapist characteristic in particular, "accurate empathy," as defined by Carl Rogers (1957), has been shown to be a predictor of therapeutic success. Within the addiction field, Miller and Sanchez (1994) identified six critical conditions, recalled using the mnemonic FRAMES, that are necessary and sufficient to induce change: 1) Feedback regarding personal risk or impairment, 2) emphasis on personal Responsibility for change, 3) clear Advice to change, 4) a Menu of alternative change options, 5) therapist Empathy, and 6) facilitation of participant optimism about the potential to change and Self-efficacy. Therapeutic interventions containing some or all of these elements have been effective in initiating change and reducing alcohol use.

Motivational interviewing (MI), known also as the motivational enhancement therapy (MET) approach (named after the MET manual developed in Project MATCH [1997] for adults with alcoholism), is further grounded in research on processes of change (Prochaska et al. 1992). The transtheoretical model describes five stages of change—precontemplation, contemplation, determination, action, and maintenance—through which people progress in modifying problem behaviors. Through the MET approach, the clinician addresses where the client is currently found in the cycle of change and assists him or her to move through the stages toward action and maintenance. Miller and Rollnick (2002) developed MI, emphasizing that the term *motivational interviewing* pertains to both a style of relating to others and a set of techniques to facilitate that process. They described five main strategies that are used in applying this approach: 1) expressing empathy, 2) developing discrepancy, 3) avoiding argumentation, 4) rolling with resistance, and 5) supporting self-efficacy. It is important to respond to a client's needs in a way that is perceived as helpful but that keeps the responsibility for change on the client. MI decreases the likelihood of being drawn into a power struggle and argument with the resistant (i.e., precontemplator) or ambivalent (i.e., contemplator) client about the need to change. More specifically, employing an empathic style is demonstrated by reflective listening techniques and a warm attitude. Developing discrepancy is achieved through asking the patient about short- and long-term goals and about how the addictive behavior affects the process of achieving these goals. Rolling with resistance and avoiding argumentation are achieved by avoiding debates about beliefs, perceptions, or behaviors, and acknowledging the differences between individuals' positions and the ability to accept and tolerate other opinions as well as to change without becoming defensive. Supporting self-efficacy is achieved by complimenting the individual for making comments on and/or progress in addressing his or her drug use in terms of quantity and frequency, or for expressing motivation to change high-risk behaviors. An intriguing issue is the matching of MI intervention to clients. Karno and Longabaugh (2005) reported that less directiveness by therapists improves drinking outcomes of patients high in reactiveness to criticism. The opposite has been found for patients low on reactiveness to directness, who appear to benefit from directiveness by therapists. Table 9–1 contrasts a directive approach with MET.

BMIs utilize a harm reduction approach that is tailored to the needs of the individual. The short course of BMI (i.e., 1–5 sessions), increased rapport, and improved commitment to change contribute to the appeal of BMI to clinicians.

The increasing interest in mechanisms of behavioral change of different psychotherapies resulted in a review of the evidence from MI studies. Apodaca and Longabaugh (2009) reviewed the literature for the following constructs of therapist behavior: MI spirit, MI-consistent behaviors, MI-inconsistent behaviors, and therapist use of specific techniques. Five constructs of client behavior were evaluated: change talk/intention, readiness to change, involvement/engagement, resistance, and the client's experience of discrepancy. The most consistent evidence was found for three constructs: client change talk/intention (Moyers et al. 2007) and client experience of discrepancy, which were both related to better outcomes, and therapist MI-inconsistent behavior, which was related to worse outcomes. Regarding use of specific techniques, use of a decisional balance exercise showed the strongest association to better outcomes. A more recent study not included in Apodaca and Longabaugh's review noted that overall MI-consistent spirit might be more important than particular MI techniques (Gaume et al. 2009).

Brief Motivational Interventions With Adolescents

Clinicians and researchers regularly note the difficulty of retaining adolescents in substance abuse treatment. Engaging adolescents in treatment has been challenging, and many adolescents have explicitly or implicitly been coerced into attending treatment. No empirical studies have provided reliable estimates of the extent and type of coercion that occurs in the process of adolescents' seeking and receiving treatment. Coercive influences can take several forms, such as exclusion from the decision-making process about seeking treatment, use of force to impose treatment on the individual, and use of restraint to retain the person in treatment (Bonnie and Monahan 2005). Coercive pressure to seek and continue treatment is not conducive to the behavior change process. Treatment providers should be sensitive to motivational barriers (Prochaska et al. 1992).

BMIs for youth with alcohol or other substance use disorders have been advocated but were not widely investigated until relatively recently (for reviews, see Monti et al. 2001; O'Leary-Tevyaw and Monti 2004). McCambridge and Strang (2004) reported a significant decrease in cannabis use at 12-week follow-up for young people ages 16–20 who participated in a single session of MI designed to reduce illicit drug use compared with nonintervention control subjects. Martin et al. (2005) conducted an uncontrolled pretest/posttest design study for 73 adolescent cannabis users. The intervention comprised an individual assessment session, followed 1 week later by a session of personalized feedback delivered in an MI style. An optional third session that focused on skills and strategies for making behavioral change was offered. Reductions were found on measures of both quantity and frequency of use and dependence; these reductions were maintained at 6-month follow-up. Regardless of the limitation of the study design, this promising approach was able to attract and retain adolescents who were not necessarily interested in change. Furthermore, the participants, most of whom perceived the intervention to be satisfactory and helpful, valued the intervention. BMI was found to be efficacious for adolescent smoking cessation (Colby et al. 1998).

Brief Motivational Interventions for Adolescents in the Emergency Department

According to the Institute of Medicine (1990), adolescents with early signs of alcohol misuse who are not seeking intervention are an important group to target in interventions because of their risk for developing significant substance abuse problems. Health care settings provide a unique opportunity to reach adolescents and are conducive to providing initial services for substance misuse and referral for additional treatment as needed. One reason to conduct interventions in medical settings, such as emergency departments, is to capi-

Table 9–1. Transcripts contrasting a directive approach with a motivational enhancement therapy (MET) approach

Assessment using a directive approach	Assessment using a MET approach	MET technique
Therapist: Tell me about your drug problem.	*Therapist:* What brings you here today?	Active listening Empathy
Tim: I don't have a drug problem.	*Tim:* I'm only here because my dad made me come.	
Therapist: What do you mean you do not have a drug problem?	*Therapist:* Tell me more about that.	Roll with resistance Maintain empathy
Tim: I use drugs, no problem…	*Tim:* My dad thinks that I have a drug problem.	
Therapist: I have reliable information in this chart about your use.	*Therapist:* Care to tell me why he thinks so?	Begin to develop discrepancy between client's understanding of his substance use disorder and the concerns of others who care for him
Tim: You sound like my dad or a probation officer.	*Tim:* I've been using and it kinda got me in trouble a couple of times.	
Therapist: Sounds like you are in denial of your drug use and consequences. We need to work on changing your negative attitude; otherwise, you could be in trouble.	*Therapist:* Sounds as if you went through some difficulties.	Active listening Empathy Further explore discrepancy
Tim: [Goes silent] I don't want to work with you.	*Tim:* I got problems in school and with the police. I don't see how coming to a place like this is gonna be helpful with that.	

Table 9–1. Transcripts contrasting a directive approach with a motivational enhancement therapy (MET) approach *(continued)*

Assessment using a directive approach	Assessment using a MET approach	MET technique
Therapist: I have a lot of experience working with teenagers like you, and I want to help you. However, you have to listen to me in order to make some changes so as not to ruin your life.	I appreciate your honesty. I am glad that we have an opportunity to talk. If you want, we can meet several times and work together to solve these problems. Shall we schedule a meeting to continue?	Roll with resistance Support self-efficacy Continue to identify opportunities to highlight discrepancy
Tim: I don't need this lecture. I'm outta here.	Well, OK.	

talize on a teachable moment or a possible window of opportunity. With respect to alcohol-abusing teens, the salience of an alcohol-related event may increase the adolescent's sense of vulnerability and thereby increase receptivity to an intervention. MI is particularly suitable for use in an emergency department due to its brevity and its fit with the teachable moment perspective.

A research group from Brown University pioneered two studies of BMI in the emergency department with adolescents and has a third study in progress. These interventions capitalized on a teachable moment; that is, the salience of an alcohol-related event may increase the adolescents' sense of vulnerability and make them more receptive to intervention (Spirito et al. 2004).

In the first study, Monti et al. (1999) evaluated the use of MI to reduce alcohol-related use and consequences among adolescents ages 18 and 19 who were being treated in an urban hospital emergency department. Ninety-four adolescents being treated in the emergency department for an alcohol-related event were randomly assigned to either a 40-minute MI intervention or a 5-minute standard care intervention (i.e., receiving a handout on avoiding drinking and driving and a substance treatment referral list). At the 6-month follow-up assessment, participants who were randomized to the MI condition were more likely to show decreased drinking and driving, traffic violations, and alcohol-related problems than were those in the standard care condition. In the second study, the same brief MI intervention was used with 152 younger adolescents (ages 13–17) treated with either brief MI or standard care in the same emergency department (Spirito et al. 2004). Both the MI and standard care resulted in reduced quantity of drinking during the 12 months of follow-up; alcohol-related negative consequences were relatively low and stayed low at follow-up in both groups. However, adolescents who screened positive for problematic alcohol use at the baseline assessment in the emergency department reported significantly more improvement in terms of average number of drinking days per month and frequency of high-volume drinking if they received MI than if they received standard care.

Components of the Motivational Interviewing Intervention

The MI intervention described in this section has been used with more than 200 adolescents recruited from the emergency department where they received care for an alcohol-related event. The intervention consists of establishing rapport, assessing drinking behavior, exploring motivation to change,

enhancing motivation with personalized feedback, establishing goals, anticipating barriers to change, and supporting coping self-efficacy.

Establishing Rapport

The MI session is introduced as an opportunity for the adolescent to talk about
his or her thoughts and feelings related to the event that resulted in the emergency department visit; to reflect on drinking and its effects; and to spend some
time, if interested, talking about ways to avoid similar negative events in the
future. The clinician should emphasize that he or she will not tell the adolescent what to do but rather that the adolescent must make his or her own choices
about drinking. The circumstances that precipitated the emergency department
visit are then reviewed, including how much the adolescent had been drinking, who was with the adolescent, and what injuries or negative consequences
resulted.

Open-ended questions are used as the primary means to develop rapport and
minimize defensiveness, thereby encouraging the adolescent to discuss recent
drinking. The clinician uses MI style (Miller 1995) to present himself or herself as empathic, concerned, nonauthoritarian, and nonjudgmental. It is important for the clinician to be respectful of the adolescent's ideas, appear
interested in hearing about the adolescent's experiences, and to not make dis-
approving statements about the adolescent's behavior.

Assessing Drinking Behavior

The assessment is used to provide personalized feedback to the adolescent
during the MI session. Measures are administered after the basic structure of
the MI session has been described to the adolescent. To provide adolescents
with a perspective on how their drinking behaviors compare with those of
other adolescents of the same gender and age, the clinician should use measures that have age and gender norms available on quantity and frequency of
drinking, such as local data and national data provided by the Monitoring the
Future survey (Johnston et al. 2008) and the Youth Risk Behavior Surveillance
survey (Centers for Disease Control and Prevention 2008).

Exploring Motivation to Change

Once the assessment is complete, the adolescent is asked what he or she likes
and does not like about drinking. Open-ended questions and reflective listening statements are used to help the adolescent generate as many likes and dis-

likes (i.e., pros and cons) about drinking as possible. The adolescent is always asked first about positive aspects of drinking (e.g., he or she is less anxious in social situations). The adolescent is also asked to elaborate on potential negative effects of such risk behaviors, including the worst thing he or she could imagine happening. Each adolescent is asked to elaborate on his or her parents' and friends' attitudes toward drinking and engaging in risky behavior while drinking. This discussion is followed by inquiring about how such attitudes might affect the youth's drinking behaviors.

This section of the MI session has several goals. First, the clinician tries to gain an understanding of how the adolescent weighs the positive and negative aspects of drinking. By listing pros and cons, the adolescent and clinician can develop a shared understanding of positive reinforcers for drinking as well as the adolescent's perceived negative consequences of drinking. Then, the clinician can tailor the MI to these personalized pros and cons, while keeping in mind the adolescent's stage of readiness for changing drinking behavior. At the end of this discussion, the clinician should also be able to identify peer and parental behaviors and attitudes that influence the adolescent's behavior and how strongly these influences affect the adolescent.

Enhancing Motivation

After exploring the adolescent's motivation to change, the clinician enhances the adolescent's understanding of his or her alcohol use, provides information about any signs of problem drinking, and encourages the adolescent in making positive changes to reduce hazardous drinking behavior. Enhancement of motivation can be done in three ways.

First, the clinician can provide personalized feedback from the assessment battery, including interpretation of the adolescent's drinking compared with age and gender norms. A computer program can be used to print a personalized feedback sheet summarizing information obtained in the assessment. Age- and gender-based normative data are used to provide feedback, in the form of percentile ranks in graphs and pie charts, on drinking frequency and quantity, frequency of drunkenness, and alcohol-related problems that have occurred with family, with friends, and at school. The printout also references signs of emotional dependence, signs of tolerance and withdrawal, and examples of risk taking related to alcohol use. The clinician decides what portions of the feedback to emphasize and what elements to de-emphasize. After providing the feedback, the clinician asks the adolescent what he or she found most surprising and what was most upsetting. The clinician needs to make sure that the adolescent interprets the meaning of the feedback correctly. For example, teens with relatively benign profiles can be encouraged to consider changes in behavior that might further limit future risk.

Second, the clinician can provide information about alcohol and alcohol's effects on adolescents in general, such as how alcohol impairs judgment and driving skills. When relevant, information about blood alcohol level and alcohol's effects on driving and other behaviors can be provided. Adolescents are tested for their blood alcohol level when admitted to the hospital, and they are typically interested in learning their blood alcohol level. They also are usually receptive to facts about the effects of alcohol at different blood alcohol levels. The fact that even very low levels of alcohol can impair driving is often a surprise to adolescents.

Finally, motivation can be enhanced by asking the adolescent to imagine the future if his or her drinking were to remain the same and if it were to change. If a discrepancy exists between an adolescent's current drinking pattern and his or her goals for the future, such a discrepancy is highlighted to try to enhance the adolescent's motivation to change. Some areas to introduce are the possible reactions of family and friends to this behavioral change. Prompts might include "What would be different (easier, harder) if you were to change your drinking?"

Establishing Goals in a Change Plan

Adolescents have a better chance of being successful at changing if they establish a plan and make a commitment to that plan. Prior to discussing a plan, the clinician should reassess the teen's interest in changing. The clinician can use open-ended questions such as "Where does this leave you now?" or "What, if anything, would you like to change?" If the adolescent is able to generate appropriate ways to reduce drinking, the clinician's main task is to help the adolescent address potential barriers to the implementation of these strategies. However, adolescents are often vague about what they will do differently, and the clinician must then help them develop a list of specific strategies. For example, an adolescent might say, "I'll just cut down on my drinking." The clinician's task in this case would be to help the adolescent specify a reduction goal that would lower the adolescent's risk. Open-ended exploration questions, such as "Tell me how you might cut down," are always tried first. If not successful, the clinician can try a more direct response: "We know that if you were to have no more than one drink an hour, your blood alcohol level would stay low. Would that be a reasonable goal?"

Developing a plan with adolescents who are not interested in making any changes in their drinking is more problematic. However, there may be some events an adolescent would like to avoid, such as getting injured after drinking. Focusing on potentially harmful behaviors, rather than alcohol consumption per se, might be a productive approach in this situation. In other cases, an adolescent may be willing to keep track of drinking, using self-monitoring procedures; this can be a useful goal, because tracking drinking may increase the adolescent's awareness of his or her drinking, especially problematic drinking.

Goal setting is most successful when goals are personalized, concrete, behavioral, and simple, and when they include a timeline. The adolescent should be encouraged to specify a time within the next few days when he or she will attempt a specific goal. A list of goals and target dates should be given to the adolescent at the end of the session. Specific and clear behavior change strategies should be listed, such as "After having an alcoholic drink, I will have a nonalcoholic drink," or "I won't 'chug' or 'shotgun' drinks." If the adolescent is unable to generate many options, the clinician can supply examples of things that other adolescents have tried. A variety of change strategies should be introduced to expose the adolescent to strategies he or she might not have envisioned but might be interested in trying. In this way, the adolescent is exposed to a number of behavior change possibilities and may use them to change behavior in the future.

Anticipating Barriers to Change

In working with the adolescent on his or her behavior change plan, the clinician should help the adolescent imagine how the change strategies might work or not work. For example, the clinician could ask how the adolescent imagines friends will react to the adolescent's decision to limit the number of drinks consumed on weekends. Asking the adolescent to anticipate what might be difficult about carrying out such a plan helps the adolescent identify ways to handle barriers to successful implementation, to refine the plan as necessary, and to develop further strategies to ensure the success of the plan. This process may also help to enhance the adolescent's feeling of self-efficacy.

Supporting Coping Self-Efficacy

Bandura (1995) defined coping self-efficacy as "one's capacity to organize and execute courses of action required to manage prospective situations" (p. 356). Coping self-efficacy has been found to increase the probability that one will resist urges and pressures to relapse. Because the adolescent needs to feel hopeful about the change plan and feel confident that it can be successful, the clinician's final task is to enhance the adolescent's sense that he or she can effectively make changes. The clinician can do this by reinforcing promising ideas, by making supportive statements about the adolescent's strengths, and by being optimistic about the adolescent's future. In addition, the clinician can state his or her belief that the adolescent has the resources to successfully carry out the change plan.

Conclusion

BMI can be a very attractive treatment option for adolescents. "It is not necessary for adolescents to admit to or acknowledge having substance use problems in order to benefit from BMI, because BMI can be applied to individuals within a range of readiness to change" (O'Leary-Tevyaw and Monti 2004, p. 65). BMI alone may not be sufficient for adolescents with high severity of alcohol or substance use disorder or with psychiatric comorbidity; however, front-loading BMI onto adolescent treatments such as CBT, as successfully reported in the Cannabis Youth Treatment study (Dennis et al. 2004), might affect proximal outcomes by improving engagement, and by providing feedback to increase readiness for change.

Cognitive-Behavioral Therapy

Cognitive-behavioral therapy approaches view substance use and related problems as learned behaviors that are initiated and maintained in the context of environmental factors. The majority of CBT approaches integrate strategies derived from classical conditioning, operant conditioning, and social learning perspectives. Experimental research within each theoretical perspective has focused on unique aspects of substance use behavior, resulting in the development of distinct intervention techniques that are often combined into a multicomponent cognitive-behavioral intervention (Dimeff and Marlatt 1995). Such interventions typically involve identifying contextual factors, such as the settings, situations, or states that may serve as potential "triggers" for abuse or relapse (Marlatt and Gordon 1985; Witkiewitz and Marlatt 2004).

Operant perspectives view substance abuse as a behavior that follows an antecedent (i.e., a trigger) and that may lead to negative consequences. This sequence is the focus of exploration in functional analysis conducted with the patient to identify triggers for substance use behavior. Intervention strategies based on operant learning often include identifying alternative reinforcers that compete with drug use and other applications of contingency management (Higgins et al. 1995). The social learning model incorporates the influence of environmental events on the acquisition of behavior, but also recognizes the role of cognitive processes in determining behavior (Bandura 1986).

Few studies have focused on the hypothesized mechanisms of change underlying CBT. Most notably, Myers and Brown (1990) found that among adolescents treated for substance use disorders, abstainers and minor relapsers were more likely to use problem-solving coping strategies than were major relapsers. Moreover, coping factors have been identified as significant predictors of treatment outcome (Myers et al. 1993). Increased self-efficacy to resist alcohol or substance use in 42 potential high-risk situations has been found to predict positive treatment outcomes in youth (Burleson and Kaminer 2005; Moss et al. 1994). The increase in self-efficacy, in addition to improved coping skills, is an important treatment objective and a proximal outcome in CBT.

Therapy sessions of CBT characteristically include modeling, behavior rehearsal, feedback, and homework assignments. It is important to take into account the adolescent's age and developmental level. Moreover, many youth may not have had sufficient opportunity to acquire certain social and coping skills normally developed during adolescence because of their heavy drug use, and components may need to be incorporated to address basic skill deficits.

Randomized Clinical Trials for Adolescent Substance Abuse Treatment

Methodological limitations characterized early treatment outcome research on cognitive-behavioral interventions for adolescent substance use disorders (Williams and Chang 2000). The mixed findings in the literature likely derived from methodological variability across studies. The emergence of formal randomized controlled trials and field experiments, however, has added significantly to the base of empirical support for CBT. These recent studies have employed more rigorous designs, with larger samples, random assignment, direct comparisons of two or more active treatments, improved measures of substance use and other variables, manual-guided interventions, and longer-term outcome assessments (Waldron and Turner 2008). These findings, taken together, establish the foundation for the effectiveness of CBT for adolescent substance use disorders.

Kaminer et al. (1998, 2002) reported on two studies evaluating a group CBT intervention for outpatient adolescent substance abusers. In the first study, adolescents were randomly assigned to 12 sessions of CBT or to a similar number of interactional group therapy sessions. Youth were all dually diagnosed. No patient-treatment matching effects between psychopathologies (i.e., externalizing disorders, internalizing disorders) and treatment modalities (i.e., CBT, interactional therapy) were found (Kaminer et al. 1998). However, the short-term efficacy of CBT was significant. Adolescents assigned to CBT showed a greater short-term improvement than those assigned to interactional therapy. As in other adolescent treatment-outcome studies, however, relapse was a problem for many youth, and differences between the groups were no longer significant a year later (Kaminer and Burleson 1999).

In a larger-scale randomized controlled trial, Kaminer et al. (2002) compared the efficacy of CBT with that of psychoeducational therapy for adolescent substance abusers. The predominantly dually diagnosed adolescents were randomly assigned to one of the two 8-week group interventions. For older youth and for males, the CBT group showed significantly lower rates of positive urinalysis than the psychoeducational therapy group at 3-month follow-up. Contrary to hypotheses, CBT did not produce any long-term differential relapse rate compared with psychoeducational therapy. However, most of the participants improved substantially in a variety of life domains. The majority of assessed substance use–related problems showed improvements at 3-month posttreatment follow-up and continued to improve at 9-month follow-up, relative to baseline, regardless of assigned treatment condition.

Marijuana use outcome was examined in a randomized clinical trial comparing individual CBT, functional family therapy (FFT), joint FFT and CBT, and group psychoeducational therapy (Waldron et al. 2001). At 4 months posttreatment, adolescents assigned to FFT and combined FFT+CBT interventions showed significant reductions in marijuana use, but at 7 months posttreatment, only those assigned to the joint and group therapy conditions showed significant reductions in use. The finding that CBT alone did not produce significant reductions in use at 4 and 7 months posttreatment is not consistent with other research (e.g., Dennis et al. 2004). However, treatment effects likely vary depending on the severity of the adolescent's use, and the form and dosage of treatment (Waldron et al. 2001).

The Cannabis Youth Treatment study was a randomized field experiment that compared a total of five interventions, in various combinations, across four implementation sites (Dennis et al. 2004). The study was designed to address the differential efficacy of the treatments implemented and the effect of treatment dosage on outcome. Two group CBT interventions were offered. Both began with two individual motivational enhancement sessions, followed by either three CBT sessions (MET/CBT-5; Sampl and Kadden 2001) or 10 CBT sessions (MET/CBT-12; Webb et al. 2002). A third intervention represented a family-based add-on intervention involving MET/CBT-12 plus a 6-week family psychoeducational intervention (Hamilton et al. 2001). In addition, a 12-session individual adolescent community reinforcement approach (Godley et al. 2006) and a 12-week multidimensional family therapy condition (Liddle 2002) were included. The five treatment models were evaluated in two arms, in a community-based program and an academic medical center. Although all five models were not implemented within a single treatment site, the replication of the MET/CBT-5 intervention across all four sites made it possible to study site differences and conduct quasi-experimental comparisons of the interventions across study arms.

Overall, 600 adolescents ages 13–18 years were randomly assigned to one of three interventions. With follow-up rates of 98% at 3 months and 94% at 12 months, Dennis et al. (2004) reported that all five interventions produced significant reductions in cannabis use and negative consequences of use from pretreatment to the 3-month follow-up, and that these reductions were sustained through the 12-month follow-up. In addition, changes in marijuana use were accompanied by reductions in behavioral problems, family problems, school problems, school absences, argumentativeness, violence, and illegal activity.

Nevertheless, these initial differences were not sustained, and the best predictor of long-term outcomes was initial level of change. The cost-effectiveness ratio was found to be higher for multidimensional family therapy than for the other interventions (French et al. 2002).

Treatment Modality: Group Versus Individual Intervention

The consistent empirical support of group CBT for substance-abusing adolescents (Burleson et al. 2006; Kaminer 2005) stands in contrast to the iatrogenic "deviant" peer-group effects reported for group interventions (Dishion et al. 1999). Neither the Cannabis Youth Treatment study group interventions nor Waldron et al.'s (2001) and Kaminer et al.'s (2002) studies in outpatient settings, which included a significant percentage of adolescents with conduct disorders, demonstrated any severe or unmanageable problems in conducting group therapy (e.g., need to eject subjects, need to discontinue a session, physical abuse). It appears that diverse referral sources allow for a mix of adolescents who are manageable in a group setting once a clearly communicated and signed behavioral contract for ground rules is introduced. Experienced therapists can competently address inappropriate behavior and other "troubleshooting," particularly in a manual-driven treatment.

Contingency Management Reinforcement Approach

Contingency management reinforcement procedures provide rewards for clean (i.e., negative) urinalysis. Drug abstinence can be improved by providing tangible incentives that are contingent on providing objective evidence of abstinence. An abstinence reinforcement system used in combination with an intensive behavioral treatment program has produced impressive outcomes in adult substance abusers (Higgins et al. 1994; Silverman et al. 1996). However, despite compelling evidence regarding the efficacy and the wide acceptability and applicability of these procedures, only limited data have been reported on testing contingency management procedures with adolescents. Noncontrolled, nonrandomized trials generated acceptable feasibility and promising efficacy of contingency management among adolescents in reducing use of cannabis (Kamon et al. 2005), tobacco (Corby et al. 2000; Roll 2005), and multiple drugs (Lott and Jenicus 2009). In randomized controlled studies of 1) contingency management in addition to multisystemic therapy compared with multisystemic therapy only in juvenile drug courts (Henggeler et al. 2006) and 2) contingency management in addition to CBT compared with CBT only (Y. Kaminer, J.A. Burleson, R. Burke, unpublished data, April 2010), no significant improvement was found for adding contingency management. These results suggest the need to continue developing contingency management–based approaches in order to improve efficacy.

Rationale and Application in Clinical Settings

Contingency management treatment is based on the scientific principles and conceptual framework of behavior analysis and behavioral pharmacology. In that framework, the use of abused drugs is considered a special case of operant behavior maintained by the reinforcing effects of the drugs involved. Higgins et al. (1994) stressed the following core strengths of contingency management: 1) conceptual clarity, 2) empiricism and operationalism, 3) compatibility with pharmacotherapies, 4) clinical breadth, and 5) demonstrable efficacy.

The strategy employed in contingency management is to rearrange the substance user's environment so that 1) drug use and abstinence are readily detected, 2) drug abstinence is positively reinforced, 3) drug use results in an immediate loss of reinforcement, and 4) the density of reinforcement derived from nondrug sources is increased to compete with the reinforcing effects of drugs.

Controlled clinical research has demonstrated the efficacy of contingency management in laboratory animals and adults with various substances of abuse. In addition to the obvious need to reduce or eliminate drug use, other behaviors to reinforce through contingency management may include clinic behavior, compliance with treatment plans, and changes in behaviors or lifestyle that may facilitate abstinence.

The treatment regimen based on contingency management procedures has shown excellent feasibility and is highly acceptable to patients. The vast majority of individuals who have been offered the treatment have accepted. Treatment acceptability is very important, in particular among individuals with substance use disorder, who are often unmotivated for initiation and/or maintenance of treatment. The contingency management treatment is also effective in retaining patients in treatment. It is noteworthy that use of marijuana (the most commonly abused drug in adolescence) is readily modifiable via a direct contingency management intervention, although such changes appear to dissipate when the contingency is removed (Stanger and Budney, in press).

Contingency management procedures can use a variety of reinforcers, many of which are commonly used in, or readily adaptable to, standard clinic settings for adolescents. These include cash, vouchers, and on-site retail items. Public opinion may be opposed to such procedures, even if efficacious, because of concerns regarding the likelihood that patients will use reinforcers to purchase drugs. However, these rewards are too little to maintain a "drug habit," and the frequent monitoring of urine for drugs precludes the possibility of continued use without detection.

A point that needs to be addressed is the cost involved in operating a contingency management system for adolescents in which cash or vouchers are used. Those who subscribe to the moral model of addiction (i.e., that addiction is a form of immoral and criminal behavior) may perceive these reinforcers as "bribes" given to bad people for compliance with treatment. However, the behavioral processes, the effectiveness of the treatment, and the economic advantage of this strategy need to be emphasized more than the nature of the incentives used. Contrary to public perception, the costs of adding contingency management to the treatment plan are small in comparison with the costs incurred with any treatment program for individuals with substance use disorder along a similar time period or the costs involved in addressing drug-related problems for the participant, family, and community. The relatively low cost of contingency management procedures ($1–$10 per day) and the reported efficacy of such programs in retaining adults in treatment suggest that contingency management procedures will be less costly to administer than standard treatment programs in both the short term and the long term. These findings lend additional support for the rationale to expand contingency management procedures to adolescent treatment settings (Stanger et al. 2009).

In conclusion, although preliminary data provide support for the feasibility and preliminary efficacy of implementing contingency management in youth with substance use disorder, additional controlled efficacy studies with larger samples are needed.

Practical Implications

Petry et al. (2000) recommended that the following checklist be used when designing and implementing contingency management procedures:

1. Target the most important behavior to be changed. Choose one that can be quantified objectively and that occurs frequently (e.g., marijuana use).

2. Choose a reinforcer. Vouchers, cash, and prizes are desirable reinforcers for clients and agreeable to staff.

3. Use behavioral principles, and keep the system simple so that staff can apply it consistently and clients can understand it.

4. Draw up a time-limited behavioral contract. Be specific regarding the targeted behavior, monitoring procedures, and reinforcement schedule.

5. Ensure consistent implementation of the contract by staff and clients.

6. Continually improve the contingency management procedures by keeping records, consulting with staff, and receiving feedback from clients regarding problems in the implementation process and what or does or does not work.

Key Clinical Concepts

- The theoretical basis of brief motivational interventions is grounded in client-centered therapy.

- The six active ingredients of effective brief interventions are represented by the acronym FRAMES: Feedback, Responsibility for change, Advice to change, Menu of alternative change options, therapist Empathy, and Self-efficacy.

- The purported mechanisms of action, or mediators, in CBT include self-efficacy and behavioral skills.

- The consistent empirical support of group CBT for substance-abusing adolescents stands in contrast to the iatrogenic "deviant" peer-group effects reported for group interventions.

- Contingency management reinforcement appears to be a promising approach for youth with substance use disorders.

References

Apodaca TR, Longabaugh R: Mechanisms of change in motivational interviewing: a review and preliminary evaluation of the evidence. Addiction 104:705–715, 2009

Bandura A: Social Learning Theory. Englewood Cliffs, NJ, Prentice Hall, 1977

Bandura A: Social Foundations of Thought and Action: A Social Cognitive Theory. Englewood Cliffs, NJ, Prentice Hall, 1986

Bandura A: Exercise of personal and collective efficacy in changing societies, in Self-Efficacy in Changing Societies. Edited by Bandura A. New York, Cambridge University Press, 1995, pp 355–394

Bonnie RJ, Monahan J: From coercion to contract: reframing the debate on mandated community treatment for people with mental disorders. Law Hum Behav 29:485–503, 2005

Bukstein OG, Winters K: Salient variables for treatment research of adolescent alcohol and other substance use disorders. Addiction 99 (suppl 2):23–37, 2004

Burleson JA, Kaminer Y: Self-efficacy as a predictor of treatment outcome in adolescent substance use disorders. Addict Behav 30:1751–1764, 2005

Burleson JA, Kaminer Y, Dennis ML: Absence of iatrogenic or contagion effects in adolescent group therapy: findings from the Cannabis Youth Treatment (CYT) study. Am J Addictions 15 (suppl 1):4–15, 2006

Centers for Disease Control and Prevention: Youth Risk Behavior Surveillance. United States, 2007. Atlanta, GA, National Center for Chronic Disease Prevention and Health Promotion, 2008

Colby SM, Monti PM, Barnett NP, et al: Brief motivational interviewing in a hospital setting for adolescent smoking: a preliminary study. J Consult Clin Psychol 66:574–578, 1998

Corby EA, Roll JM, Ledgerwood DM, et al: Contingency management interventions for treating the substance abuse of adolescents: a feasibility study. Exp Clin Psychopharmacol 8:371–376, 2000

Dennis M, Godley SH, Diamond G, et al: The Cannabis Youth Treatment (CYT) study: main findings from two randomized trials. J Subst Abuse Treat 27:197–213, 2004

Dimeff LA, Marlatt GA: Relapse prevention, in Handbook of Alcoholism Treatment Approaches: Effective Alternatives. Edited by Hester RK, Miller WR. Boston, MA, Allyn & Bacon, 1995, pp 176–194

Dishion TJ, McCord J, Poulin F: When interventions harm: peer groups and problem behavior. Am Psychol 54:755–764, 1999

French MT, Roebuck MC, Dennis ML, et al: The economic cost of outpatient marijuana treatment for adolescents: findings from a multi-site field experiment. Addiction 97 (suppl 1):84–97, 2002

Gaume J, Gmel G, Faouzi M, et al: Counselor skill influences outcomes of brief motivational interventions. J Subst Abuse Treat 37:151–159, 2009

Gil AG, Wagner EF, Tubman JG: Culturally sensitive substance abuse intervention for Hispanic and African American adolescents: empirical examples from the Alcohol Treatment Targeting Adolescents in Need (ATTAIN) project. Addiction 99 (suppl 2):140–150, 2004

Godley SH, Meyers RJ, Smith JE, et al: The adolescent community reinforcement approach for adolescent cannabis users (DHHS Publ No SMA-01-3489). Cannabis Youth Treatment (CYT) Manual Series, Vol 4. Rockville, MD, Center for Substance Abuse Treatment, Substance Abuse and Mental Health Services Administration, 2006. Available at: http://www.chestnut.org/li/cyt/products/acra_cyt_v4.pdf. Accessed January 2, 2010.

Hamilton N, Brantly L, Tims F, et al: Family support network (FSN) for adolescent cannabis users (DHHS Publ No SMA-01-3488). Cannabis Youth Treatment (CYT) Manual Series, Vol 4. Rockville, MD, Center for Substance Abuse, Substance Abuse and Mental Health Services Administration, 2001

Henggeler SW, Halliday-Boykins CA, Cunningham PB, et al: Juvenile drug-court: enhancing outcomes by integrating evidence-based treatments. J Consult Clin Psychol 74:42–54, 2006

Higgins ST, Budney AJ, Bickel WK: Applying behavioral concepts and principles to the treatment of cocaine dependence. Drug Alcohol Depend 34:87–97, 1994

Higgins ST, Budney AJ, Bickel WK, et al: Outpatient behavioral treatment for cocaine dependence: one-year outcome. Exp Clin Psychopharmacol 3:205–212, 1995

Hill KG, White HR, Chung I, et al: Early adult outcomes of adolescent binge drinking: person- and variable-centered analyses of binge drinking trajectories. Alcohol Clin Exp Res 24:892–901, 2000

Institute of Medicine: Broadening the Base of Treatment for Alcohol Problems. Washington, DC, National Academy Press, 1990

Johnston LD, O'Malley PM, Bachman JG, et al: Monitoring the Future National Survey Results on Drug Use, 1975–2007, Volume I: Secondary School Students (NIH Publ No 08-6418A). Bethesda, MD, National Institute on Drug Abuse, 2008

Kaminer Y: Challenges and opportunities of group therapy for adolescent substance abuse: a critical review. Addict Behav 30:1765–1774, 2005

Kaminer Y, Bukstein OG: Adolescent Substance Abuse: Psychiatric Comorbidity and High-Risk Behavior. New York, Routledge/Taylor & Francis, 2008

Kaminer Y, Burleson J: Psychotherapies for adolescent substance abusers: 15-month follow-up of a pilot study. Am J Addict 8:114–119, 1999

Kaminer Y, Blitz C, Burleson J, et al: Psychotherapies for adolescent substance abusers: treatment outcome. J Nerv Ment Dis 186:684–690, 1998

Kaminer Y, Burleson J, Goldberger R: Psychotherapies for adolescent substance abusers: short- and long-term outcomes. J Nerv Ment Dis 190:737–745, 2002

Kamon J, Budney A, Stanger C: A contingency management intervention for adolescent marijuana abuse and conduct problems. J Am Acad Child Adolesc Psychiatry 44:513–521, 2005

Karno MP, Longabaugh R: Less directiveness by therapists improves drinking outcomes of reactant clients in alcoholism treatment. J Consult Clin Psychol 73:262–267, 2005

Liddle HA: Multidimensional family therapy treatment (MDFT) for adolescent cannabis users (DHHS Publ No 02-3660). The Cannabis Youth Treatment (CYT) Manual Series, Vol 5. Rockville, MD, Center for Substance Abuse, Substance Abuse and Mental Health Services Administration, 2002

Lott DC, Jenicus S: Effectiveness of very low-cost contingency management in a community adolescent treatment program. Drug Alcohol Depend 102:162–165, 2009

Maisto SA, Conigliaro J, McNeil M, et al: Factor structure of the SOCRATES in a sample of primary care patients. Addict Behav 24:879–892, 1999

Marlatt GA, Gordon JR: Relapse Prevention: Maintenance Strategies in the Treatment of Addictive Behaviors. New York, Guilford, 1985

Martin G, Copeland J, Swift W: The Adolescent Cannabis Check-Up: feasibility of a brief intervention for young cannabis users. J Subst Abuse Treat 29:207–213, 2005

McCambridge J, Strang J: The efficacy of single-session motivational interviewing in reducing drug consumption and perceptions of drug-related risk and harm among young people: results from a multi-site cluster randomized trial. Addiction 99:39–52, 2004

McLellan AT, Woody GE, Luborsky L: Increased effectiveness of substance abuse treatment: a prospective study of patient-treatment matching. J Nerv Ment Dis 171:597–605, 1983

Miller WR: The ethics of motivational interviewing revisited. Behav Cogn Psychother 23:345–348, 1995

Miller WR, Rollnick S: Motivational Interviewing: Preparing People for Change, 2nd Edition. New York, Guilford, 2002

Miller WR, Sanchez V: Motivating young adults for treatment and lifestyle change, in Issues in Alcohol Use and Misuse by Young Adults. Edited by Howard G, Nathan P. Notre Dame, IN, University of Notre Dame Press 1994, pp 51–81

Monti PM, Colby SM, Barnett NP, et al: Brief intervention for harm reduction with alcohol-positive older adolescents in a hospital emergency department. J Consult Clin Psychol 67:989–994, 1999

Monti PM, Colby SM, O'Leary TA: Adolescents, Alcohol, and Substance Abuse: Reaching Teens Through Brief Interventions. New York, Guilford, 2001

Moss HB, Kirisci L, Mezzich AC: Psychiatric comorbidity and self-efficacy to resist heavy drinking in alcoholic and nonalcoholic adolescents. Am J Addict 3:204–212, 1994

Moyers TB, Martin T, Christopher PJ, et al: Client language as a mediator of motivational interviewing efficacy: where is the evidence? Alcohol Clin Exp Res 31 (suppl 10):40S–47S, 2007

Myers MG, Brown S: Coping and appraisal in relapse risk situations among substance abusing adolescents following treatment. J Adolesc Chemical Dep 1:95–105, 1990

Myers MG, Brown S, Mott V: Coping as a predictor of adolescent substance abuse treatment outcome. J Subst Abuse 5:15–29, 1993

O'Leary-Tevyaw T, Monti PM: Motivational enhancement and other brief interventions for adolescent substance abuse: foundations, applications and evaluations. Addiction 99 (suppl 2):63–75, 2004

Petry NM, Petrakis I, Trevisan L: A comprehensive guide to the application of contingency management procedures in clinical settings. Drug Alcohol Depend 58:9–25, 2000

Prochaska JO, DiClemente CC, Norcross JC: In search of how people change: applications to addictive behaviors. Am Psychol 47:1102–1114, 1992

Project MATCH: Matching alcoholism treatments to client heterogeneity: Project MATCH posttreatment drinking outcomes. J Stud Alcohol 58:7–29, 1997

Rogers CR: The necessary and sufficient conditions of therapeutic personality change. J Consult Psychol 21:95–103, 1957

Roll JM: Assessing the feasibility of using contingency management to modify cigarette smoking by adolescents. J Appl Behav Anal 38:463–467, 2005

Sampl S, Kadden R: Motivational enhancement therapy and cognitive behavioral therapy for adolescent cannabis users: 5 sessions (DHHS Publ No SMA-01-3486). Cannabis Youth Treatment Series, Vol 1. Rockville, MD, Center for Substance Abuse Treatment, Substance Abuse and Mental Health Services Administration, 2001

Silverman K, Higgins ST, Brooner RK, et al: Sustained cocaine abstinence in methadone maintenance patients through voucher-based reinforcement therapy. Arch Gen Psychiatry 53:409–415, 1996

Spirito A, Monti PM, Barnett NP, et al: A randomized clinical trial of a brief motivational intervention for alcohol-positive adolescents treated in an emergency department. J Pediatr 145:396–402, 2004

Stanger C, Budney AJ: Contingency management approaches for adolescent substance use disorders. Child Adolesc Psychiatr Clin N America (in press)

Stanger C, Budney AJ, Kamon JL, et al: A randomized trial of contingency management for adolescent marijuana abuse and dependence. Drug Alcohol Dep 105:240–247, 2009

Waldron HB, Turner CW: Evidence-based psychosocial treatments for adolescent substance abuse. J Clin Child Adolesc Psychol 37:238–261, 2008

Waldron HB, Slesnick N, Brody J, et al: Treatment outcomes for adolescent substance abuse at 4- and 7-month assessments. J Consult Clin Psychol 69:802–813, 2001

Webb C, Scudder M, Kaminer Y, et al: The motivational enhancement therapy and cognitive behavioral therapy supplement: 7 sessions of cognitive behavioral therapy for adolescent cannabis users. Cannabis Youth Treatment (CYT) Series, Vol 2 (DHHS Publ No SMA-02-3659). Rockville, MD, Center for Substance Abuse Treatment, Substance Abuse and Mental Health Services Administration, 2002

Williams RJ, Chang SY: A comprehensive and comparative review of adolescent substance abuse treatment outcome. Clinical Psychology: Science and Practice 7:138–166, 2000

Witkiewitz K, Marlatt GA: Relapse prevention for alcohol and drug problems: that was Zen, this is Tao. Am Psychol 59:224–235, 2004

Relevant Website

Motivational Interviewing (resources for clinicians, researchers, and trainers): http://www.motivationalinterview.org/

10

The Adolescent Community Reinforcement Approach and Multidimensional Family Therapy

Addressing Relapse During Treatment

Gayle A. Dakof, Ph.D.

Susan H. Godley, Rh.D.

Jane Ellen Smith, Ph.D.

Adolescent substance abuse treatments that involve family members and that seek to change or influence an adolescent's environment have demonstrated considerable efficacy in numerous randomized clinical trials (Austin et al. 2005; Dennis et al. 2004; Rigter et al. 2005; Vaughn and Howard 2008; Waldron and Turner 2008). Compared with standard care, these treatments have demonstrated superiority in enrolling and retaining youth in substance abuse treatment, and in reducing not only drug use but also psychiatric comorbidity. A shared assumption among approaches is that adolescents are part of multiple systems, which are critical to incorporate as change agents or to address during treatment. In this chapter, we highlight two of these approaches, the adolescent community reinforcement approach (A-CRA) and multidimensional family therapy (MDFT), by presenting certain core interventions, practice guidelines, and principles of A-CRA and of MDFT in the context of case illustrations of how each approach addresses relapse during a treatment episode.

Few would deny that the prevention of relapse is an important goal of substance abuse treatment or that the probability of relapse or continued use among adolescents is extremely high (e.g., Brown et al. 2001; Dennis et al. 2004; Williams and Chang 2000; Latimer et al. 2000). Research has identified pretreatment, during-treatment, and posttreatment factors that may influence relapse, and although this research has been very illuminating, we argue that during-treatment factors have been unnecessarily narrow (i.e., length of treatment, extent of family involvement) and suggest that investigating how specific treatment approaches address relapse during treatment may offer insight into heretofore unidentified or underinvestigated factors. Family-based models and community reinforcement approaches generally, and MDFT and A-CRA in particular, acknowledge that relapse is an expected occurrence during adolescent substance abuse treatment, as well as an opportunity for growth and learning. Both A-CRA and MDFT delineate specific guidelines and procedures to address relapse that occurs during a treatment episode, and to prevent and minimize the harm of posttreatment relapse.

The Adolescent Community Reinforcement Approach

A-CRA is a behavioral intervention developed to treat adolescents with substance use disorders. It has been widely implemented through funding from the Center for Substance Abuse Treatment (Center for Substance Abuse Treatment 2006, 2009) and other sources in more than 50 treatment agencies in 20 states. Originally developed in the 1970s and 1980s as an approach to treat adults with alcohol disorders (Azrin 1976; Azrin et al. 1982; Hunt and Azrin 1973), the intervention was adapted for adolescents, manualized, and evaluated as part of the Cannabis Youth Treatment study (Dennis et al. 2004; Godley et al. 2001). A-CRA also has been evaluated in randomized clinical trials of assertive continuing care (Godley et al. 2007) and as an intervention with homeless adolescents in the southwestern United States (Slesnick et al. 2007).

The overall style of A-CRA is behavioral or cognitive-behavioral. Therapists are trained to identify an adolescent's individual reinforcers and those of his or her caregivers. Once these reinforcers are identified, the therapist helps the adolescent and family draw the relationships between attaining reinforcers and reducing or stopping substance use. For example, an adolescent may want to "get off" probation or attend college. A parent may want his or her adolescent to get a good job one day or just stop "getting in trouble." These reinforcers can be used as therapists discuss with adolescents and parents why it is important to attend sessions, learn and practice new skills, and sample periods of not using substances. Another primary goal of A-CRA is to increase the family, social, and educational or vocational reinforcers of an adolescent, so that the adolescent's environment will increasingly support recovery. Conversely, if an adolescent uses alcohol or other drugs, then a time-out from these reinforcers occurs (based on Hunt and Azrin 1973). To facilitate engagement and retention, the therapist uses warmth, uses understanding statements, and is nonjudgmental.

The A-CRA manual (Godley et al. 2006) developed for the Cannabis Youth Treatment study outlines an outpatient program that targets youth ages 12–18 years with cannabis, alcohol, and/or other substance use disorders, as diagnosed using the *Diagnostic and Statistical Manual of Mental Disorders*, 4th Edition, Text Revision (American Psychiatric Association 2000). However, A-CRA also has been implemented in intensive outpatient and residential treatment settings (Godley et al. 2009). A-CRA includes guidelines for three types of sessions: adolescents alone, parents/caregivers alone, and adolescents and parents/caregivers together. Treatment begins with an overview of what the adolescent can expect and emphasizes that the goal of therapy is to help the adolescent have a more satisfying life.

Subsequent sessions are very flexible, and the clinician draws from a toolbox of 17 treatment procedures to help adolescents improve their quality of life and decrease or eliminate alcohol and/or drug use. Clinicians are taught to introduce each procedure with a rationale so the adolescent can understand how the techniques will be beneficial. One group of these procedures facilitates ongoing assessment and goal setting. For example, the Functional Analysis of Substance Use and the Functional Analysis of Prosocial Behaviors help the adolescent understand what patterns are associated with those behaviors and their positive and negative consequences. Then, the clinician and adolescent can discuss how these patterns might be changed. The Happiness Scale and the Goals of Counseling show that the therapist cares about the adolescents' happiness in important life areas and wants to help them achieve the goals they care about. Other procedures target skill building, including Problem Solving and Communication Skills to help adolescents learn how to address challenges and enhance their relationships. Because it is important for adolescents to engage in enjoyable activities without alcohol or drugs, there are procedures for increasing these activities, as well as a procedure called Systematic Encouragement to help the adolescent break down what will be needed to try out a new skill or activity and provide the adolescent the opportunity to try a first step during a therapy session. Some procedures, such as Anger Management and Job Seeking Skills, will be used only if needed by a particular adolescent. Two sessions are designed for caregivers alone, and two more are for caregivers and adolescents to work together on improving their relationship(s). These four sessions with caregivers are considered the minimum number; more can be added if needed. Role-playing/behavioral rehearsal is a critical component of the skills training components (e.g., Drug Refusal, Problem Solving).

Every session ends with a mutually agreed-upon homework assignment to either practice skills learned during sessions or engage in a new prosocial activity after potential barriers to completing the assignment are discussed and addressed through problem solving. To reinforce completion of homework, which helps ensure generalization of skills learned in sessions to the adolescent's natural environment, the clinician begins each session with a review of the homework assignment from the previous session.

Case Illustration

The following case illustrates how an A-CRA therapist would work with a youth who has had a relapse. Most A-CRA sessions are with the adolescent alone, and it is most often in this context that the therapist recognizes that an adolescent has had a relapse. Parents or others may ultimately play an important role in the relapse prevention plan, as described below. The clinician follows a

Table 10–1. Therapist guidelines for adolescent community reinforcement approach (A-CRA) sessions

1. The A-CRA clinician is positive, enthusiastic, and nonjudgmental during interactions with adolescents and caregivers. At the same time, the clinician provides guidelines and direction during sessions.

2. The clinician consistently identifies the adolescent's and caregivers' reinforcers and helps them see how changes in their behavior can help attain these reinforcers. A behavioral approach is based on the premise that reinforcers will, by definition, be potent motivators for change. A prime example of this is A-CRA's emphasis on a satisfying but healthy social and recreational life to replace activities that have been dominated by substance use.

3. The clinician understands the importance of checking for generalization of newly learned behaviors in the adolescent's and caregivers' lives outside of the session. This is why A-CRA clinicians work with the adolescent and caregivers to design homework assignments at the end of each session and check back regarding homework completion during each session.

4. Procedures are introduced at clinically meaningful times for the most impact. Clinicians are expected to "weave" procedures into the session based on the adolescent's needs, rather than awkwardly announcing, "Today, we are going to do such and such procedure." Appropriate introduction of procedures translates into their having more meaning for the participant and greater generalization to real-world applications.

5. Caregivers and other individuals who are important in the adolescent's life are involved in sessions or as part of case management activities. These individuals can help create either a positive and supportive environment for the adolescent or one that is negative and punishing. The A-CRA caregiver procedures are designed to increase the positive nature of these relationships.

number of guidelines (see Table 10–1) during a session, regardless of the session content, and many of these are illustrated in the sample session dialogue that follows.

The youth in this case example, Tom, is 15 years old. He lives with his mother and sister. His drug of choice is marijuana, and he has struggled in school and been referred for treatment by the juvenile justice authority. Before the session described below, the therapist met with Tom several times. They have already completed a Functional Analysis (of Substance Use and Prosocial Behaviors) and the Happiness Scale, worked together on Goals of Counseling, and learned and practiced communication and problem-solving skills. The therapist also has had two sessions with Tom's mother, during which the therapist described the A-CRA intervention, provided her the opportunity to talk about what she wanted for her son and her frustrations related to her son's behaviors, and reviewed important parenting skills (with an emphasis on what Tom's mother was already doing well). Prior to the session described below, Tom provided a urine test, and it was positive for marijuana.

First Session

> THERAPIST: I'm really glad that you came to your session today. You knew there was a possibility that we would do a drug screen, and I'm guessing you also knew how it would turn out, so I think it is really good that this didn't keep you from coming.
>
> TOM: Yeah. I had a relapse.
>
> THERAPIST: What do you think about us talking about that—you know, looking at what happened, and thinking of ways you can avoid future relapses? Are you okay with that?
>
> TOM: Yeah.
>
> THERAPIST: Let's talk about what happened. I'll fill in another road map [Functional Analysis], and we can see if it adds anything to the one we did during your first session.
>
> TOM: There's not much to say. My girlfriend broke up with me. On my way home, J.T. was feeling sorry for me and offered me some weed. When I got home, I smoked it.
>
> THERAPIST: Gee, I'm really sorry about your girlfriend—that's really tough. We can definitely talk more about that if you'd like to. If it's OK with you, I'd like to just stick with the relapse for a minute though. You said J.T. was feeling sorry for you. What were you doing or saying that made him feel sorry for you? Looking at your prior road map, you said that your internal triggers were feeling sad and lonely. Do you think he was responding to that?
>
> TOM: I guess so. I was pretty mad too.
>
> THERAPIST: I understand. That makes sense. So I'm listing all of these feelings in the Internal Triggers column on your new road map [see Column 2 of Figure 10–1]. Do you remember why we try to identify internal triggers?
>
> TOM: So I don't keep smoking every time I feel upset.
>
> THERAPIST: That's correct. You were definitely right on target a few weeks ago when you said that feeling sad and lonely could lead you to a relapse. And here's some new information you've just come up with: feeling mad can set you up to smoke too. So we have to help you figure out a way to

do something different the next time you feel sad, lonely, or mad—so that you have more options to start feeling better besides smoking.

TOM: I could use more options. I can't keep getting in trouble.

THERAPIST: Before we figure out options, let's make sure we have the whole picture of what was going on when you decided to get high. Let's look at the external triggers now [Column 1 of Figure 10–1]. Like you told me before, you smoke alone at home after school. Now you mentioned that J.T. gave you the weed.

TOM: Yes. And I even told him that I'd better not. But when he kept pushing it my way, I just took it. I'm not saying it's his fault though. He didn't force me to smoke.

THERAPIST: He didn't force you to smoke, but he made it *easier* for you to smoke. It will be important for us to practice some drug refusal skills before we're done today. These are assertiveness skills that focus on ways to turn down offers of drugs from friends.

I've already listed the using behavior [Column 3 of Figure 10–1]. Let's go over the positive consequences of your smoking in this specific situation [Column 4 in Figure 10–1]. When we did your first road map, you said that some of the things you liked about getting high were feeling relaxed and mellow. Do these fit here?

TOM: Yes. But I especially like what I *don't* feel—or think—when I'm high: I don't think about or feel much of anything, which is *exactly* what I wanted. I didn't want to be thinking about my girlfriend.

THERAPIST: OK. And when you aren't having any unpleasant thoughts or feelings, are you having any positive feelings that you can identify? Think back to when you were physically feeling relaxed and mellow in that situation. What were some positive feelings?

TOM: Maybe I was feeling...I don't know...content? Not sure I'd say happy.

THERAPIST: I'll put "happy" with a question mark then. And I bet you can tell me *why* we're looking at the positive things you associate with smoking weed. Do you remember why we spend time on this?

TOM: I think you said it has something to do with why I get high in the first place.

THERAPIST: Good! We figure that you keep choosing to smoke in these situations because it gives you a number of positive things, like it helps you feel relaxed and content, and you don't have to think about unpleasant things. And so what do we need to do?

TOM: I need to not smoke.

THERAPIST: Yes, I'm hoping you continue to think that way. But it seems like we'd better come up with a plan so that you can get some of these positive things the next time you're sad or mad—but without your having to smoke.

External triggers	Internal triggers	Using behavior
1. *Who* were you with when you used? Nobody—but had just seen JT	1. What were you *thinking* about right before you used? Was thinking all sorts of things— like why my girlfriend broke up with me	1. *What* did you use? Marijuana
2. *Where* did you use? Home-bedroom	2. What were you *feeling physically* right before you used? Don't know	2. *How much* did you use? 1 small blunt
3. *When* did you use? After school	3. What were you *feeling emotionally* right before you used? Mad, sad, lonely	3. Over *how long* a period of time did you use? 1 hour

Short-term positive consequences	Long-term negative consequences
1. What did you like about using with (*nobody*)? *Nobody bothered me*	1. What are the negative results of your using in each of these areas? a. Interpersonal *Mom will be really upset; a little mad at JT for giving me marijuana (he knows I've gotten in trouble for it already)*
2. What did you like about using (*in bedroom*)? *Wouldn't get caught*	b. Physical *Nothing*
3. What did you like about using (*after school*)? *I needed to do something then because I was upset and I knew my mom was at work*	c. Emotional *Problem didn't go away—I still feel upset, and now I'm mad at myself for relapsing*
4. What were the pleasant *thoughts* you had while using? *I wasn't thinking much of anything, which is exactly what I wanted; I wasn't thinking about my girlfriend*	d. Legal *Not sure—but it can't be good*
5. What were the pleasant *physical feelings* you had while using? *Relaxed, mellow*	e. Job/School *Didn't study that night and so failed a test the next day*
6. What were the pleasant *emotions* you had while using? *Content, happy?*	f. Financial *None* g. Other

Figure 10–1. Adolescent community reinforcement approach (A-CRA) functional analysis for relapse.

TOM: Sounds good to me.

THERAPIST: I'm glad you're on board. Let me ask first, though, if you remember talking about the negative or the "not-so-good" consequences associated with smoking?

TOM: Yup. We can start again with my mom being upset with me. Oh, and I didn't study that night when I was high, so I failed a test the next day.

THERAPIST: I'm going to add these to your new road map [Column 5 of Figure 10–1].

The therapist then discusses additional negative consequences and works with Tom to develop a relapse prevention plan. Some refusal skills training is included. In this case, the therapist believes that Tom's mother could be a helpful part of this plan. The conversation resumes at this point in the session.

THERAPIST: Based on what we know from this new road map and the earlier one, it looks like we need to find some things for you to do when you get upset so that you don't have to smoke. We'll probably have to find some immediate thing you can do, but I am also wondering about all the time you spend alone in your room in the evenings. We have talked a little about this before, and about how being lonely might set you up to relapse.

TOM: That's why I liked talking to my girlfriend at night—I mean my ex-girlfriend.

THERAPIST: Yes, and it looks like that might have helped for a while. But let's do one thing at a time. First let's concentrate on what you can do the next time you feel really sad or mad about something. Let's narrow it down further and say you get upset by something that happens in school. And remember that you're going to run into a number of your external triggers right after school.

TOM: Like J.T.

THERAPIST: Yes. So as for J.T.—let's take some time and do that assertive exercise I mentioned before.

At this time, the therapist reviews A-CRA's Drink/Drug Refusal Skills. The fact that Tom spends a lot of time home alone is also addressed in this session, in part because that behavior appears to be a trigger for relapse, but also because A-CRA stresses the importance of a satisfying social life that does not revolve around drugs.

THERAPIST: OK. So that deals with one trigger, J.T. What about another trigger: going home alone to your room?

TOM: Well, sometimes I like to be home alone. And I don't smoke *every* time I'm home alone—or upset.

THERAPIST: I'm sure that's true. But it seems like we have to be extra careful right now. One option would be for you to go somewhere else when you're upset so that you're around people—nonusing people. What do you think about that?

TOM: I think I'd like to be able to go home after school! I don't want to feel like it isn't safe for me to go home just because I'm upset.

THERAPIST: Fair enough. So what would make it safe for you to go home even if you were upset?

TOM: I don't know. I guess maybe it helps for me to talk to someone. But I could call or text them and still be at home.

THERAPIST: OK. And who would be a good person to talk to or text when you're upset? Of course, it should be somebody who won't give you weed to feel better!

TOM: I'm not sure. I have a few friends who don't get high, but I wouldn't want to whine to them about being upset.

THERAPIST: What about talking to your mom?

TOM: But she's not home then. She's at work until 6:00.

THERAPIST: Have you ever called her at work for an emergency? Can she take just a few minutes to talk?

TOM: But this wouldn't exactly be an emergency. Or maybe it would be…

THERAPIST: Oh, I bet your mom would consider this an emergency. It wouldn't have to be a long conversation. Maybe you could just let her know that you're upset and need someone to talk to for a few minutes. You could clear this plan with her ahead of time. Would your mom be up for this?

TOM: I think she'd make time to talk if she knew it was important. She can be real calm with me when I'm upset about stuff at school, so she might actually be a good person to talk to.

THERAPIST: Sounds like your mom would help you feel relaxed. Do you think you'd end up feeling content? This is important, because remember that we're trying to allow you to have some of those same positive things that you get from smoking when you're upset—but *without* smoking.

TOM: If I give it a chance, I think it might help. It's worth a try.

THERAPIST: Excellent. Let's practice the conversation you might have with your mom over the phone when you are in a situation where you're at risk for smoking and nobody is around to talk to you. We can use the communication skills we've been practicing.

The therapist reviews the A-CRA Communication Skills and applies them in this situation. Role-plays are used, and feedback is given. A backup plan using A-CRA's Problem-Solving procedure would also be developed in the event that the mother is unavailable to speak during a high-risk time. Once the immediate high-risk triggers have been addressed, the issue of Tom's spending a lot of time home alone is raised again.

THERAPIST: Now we have a solid plan for those times when you're really upset. But I want to get back to this idea of your loneliness in general being a trigger for relapse. I recall that we talked a few sessions ago about your going to work out with your friend as a way to stay out of the house some. What else can you do? Remember that these kinds of activities can help you not think about using, distract you, and keep you busy. For now, how about we focus on some things you might want to do over the weekend?

The therapist and Tom spend time coming up with a specific plan for engaging in a pleasant activity with a friend. As with all assignments, obstacles that might interfere with executing the plan are identified and addressed. Next, the therapist raises the possibility of Tom's spending some time with his mother as well.

THERAPIST: You've come up with a great plan for a fun activity with a non-using friend. I support you 100% for that! I'm also thinking, though, that one of the goals you mentioned when we did the Goals of Counseling exercise last week was to spend time doing fun things with your mom like you used to. What do you think about that as an option for this weekend too? The activity with your friend is for Saturday night. What about the rest of the weekend?

TOM: I don't know if my mom would want to. It's been a long time since we've done anything fun together.

THERAPIST: I can understand why you might wonder. What do you think about asking her?

TOM: I guess I could ask. But I don't even know what I'd be asking her to do.

THERAPIST: Good point. We can either figure that out here and you can ask your mom if she's interested, or you can go home and discuss it with her. You could even do a Problem-Solving exercise with her; I taught her how to do that when she came in here by herself last week.

TOM: I think I should first ask her if she has time to do something, and if she even wants to. She might not want to if she finds out I relapsed. Anyway, if she wants to do something, I think it might be good to do some problem solving with her to come up with an idea.

THERAPIST: So how do you want to handle the relapse news?

TOM: I figure she'll find out one way or another, so I'd rather just tell her.

THERAPIST: Let's practice what you'll say to her. We can rely on the communication skills you've learned. Go ahead and give it a try. How would you start the conversation about the relapse?

TOM: Well, I'd say, "Mom, I know you've gotten upset before when I've had a relapse. I need you to know that I'm in control—I'm taking care of it—but I need you to help me this weekend. Do you want to do something this weekend—if you have time?"

THERAPIST: That's great. You used many of the elements of the communication skills we've been practicing. You told her that you *understood* how she felt about your relapse, and you even *understood* that she might be busy this weekend. Excellent! You also took some *responsibility* for your difficulties. And I liked how you made a request for help. Can you think of a way to make that request a little more specific? You mentioned earlier that you might like to do some problem solving with her to come up with an idea. You could even suggest doing that so there isn't pressure to come up with a specific activity on the spot. Or you could suggest a few activities.

The therapist uses A-CRA's Communication Skills training to help Tom shape how he talks to his mother. The role-play is repeated several times, with praise and specific suggestions offered. In an effort to increase the likelihood that Tom will actually have the conversation with his mother, the therapist encourages Tom to make the call to the mother during the session (i.e., using A-CRA's Systematic Encouragement procedure).

THERAPIST: You're doing a great job here today. It shows how committed you are to your goal of not smoking anymore. I'd like to mention one more strategy that's been helpful to people in your situation: an *Early Warning System*. This is an agreement you would set up in advance with a friend or family member—an agreement that the person would help you anticipate high-risk situations and be available to you in the event that you find yourself in one.

The therapist works with Tom to get specific about who Tom could ask to be part of his Early Warning System and what that individual would do, and to determine alternative plans (e.g., calling the therapist) if this person could not be contacted. Then the therapist has Tom role-play asking the person to help.

Second Session

At the next session, the therapist asks whether Tom needed to call his mom as they had practiced, and how it went. They review if Tom did the pleasant activity with his friend and if he enlisted the person identified to be part of his Early Warning System. Within the A-CRA framework, checking on homework (which is often called something else) helps the therapist know if a young person is learning to generalize the skills that he or she is learning within the sessions and that lead to sustainable behavior change. The therapist understands that completing homework is challenging for most adolescents. To increase the probability of success, the therapist and adolescent thoroughly discuss and problem-solve around barriers that might get in the way. If the homework is not completed, the therapist and youth work collaboratively to design another attempt for the following week, again problem-solving regarding potential barriers.

In this case, the therapist worked with Tom and his mother for about another month. The therapist had one more individual session with the mother to help her learn communication and problem-solving skills, and then two sessions with Tom and his mother together, during which they practiced these skills and completed Adolescent-Caregiver Happiness Scales, so they could talk about how to make their relationship more satisfying. Tom greatly reduced his marijuana use and improved his school attendance, and both Tom and his mother reported that they got along better.

Multidimensional Family Therapy

MDFT is a family-based, comprehensive treatment system for adolescent drug abuse and related behavioral and emotional problems (Liddle et al. 1991). The model is widely recognized in the United States and abroad as an effective science-based treatment for adolescent substance use disorders and delinquency (e.g., Liddle et al. 2008, 2009; Rigter et al. 2005; Vaughn and Howard 2004; Waldron and Turner 2008). MDFT is theory driven, combining aspects of several theoretical frameworks (i.e., family systems theory, developmental psychology, and the risk and protective model of adolescent substance abuse). It incorporates key elements of effective adolescent drug treatment, including comprehensive assessment; an integrated treatment approach; family involvement; developmentally appropriate interventions; specialized engagement and retention protocols; attention to qualifications of staff and their ongoing training; gender and cultural competence; and focus on a broad range of outcomes (Austin et al. 2005; Brannigan et al. 2004; Jackson-Gilfort et al. 2001; Liddle et al. 2006).

MDFT is both a tailored and a flexible treatment delivery system. Depending on the needs of the youth and family, MDFT can be conducted from one to three times per week over the course of 3–6 months, both in the home and in the clinic. Therapists work simultaneously in four interdependent treatment domains—adolescent, parent, family, and extrafamilial domains—each of which is addressed in three stages: Stage 1, build a foundation for change; Stage 2, facilitate individual and family change; and Stage 3, solidify changes and launch. At various points throughout treatment, therapists meet alone with the adolescent, alone with the parent(s), or conjointly with the adolescent and parent(s), depending on the treatment domain and specific problem being addressed.

In Stage 1, overall therapeutic goals are similar for both the adolescent and parent domains. For example, in Stage 1, goals for both the adolescent and parent are to develop a therapeutic alliance and enhance motivation to participate in treatment and to change their behaviors. In this stage, the therapist creates an environment in which both the youth and parents feel empowered, respected, understood, and esteemed. The primary goals of Stage 1 are to develop a strong therapeutic alliance with youth and parents, and to enhance in each the motivation to truthfully examine oneself and be willing to change one's behavior. Accomplishment of these goals set the foundation for Stage 2, where the emphasis is on behavioral and interactional change.

In Stage 2, the longest stage in MDFT, most of the action takes place, and there are distinctive goals for each of the four domains. In the *adolescent domain*, the therapist works collaboratively with the parents and youth to help the youth communicate effectively with parents and other adults; develop coping, emotion regulation, and problem-solving skills; improve social competence; and establish alternatives to substance use and delinquency. For the youth, in particular, the therapist helps him or her feel safe to reveal the truth about his or her life generally, and about substance use in particular, to his or her parents and the therapist. The therapist must be nonpunitive and nonmoralistic about drug use; help the parents control their anger and disappointment and move to a more sympathetic and problem-solving stance; and encourage the youth to have positive goals (to dream and hope) for himself or herself, and then highlight for the youth the discrepancy between those goals (e.g., graduate from high school, go to college, get a good job, avoid going to jail, get his or her own apartment) and continued drug use. In the *parent domain*, MDFT focuses on increasing the parents' behavioral and emotional involvement with their teen and on improving parenting skills, especially monitoring their teen's activity, clarifying expectations, limit setting, and articulating both negative and positive consequences. Work within the *family domain* focuses on decreasing family conflict, deepening emotional attachments, and improving communication and problem-solving skills. The MDFT therapist helps youth and parents see substance use as a health and lifestyle problem (e.g., it can interfere with the youth's getting what he or she wants out of life). Drug tests are used in the treatment as a way to encourage open communication about substance use, and to avoid the debate about whether or not the youth is using. Within the *extrafamilial domain*, MDFT fosters family competency in interactions with social systems (e.g., school, juvenile justice, recreational). The MDFT treatment team typically includes a therapist assistant who, in a highly coordinated collaboration with the therapist, works with the family members in the context of important institutions that influence their lives. For example, the therapist assistant might help the parents find a more appropriate school placement for their teen; obtain needed economic assistance, such as food stamps and Medicaid; or procure mental health or substance abuse treatment services for themselves or other children in the family.

Stage 3 helps parents and teens strengthen their accomplishments in treatment to facilitate lasting change, create concrete plans addressing how each will respond to future problems (bumps in the road, such as relapse, family arguments, and disappointments), and reinforce strengths and competencies necessary for a successful launch from treatment.

Planning Sessions and Setting Goals

Session planning and preparation is an important objective for the MDFT therapist. On a weekly basis, the therapist reviews, and modifies if necessary, the overarching therapeutic goals for each case, and then the specific goals for the upcoming week. Once the goals are established, the therapist can determine the focus of the sessions for the week, including how many sessions to hold, location of the session (home, school, clinic), and the individuals who should attend each session (e.g., parents, youth, parent and youth, whole family). Goals are articulated in clear behavioral terms: what the youth and parents will do or say both within the session and outside the session. Session goals designed to address relapse are presented in Table 10–2. As is typical in MDFT, the goals have a temporal sequence; the goals cover the four domains of MDFT intervention (youth, parent, family, and extrafamilial); and these goals are accomplished over two to three sessions.

Interventions Designed to Meet Therapeutic Goals of Relapse Sessions

In the sequence of sessions designed to address relapse, typically the MDFT therapist begins with the parents alone. This could be a whole session of 45–60 minutes or part of a session (approximately 20 minutes). The length of the session and whether it is a whole session or part of a multipart session are determined by the therapist, based on his or her understanding of what is needed to accomplish the articulated therapeutic goals. For instance, if the therapist believes, based on prior work with the family, that the parents have a tendency to react in a very harsh manner, or that their disappointment and anger about the relapse will be tremendously deep, the therapist might decide that he or she needs a whole session to help the parents address these issues fully. If, on the other hand, the therapist determines that he or she can help the parents deal with their disappointment and set the foundation for having a productive conversation with their teen more quickly, then the therapist might begin by having the first part of a 90-minute multipart session alone with the parents. In this situation, the therapist first works alone with the parents, and then brings the youth into the session for a family discussion. The therapist's knowledge about the family and the MDFT model guides clinical decision making.

In that first full- or partial-session intervention with the parents, the therapist encourages the parents to fully discuss the situation, expressing their thoughts and feelings about the relapse, including their frustration, disappointment, hopelessness, and anger. The therapist aims to end this session or part of a session with the parents understanding that relapse is part of the recovery process and to be ready to address the relapse in a therapeutic instead of a punitive way. After a youth's relapse, especially if it is not the first relapse or if it is a particularly long-lasting or severe relapse, the parents may feel hopeless and want to give

Table 10–2.   Therapeutic goals for multidimensional family therapy sessions addressing relapse

1. Parents understand the naturalness (a "law of life") that relapse is part of the recovery process (two steps forward and one step backward).

2. Parents agree to address the relapse in a therapeutic instead of a punitive way. They agree that their objective is to help the youth recover from the relapse, and to set in motion action to prevent further relapses.

3. The youth describes the relapse (e.g., how it came about, what happened, what he or she was thinking or feeling, whether he or she tried to stop or prevent it, what is going on with him or her now).

4. Parents listen to the youth and encourage him or her to feel comfortable revealing this information to them. Parents express to the youth their thoughts and feelings about the relapse, and agree that this means everybody must work harder to figure out how to best prevent future relapse.

5. The youth agrees with the idea that everybody (parents, youth, therapist, and perhaps other family members) must work harder or differently to help prevent relapse.

6. The youth and parents agree on a behavioral plan to prevent relapse.

7. The youth and parents have reduced feelings of failure, frustration, shame, guilt, and anger toward self and each other.

8. The youth and parents will continue to conceive of the solution to their problems from a developmental–family perspective.

9. The youth and parents recognize the seriousness of the situation, but also realize that this is not the end of the world, and feel confident that the new plan to prevent relapse will work.

10. The youth and parents continue to talk openly about substance use, relapse, and recovery, and to implement the behavioral plan, including refining and changing components as needed to be successful.

11. The youth and parents consider whether or not increasing the youth's involvement in prosocial activities, such as employment, tutoring, volunteer work, or sports, might help to crowd out opportunities for drug use. The therapeutic team works to assist the youth and family to locate such activities.

up on their child and either send the child to residential treatment or, if the juvenile justice system is involved, let the court place the youth in a long-term commitment facility. The therapist's job is to sympathize with the parents' disappointment, frustration, hopelessness, and pain, as well as to help parents recommit to help their child through this outpatient treatment. Of course, if the therapist believes that the teen cannot stop using drugs on an outpatient basis because of repeated relapses and if the youth is using substances to the extent that his or her life is in danger, then the MDFT therapist will recommend residential treatment and work with the youth and family to facilitate such treatment. In the case illustration that follows, the therapist has determined that the prognosis for the youth in an outpatient setting is favorable.

Case Illustration

Session With Mother

The following is a transcript illustration of how an MDFT therapist works with a parent who is hopeless following multiple relapses on the part of her son. The youth, Alex, is 16 years old, has been using drugs (primarily marijuana) and alcohol since he was 12, and at the time of treatment was on probation for repeated criminal offenses. Prior to this session, the mother called the therapist to say that she wanted to stop treatment. Her plan was to speak to Alex's probation officer and request incarceration for Alex. On the telephone, the therapist sympathized with the mother's position but also asked her to come into the clinic for one last session. After some reluctance, the mother agreed to one last session.

At the beginning of the session, the mother expresses her frustration: "I recommend harsher punishment. I mean, I am his mother but I can only do so much with a 16-year-old boy. He's gonna do whatever the hell he wants to do.…Well, just like anybody who has an addiction, they're not going to quit until they're ready to quit. Whatever addiction, you can't make someone quit."

The therapist starts by simultaneously recognizing the mother's pain and hopelessness, and the seriousness of her son's situation:

> THERAPIST: I see you feel hopeless. You've done a lot, I understand, and now you are thinking that you don't know what more you can do. I know. And I agree you have done a lot. You've been here in treatment. You've been in court and at meetings with his probation officer. You've

tried everything you can think of and beyond, and there were times when he was doing OK, but now we are here, and you think, What more can I do? I understand that, and I don't have the answer, but I know he is in a real dangerous situation, and now he is saying he doesn't care if he goes to prison.

MOTHER: Yeah.

While staying with the mother's hopelessness, the therapist highlights the seriousness of her son's situation.

THERAPIST: And that bothers me because it is a big deal, and he probably doesn't realize that we're talking about his whole life. I know kids who go to prison for 6 months, and then they do something wrong—and it's a setup for messing up—and then the 6 months turns into 9 months. Then they get released and are on probation, and they have to be angels on probation. Nobody can do it. I couldn't do it. So they mess up in some way, and it's a probation violation; then they're back in prison for a few months, and so on and so forth. Then they turn around, and they're 25 years old, and from 16 to 25 this has been their life—in and out of detention and probation. I'm not trying to be melodramatic but...

MOTHER: You're right, and he has been told that. A very, very good friend of mine from high school has been in and out of prison, and it started with a little pot. Alex knows this. And it's like, "Well, it ain't gonna happen to me. I'm not that stupid. I'm not going to get caught."

A little later in the session, the mother agrees with the therapist about the danger her son faces—drug addiction and incarceration. The therapist responds by highlighting the seriousness of the problem, offering a solution, and once again acknowledging the mother's feelings of emotional depletion.

THERAPIST: Yeah, but that's what he doesn't understand. I told you I've seen this I don't know how many times. And then they're crying, but then it's too late. But now it's *not* too late. He can, you can, we can stop that from happening. There will come a point, though, when it will be too late, and then he'll cry, but then it's done....The only thing I can think of goes back to you: that you are really the only one who can save him. Maybe a new or a renewed commitment from you will help. I'm thinking that is what needs to happen now. But I know you have so much on your plate, and I know what I am suggesting is not easy, and you've tried a lot and you feel like you've done a lot already, don't know how much more you have to give....But...

MOTHER: This is my son.

THERAPIST: Exactly.

MOTHER: I mean, do I use tough love, do I become a little Hitler, or do I just smother him with kindness and love?

THERAPIST: Well, that's what we are here to figure out. But I do think, I mean, it's the only option: you're the mother, you're the parent. You are the only one who has influence on him. And when you start to give up, he will really give up. Look, I completely understand your feeling of wanting to give up. I know, because you've tried everything. And that's why it is so hard to be a parent, because you want to give up, you're tired, you've tried and tried, but you can't give up because there is nobody else.

MOTHER: So what do I do? There's like a thousand things going through my mind.

The MDFT therapist does not want to go to problem solving too quickly. In this situation, the therapist decides not to do any problem solving in the session, and instead to spend more time alone with the mother, allowing her to fully explore the issues at hand—the mother's feelings of emotional depletion ("can't do this anymore") and her son's jeopardy—and ultimately resurrecting the mother's commitment to keep working in treatment to help her son. To go to problem solving too quickly runs the risk that the mother's commitment will be only fleeting or inconsistently manifested, and of course, a commitment and solid foundation are necessary for the remainder of the therapeutic work.

The therapist stays with the topic of the mother's hopelessness, and offers the mother total support and understanding.

THERAPIST: I know you've done a lot. You told me about the problems in your marriage, and I know how draining that is. It's very hard to give as much as you need to give to your kids when you're in the middle of all of this relationship stuff. And you have a child who is in trouble, who needs even more. Right? So that's doubly hard. I don't know, I thought I heard you say at the beginning of the session that you don't have enough energy. That you can't dig down and find the energy that is needed to give to Alex now. What do you think?

MOTHER: Probably.

THERAPIST: That you do or you don't?

MOTHER: Remember that phrase I said to you a while back, that outward appearances are not inward reality? On the outside I'm happy and energetic, but on the inside I struggle....My mind is going 1,000 miles an hour, and I can't stop and focus on one thing because there are so many things that need to be attended to.

THERAPIST: But the thing is, you can't do everything. You're only one human being.

MOTHER: I think everybody thinks I'm supermom.

The session continues with the therapist sympathizing with the mother's burden, highlighting the seriousness of the situation for her son, and empowering the mother.

THERAPIST: I can see, as I said before, that you are a very smart person and you have a powerful personality. You can influence Alex. I know you can get him on the right track and then you'll look back and you'll say, "You know, I saved his life. I'm the one who did it. I made a difference. It was me." I can help, but it's really you. What you say here—the decision about putting your kids first, I mean—it's great. I really admire you for that.

At the very end of the session, Alex's mother stands up and looks the therapist directly in the eyes.

MOTHER: So when do you want to see him? If I have to go duct-tape his legs together and put him in the car, he will be here.

The therapist and parent agree to have a session as soon as possible with Alex, to hear from him and to begin developing a family-centered behavioral plan for how to help Alex stop using drugs and alcohol.

Session With Parent and Youth

The next core area of work is to facilitate an extended conversation between a youth and his or her parents, focusing specifically on what happened and why, and allowing the youth and parents to explore their feelings and thoughts about the relapse. The therapist needs to facilitate a focused discussion between the youth and parents in which the teen has sufficient time to fully voice his or her experience to the parents, and in which the parents listen and express themselves but at the same time refrain from excessive criticism and judgment— actions that can serve to push their child further away from them. This discussion should end in an agreement between the youth and parents 1) that this relapse is serious but not the end of the world, 2) that what matters is how the youth and parents deal with the relapse, and 3) that they have to work harder or differently to prevent further relapses. If it has not been done already, this is a good time to drug-test the youth. In MDFT, the drug test is used not to catch or punish the youth but to encourage open communication between parents and child about the youth's use. Positive urine screens are defined not as evidence of the teen's addiction but instead as proof that continued and perhaps increased effort on everyone's part is required.

In the case of Alex, the next session, which involved Alex and his mother, occurred 2 days after the therapist's session with the mother. The therapist started the session by asking the mother to talk to Alex about some of the things that the therapist and the mother had discussed in the previous session, specifically the mother's decision not to give up on her son and not to let him give up on himself. The son was moved by the mother's strong commitment to not let him ruin his life. He cried and talked about his own struggles and disappointment in himself, and his desire to just go to jail to serve his sentence because he felt staying clean was too difficult. He said, "I just want to go to jail and get it over with. I can't do it.... I'm going to fail probation anyway. I can't stay clean. So why not just go to jail now? It will be easier." At the end of this sequence, the therapist asked both mother and son to verbally state their new commitment to see Alex clean from drugs, back in school, and off probation.

The next part of the session was focused on problem solving, and Alex, his mother, and the therapist talked together about what they and others in the family could do to help Alex meet his goals. In MDFT, the family-centered behavioral plan is developed collaboratively and is conceived as just a beginning plan. It may work, but it may not work, and then the family and therapist will meet to revise the plan collaboratively. This prevents disappointment and extreme action (e.g., kicking the youth out of the house) if the plan does not work initially.

After this second relapse session, the therapist continued to work with the youth and family, addressing any problems and challenges they had in following their plan, adjusting the plan so it would work better for them, praising them for all their good work and accomplishments, and facilitating conversations about how much they love and appreciate each other. Alex was able to meet his goals of remaining drug free. He successfully completed probation and 2 years later graduated from high school.

Conclusion

The descriptions of the adolescent community reinforcement approach and multidimensional family therapy in this chapter reveal several ways in which they are similar, even though some of the underlying theories, therapeutic guidelines, and methods differ. (For more specific details about A-CRA and MDFT, see Godley et al. 2001 and Liddle et al. 2005, respectively.) Although A-CRA, MDFT, and other efficacious treatments for adolescent substance abuse have distinct therapeutic formats and methods, it has been suggested that carefully designed and implemented interventions will result in generally favorable outcomes regardless of specific therapeutic model, techniques, or methods (cf. Dennis et al. 2004). This view and the ensuing debate are not unlike the well-established debate in the broader field of psychotherapy, generally framed as follows: Do certain specific elements that are unique to different therapies make them more effective than others, or are the shared features across approaches responsible for treatment effects (DeRubeis et al. 2005; Norcross et al. 2006; Wampold et al. 1997)? It is possible that the similarities in certain therapeutic methods between A-CRA and MDFT illustrate certain important shared features.

Therapists implementing both approaches are highly nonpunitive and nonjudgmental toward youth and parents; in fact, this is one of the first instructions given to new therapists. In each approach, therapists are trained to 1) be aware of how their statements, in both content and tone, can be interpreted by youth and parents as judgmental; 2) desist from making such statements; and 3) pay attention to and comment on client strengths. Both approaches, then, are strength based, acknowledging strengths that are present, for example, in the existing parent-child relationship or in the adolescent's life. Both MDFT and A-CRA value the importance of therapeutic alliance and promote interactions between the therapist and the adolescents and caregivers that enhance this alliance. This focus on therapeutic alliance is consistent with the robust findings concerning the importance of therapeutic alliance to psychotherapeutic outcome across patient populations and treatments (see Horvath et al. 1993).

Although not evident in the clinical illustrations in this chapter, but as is well documented in other chapters in this book, comorbid disorders are very common among adolescents entering substance abuse treatment. Both A-

CRA and MDFT are behavioral interventions that do not exclude the use of pharmacotherapy when indicated. For clinicians who are not psychiatrists, both approaches have guidelines or procedures that can be helpful in working with disorders that co-occur with substance use. At a minimum, therapists are expected to screen youth for co-occurring problems and, when warranted, make appropriate referrals to a psychiatrist for evaluations and any indicated pharmacotherapy treatment and then work closely with the psychiatrist during subsequent treatment. For example, therapists can help support medication compliance and watch for medication side effects that can be reported to the psychiatrist.

Another commonality between these two approaches is that they are flexible and allow therapists to individualize processes or procedures. Qualitative interviews with therapists trained in these approaches have revealed that these attributes of MDFT and A-CRA are highly valued by therapists (Godley et al. 2001). In the case examples above, the specific content of the sessions was based on what was happening in the specific adolescent's or family's life, and both therapists helped the adolescents identify ways to replace substance use behavior specific to their interests. Both therapies acknowledge that plans or homework may not be completed as originally conceived, and require the therapist to work collaboratively with the youth and family to outline other plans or homework, while trying to discover and problem-solve barriers to success. Whereas the A-CRA therapist might talk about an individual youth's "reinforcers," and an MDFT therapist might talk about a youth's "hopes and dreams," these labels refer to the same constructs—that is, the importance of identifying what is individually meaningful for each youth.

Both approaches have sessions with the youth alone, with the parent(s) alone, and with the parent(s) and youth together. Although A-CRA may have more individual sessions with adolescents than does MDFT, and MDFT may have more family sessions, each approach recognizes that parents are critical in an adolescent's life. MDFT involves the family as a key agent of change, whereas A-CRA recognizes the family as crucial to creating a more positive environment for the adolescent, including one that is conducive to recovery. Likewise, both approaches recognize that other systems or parts of the adolescent's environment are also critical in facilitating recovery, including the school, peer group, other social services with which he or she might be involved, and even the work environment.

In this chapter, we have briefly described these two different adolescent treatment and family approaches. It is important to note that implementing these approaches with fidelity requires more than reading this chapter or the respective treatment manuals (see Godley et al., in press). Both approaches have been replicated often, and the development teams have learned that replication with fidelity takes much work from the trainers and developers, managers at replication sites, and therapists. A review of implementation research (Fixsen et al. 2005; Miller et al. 2006; Roman and Johnson 2002) reveals that this is true not only for these approaches, but for the now growing array of evidence-based approaches. A combination of training and ongoing support through coaching, expert reviews, and feedback on actual sessions is needed to ensure accurate implementation of the models. It is clear, however, that many adolescent substance abuse treatment therapists welcome evidence-based approaches that are individualized and flexible, that share a common language, and that focus on the strengths of adolescents and their families.

Key Clinical Concepts

Both A-CRA and MDFT share the following features, which perhaps form the outline of core features of efficacious adolescent substance abuse treatment generally:

- Relapse, an expected occurrence during adolescent substance abuse treatment, can be an opportunity for growth and learning if directly and systematically addressed in treatment.
- Therapists should be nonjudgmental and nonpunitive, and adopt a decidedly strength-based orientation to youth and families.
- Therapists should collaborate with youth to develop meaningful adolescent-driven goals.
- Family and other social systems are important to recovery.
- Manualized interventions should be both systematic and flexible, requiring therapist judgment, creativity, and clinical decision making.
- Successful implementation of evidence-based treatments requires therapists to participate in systematic and intensive training.

References

American Psychiatric Association: Diagnostic and Statistical Manual of Mental Disorders, 4th Edition, Text Revision. Washington, DC, American Psychiatric Association, 2000

Austin AM, Macgowan MJ, Wagner EF: Effective family based interventions for adolescents with substance use problems: a systematic review. Res Soc Work Pract 15:67–83, 2005

Azrin NH: Improvements in the community reinforcement approach to alcoholism. Behav Res Ther 14:339–348, 1976

Azrin NH, Sisson RW, Meyers R, et al: Alcoholism treatment by disulfiram and community reinforcement therapy. J Behav Ther Exp Psychiatry 13:105–112, 1982

Brannigan R, Schackman BR, Falco M, et al: The quality of highly regarded adolescent substance abuse treatment programs: results of an in-depth national survey. Arch Pediatr Adolesc Med 158:904–909, 2004

Brown SA, D'Amico EJ, McCarthy DM, et al: Four-year outcomes from adolescent alcohol and drug treatment. J Stud Alcohol 62:381–388, 2001

Center for Substance Abuse Treatment, Substance Abuse and Mental Health Services Administration: Family centered substance abuse treatment grants for adolescents and their families (Publ No RFA-TI-06-007). Rockville, MD, Center for Substance Abuse Treatment, Substance Abuse and Mental Health Services Administration, 2006

Center for Substance Abuse Treatment, Substance Abuse and Mental Health Services Administration: Family centered substance abuse treatment grants for adolescents and their families (Publ No RFA-TI-09-002). Washington, DC, Center for Substance Abuse Treatment, Substance Abuse and Mental Health Services Administration, 2009

Dennis ML, Godley SH, Diamond G, et al: The Cannabis Youth Treatment (CYT) study: main findings from two randomized trials. J Subst Abuse Treat 27:197–213, 2004

DeRubeis RJ, Brotman MA, Gibbons CJ: A conceptual and methodological analysis of the nonspecifics argument. Clinical Psychology: Science and Practice 12:174–183, 2005

Fixsen DL, Naoom SF, Blasé KA, et al: Implementation Research: A Synthesis of the Literature (FMHI Publ No 231). Tampa, FL, University of South Florida, Louis de la Parte Florida Mental Health Institute, The National Implementation Research Network, 2005

Godley MD, Godley SH, Dennis ML, et al: The effect of assertive continuing care (ACC) on continuing care linkage, adherence and abstinence following residential treatment for adolescents. Addiction 102:81–93, 2007

Godley SH, White WL, Diamond G, et al: Therapists' reactions to manual-guided therapies for the treatment of adolescent marijuana users. Clinical Psychology: Science and Practice 8:405–417, 2001

Godley SH, Meyers RJ, Smith JE, et al: The adolescent community reinforcement approach for adolescent cannabis users (DHHS Publ No SMA-01-3489). Cannabis Youth Treatment Series, Vol 4. Rockville, MD, Center for Substance Abuse Treatment, Substance Abuse and Mental Health Services Administration. 2006. Available at: http://www.chestnut.org/li/cyt/products/acra_cyt_v4.pdf. Accessed January 2, 2010.

Godley SH, Smith JE, Meyers RJ, et al: Adolescent community reinforcement approach (A-CRA), in Substance Abuse Treatment for Youth and Adults: Clinician's Guide to Evidence-Based Practice Series. Edited by Springer DW, Rubin A. New York, Wiley, 2009, pp 109–201

Godley SH, Garner BR, Smith JE, et al: A large-scale dissemination and implementation model. Clinical Psychology: Science and Practice (in press)

Horvath AO, Gaston L, Luborsky L: The alliance as predictor of benefits of counseling and therapy, in Psychodynamic Treatment Research: A Handbook for Clinical Practice. Edited by Miller N, Luborsky L, Barber J, et al. New York, Basic Books, 1993, pp 247–274

Hunt GM, Azrin NH: A community-reinforcement approach to alcoholism. Behav Res Ther 11:91–104, 1973

Jackson-Gilfort A, Liddle HA, Tejeda MJ, et al: Facilitating engagement of African American male adolescents in family therapy: a cultural theme process study. J Black Psychol 27:321–340, 2001

Latimer WW, Newcomb M, Winters KC, et al: Adolescent substance abuse treatment outcome: the role of substance abuse problem severity, psychosocial and treatment factors. J Consult Clin Psychol 68:684–696, 2000

Liddle HA, Dakof GA, Diamond GS: Adolescents and substance abuse: multidimensional family therapy in action, in Family Therapy of Drug and Alcohol Abuse, 2nd Edition. Edited by Kaufman E, Kaufman P. Boston, MA, Allyn & Bacon, 1991, pp 120–171

Liddle HA, Rodriguez RA, Dakof GA, et al: Multidimensional family therapy: a science-based treatment for adolescent drug abuse, in Handbook of Clinical Family Therapy. Edited by Lebow J. New York, Wiley, 2005, pp 128–163

Liddle HA, Rowe CL, Gonzalez A, et al: Changing provider practices, program environment, and improving outcomes by transporting multidimensional family therapy to an adolescent drug treatment setting. Am J Addict 15 (suppl 1):102–112, 2006

Liddle HA, Dakof GA, Turner WM, et al: Treating adolescent drug abuse: a randomized trial comparing multidimensional family therapy and cognitive behavior therapy. Addiction 103:1660–1670, 2008

Liddle HA, Rowe CL, Dakof GA, et al: Multidimensional family therapy for early adolescent substance abusers: twelve month outcomes of a randomized controlled trial. J Consult Clin Psychol 77:12–25, 2009

Miller WR, Sorensen JL, Selzer JA, et al: Disseminating evidence-based practices in substance abuse treatment: a review with suggestions. J Subst Abuse Treat 31:25–39, 2006

Norcross JC, Beutler LE, Levant RF (eds): Evidence-Based Practices in Mental Health: Debate on the Fundamental Questions. Washington, DC, American Psychological Association, 2006

Rigter H, Van Gageldonk A, Ketelaars T: Treatment and Other Interventions Targeting Drug Use and Addiction: State of the Art 2004. Utrecht, The Netherlands, National Drug Monitor, 2005

Roman PM, Johnson JA: Adoption and implementation of new technologies in substance abuse treatment. J Subst Abuse Treat 22:210–218, 2002

Slesnick N, Prestopnik JL, Meyers RJ, et al: Treatment outcome for street-living, homeless youth. Addict Behav 32:1237–1251, 2007

Vaughn MG, Howard MO: Adolescent substance abuse treatment: a synthesis of controlled evaluations. Res Soc Work Pract 14:325–335, 2004

Vaughn MG, Howard MO: Adolescent substance abuse treatment, in Readings in Evidence-Based Social Work: Syntheses of the Intervention Knowledge Base. Edited by Vaughn MG, Howard MO, Thyer BA. Thousand Oaks, CA, Sage, 2008, pp 171–187

Waldron HB, Turner CW: Evidence-based psychosocial treatments for adolescent substance abuse. J Clin Child Adolesc Psychol 37:1–24, 2008

Wampold BE, Mondin GW, Moody M, et al: A meta-analysis of outcome studies comparing bona fide psychotherapies: empirically, "all must have prizes." Psychol Bull 122:203–215, 1997

Williams RJ, Chang SY: A comprehensive and comparative review of adolescent substance abuse treatment outcome. Clinical Psychology: Science and Practice 7:138–166, 2000

Suggested Readings

Deas D, Thomas SE: An overview of controlled studies of adolescent substance abuse treatment. Am J Addict 10:178–189, 2001

Rowe CL: Family therapy for drug abuse: review and updates 2003–2010. J Marital Fam Ther (in press)

Waldron HB, Turner CW: Evidence-based psychosocial treatments for adolescent substance abuse. J Clin Child Adolesc Psychol 37:1–24, 2008

Winters KC, Botzet AM, Fahnhorst T, et al: Adolescent substance abuse treatment: a review of evidence-based research, in Handbook on the Prevention and Treatment of Substance Abuse in Adolescence. Edited by Leukefeld C, Gullotta T, Staton Tindall M. New York, Springer, 2009

Relevant Websites

Adolescent community reinforcement approach (A-CRA): http://www.chestnut.org/LI/acra-acc/index.html

Multidimensional family therapy (MDFT): www.ctrada@med.miami.edu

National Registry of Evidence-based Programs and Practices (NREPP): http://www.nrepp.samhsa.gov

11

Twelve-Step Mutual-Help Programs for Adolescents

Steven L. Jaffe, M.D.

John F. Kelly, Ph.D.

Alcohol and other drug use disorders often emerge during adolescence and can have lasting developmental ramifications that can affect mental and physical health, and delay the achievement of important developmental milestones (Substance Abuse and Mental Health Services Administration [SAMHSA] 2008). During the past 20 years, professional efforts have focused on developing and testing effective interventions specifically with young people in an attempt to minimize the duration and impact of substance-related problems (Vaughn and Howard 2004; Winters et al. 2009). However, in spite of highly rigorous treatment implementation efforts, relapse is common when treatment ends (Dennis et al. 2004). To help extend the benefits of professional interventions, both adult and adolescent treatment programs typically refer patients to community recovery-focused groups, such as Alcoholics Anonymous (AA) and Narcotics

Anonymous (NA) (Humphreys 1991; Kelly and Yeterian, in press; Kelly et al. 2008c; Knudsen et al. 2008). Youth have been shown to benefit from AA and NA participation (Kelly and Myers 2007). However, given that these mutual-help groups were developed for and consist mostly of adults, adolescents may face additional barriers to engagement that may compromise any potential benefits.

Our main aim in this chapter is to describe ways clinicians can facilitate the use of these freely available community resources and maximize any potential therapeutic gains. We briefly provide the historical context and origin of 12-step fellowships; describe the fundamental elements of such programs and ways to adapt these specifically for youth; provide a brief overview of the evidence of effectiveness of adolescent participation in 12-step groups; and describe some 12-step facilitation strategies and describe future directions for research and practice.

History and Development of 12-Step Mutual-Help Programs

Twelve-step recovery group programs commenced with the development of AA in 1935. Bill Wilson, a New York stockbroker who was later to become a co-founder of AA, was attending meetings of the Oxford Group in an attempt to stop drinking and live a better life. The Oxford Group was a nondenominational but Christian-focused group that attempted to practice a simple Christianity without fanfare (Oxford Group 1933). The Oxford Group's philosophy involved surrendering one's will to God, taking a personal moral inventory, confessing past crimes, making amends, and helping others. During Wilson's fourth hospitalization for alcoholism treatment, while trying to practice the principles of the Oxford Group and being medicated for alcohol withdrawal, he experienced an overwhelming spiritual exaltation. He continued to attend Oxford Group meetings and discovered that trying to help other alcoholics often helped him not to drink.

In 1935, on an unsuccessful business trip in Akron, Ohio, and at risk of resuming drinking again, Wilson connected with Dr. Robert Smith, an alcoholic physician, who also was struggling not to drink using the same Oxford Group methods and support. Wilson and Smith spent 6 hours discussing their plight. From this unique 6-hour "sharing" of one alcoholic helping another, the movement began, splitting off from the Oxford Group to form an organization focused purely on alcoholism recovery. The sharing ideology subsequently developed into today's AA, where millions of people find help and support for their addiction recovery. This community-based peer-run recovery strategy has extended to other addictions—drugs (e.g., Narcotics Anonymous, Marijuana Anonymous), food (e.g., Overeaters Anonymous), sex (e.g., Sex and Love Addicts Anonymous), and gambling (Gamblers Anonymous)—and to participants' significant others (e.g., Al-Anon, Alateen) (Kelly and Yeterian 2008). Membership has extended to an increasing number of women, who now make up one-third of AA members, and in recent years to young people (Alcoholics Anonymous 2008).

Fundamental Elements of 12-Step Community Programs and Adaptation for Youth

The remarkable growth and development of AA stems from the guidelines detailed in Alcoholics Anonymous' (1952) *Twelve Steps and Twelve Traditions*. AA is a unique organization in that it owns no property, does no fund-raising, avoids politics, and does not accept outside contributions. No member of AA can give more than $1,000 per year to the organization. Membership in AA is open to anyone who wants to stop drinking. This free and open decentralized structure enables AA to avoid the problematic issues of finances and politics, and no one individual can emerge to corrupt its purpose.

AA and other 12-step organizations might be said to contain eight core elements: 1) the 12 steps, 2) the 12 traditions, 3) meetings, 4) sponsorship and fellowship, 5) "higher power," 6) slogans, 7) service, and 8) literature. Kelly and McCrady (2009) provide detailed explanations of each of these.

In addition to attendance at meetings, which occur daily in almost every city and town in the United States, sponsorship is an integral and essential component of a 12-step program. A sponsor is a member of a stable 12-step program who forms a special relationship with the new member. Frequent telephone contact and individual meetings with the sponsor create a positive supportive relationship that focuses on skills to stay sober and how to "work" the 12 steps.

Another component unique to AA and other 12-step organizations is connecting to recovering peers. This aspect is especially useful to adolescents working the program because they are likely to relapse if they continue to associate with former alcohol- or drug-using friends (Brown 1993). Mutual-help programs, such as AA and NA, provide the opportunity for the adolescent to create and foster a new sober peer group while attending meetings (Kelly et al. 2008b).

Many adolescent substance abuse hospital, partial hospital, residential, and outpatient programs integrate 12-step mutual-help program components into their professionally led individual and group therapies (Drug Strategies 2003). Thus, treated youth may begin to work some of the 12 steps with the counselors of treatment programs and often begin to attend community AA or NA meetings under staff supervision (Knudsen et al. 2008). This enhances the adolescent's connection to the 12-step program while he or she is in the most intensive part of treatment. A passive referral to 12-step groups at the end of treatment is not as effective as beginning to facilitate and monitor attendance during treatment (Kelly and Yeterian, in press).

We present below the first five steps and describe ways they can be modified to make them meaningful for adolescents. The recommendations are based on Jaffe's (1990) workbook about the first five steps, in which the adolescent responds to specific questions by writing answers, which are reviewed by counselors and then may be presented to a group.

1. *We admitted we were powerless over our addiction—that our lives had become unmanageable.* The workbook instructs the adolescents to examine in detail the negative consequences of their alcohol and drug use. Various issues are explored, such as the ways in which drug and alcohol use puts their own and others' lives in danger and the effects it has on family, school, work, mood, and self-esteem. The major goal is to accurately appraise whether drugs and alcohol are destroying their lives such that they need to stop in order to make their lives better. Because adolescents often desire to feel powerful, the workbook emphasizes that by abstaining from alcohol and drugs, individuals become more empowered to have greater confidence and control in their lives. Although many adult programs emphasize the concept of surrendering and admitting that one is an addict, these emphases tend to be not as useful for adolescents. Instead, the emphasis is on enhancing power by doing what one needs to do (i.e., stop using alcohol and drugs).

In addition to Jaffe's 1990 workbook, he developed another workbook, the *Adolescent Substance Abuse Intervention Workbook* (Jaffe 2000). In this workbook, he modified the first step to concretely guide the adolescent in exploring how 12 areas of the adolescent's life may have been negatively affected by alcohol or drugs. This helps the adolescent to move from pre-contemplation to contemplation according to the stages of change (Prochaska and DiClemente 1982). This workbook becomes the basis for a 2-hour intervention: an hour to complete the questions and checklists and another hour to present to a group or counselor. In addition to using the strategies of motivational enhancement therapy, completing this intervention also corresponds to working the first step of AA or NA. A pilot study of this workbook intervention with substance-using adolescents in juvenile detention showed increased recognition of the harm drugs may cause (Jaffe et al. 2008).

2. *We came to believe that a Power greater than ourselves could restore us to sanity.* This step is approached in the adolescent workbook (Jaffe 1990) by recognizing that the first higher power in a child's life is the person who raised him or her. For many drug-abusing or drug-addicted adolescents, parental figures were neglectful or abusive. Mourning—eliciting the pain and sadness caused by the disappointments in their childhood higher powers—enables them to begin to develop a sense of something positive in the universe that they can turn to for help. The concept of a higher power is not a religious belief but a spiritual feeling that one can trust something positive (e.g., the group, another person, nature) to take care of those aspects of one's life that one cannot control: one needs to have trust in the stability of the world and realize that one controls one's own behavior but not what others say or do. For many adolescents, the concrete positive feeling of their relationships with other members becomes their 12-step higher power.

3. *We made a decision to turn our will and our lives over to the care of God as we understood God.* The adolescent workbook (Jaffe 1990) presents an interpretation of this step that involves having the adolescents make a decision to commit themselves to working the steps and having a positive spiritual power. The teenagers are helped to recognize that they turned over their lives to alcohol and drugs. Now they are being asked to turn their lives over to a positive program.

4. *We made a searching and fearless moral inventory of ourselves.* The workbook (Jaffe 1990) instructs the adolescents to answer numerous detailed questions covering all aspects of their childhood and present life.
5. *We admitted to God, to ourselves, and to another human being the exact nature of our wrongs.* At this point, the adolescents discuss their inventories with a counselor or their sponsor.

Although at first glance, the language and terminology of 12-step treatment may look peculiar and overtly religious, many of the same strategies of present-day evidence-based treatments are inherent in this treatment modality. An empathic, nonconfrontational approach using feedback and an emphasis on individual responsibility are fundamental to both motivational enhancement therapy and 12-step treatment. The coercive approaches of the 1990s, including programs such as Scared Straight, were a misinterpretation of 12-step recovery. Cognitive-behavioral therapy strategies, such as the use of distraction and calling one's sponsor to deal with thoughts and urges to use a substance, are integral parts of a 12-step program. Contingency management–type reinforcers in the form of chips are awarded for periods of sober time. Also, meetings and sponsor relationships contain large amounts of positive reinforcement. Parental management techniques and family issues are part of Al-Anon and Alateen. In addition, the 12-step programs' concepts of a higher power are contained in the mindfulness concept of dialectical behavior therapy. Thus, although the language may differ, underneath 12-step methods are elements of many commonly used contemporary treatments (McCrady 1994). In addition, a recent systematic review of the mechanisms of behavior change through which AA has been shown to work revealed that AA works by enhancing abstinence self-efficacy and active coping efforts, and through maintaining and enhancing motivation for abstinence within a supportive peer recovery context (Kelly et al. 2009)—all purported mechanisms of commonly used cognitive and behavioral interventions.

Evidence of Effectiveness of Adolescent Participation in 12-Step Groups

Although research on adolescent 12-step mutual-help participation has been sparse, a number of outcome studies have examined the utility of such participation among youth (for a detailed review, see Kelly and Myers 2007). Alford et al. (1991) followed up 157 chemically dependent adolescents and found significantly increased abstinence at 6 months for those who completed AA- and NA-based treatment programs. Kennedy and Minami (1993) reported an abstinence rate of 47% at 1 year for participants in a 3-day inpatient program followed by a 22-day wilderness AA- and NA-based program. The Chemical Abuse Treatment Outcome Registry (Harris and Hoffman 1989; Hsieh et al. 1998), which included over 2,300 adolescents treated in 24 AA- and NA-based residential programs, demonstrated an abstinence rate of 50% at 1-year follow-up. Attending two or more AA or NA meetings in a week was the most significant variable for positive outcome. Winters et al. (2000) used improved scientific methodology with a good follow-up contact rate, standardized measures, and confirmation of self-reports to study 179 adolescents who received 12-step-based residential treatment compared with 66 similar adolescents who needed treatment but lacked insurance coverage. At 1-year follow-up, those who had completed treatment had an abstinent/minor relapse rate of 53%, compared with 28% for those who needed but did not receive treatment. The favorable outcome continued at 5-year follow-up for the treatment group, especially for those individuals who attended aftercare AA or NA meetings (Winters et al. 2007).

Kelly et al. (2000) studied 99 adolescents following 12-step-based residential substance use disorder treatment, with an average length of stay of 12.5 days. At the 3-month follow-up, 31% were abstinent, and 30.3% were abstinent at 6 months. AA or NA attendance was found to uniquely contribute to the maintenance and enhancement of motivation for abstinence. A further analysis showed that active involvement, including use of a sponsor and working the 12 steps, was associated with increased motivation for abstinence above that attributable to attendance alone (Kelly et al. 2002). Significant limitations of these studies included lack of random assignment and the fact that only post-inpatient/residential treatment programs were studied (Kelly and Myers 2007). Two further long-term studies both showed benefits of AA or NA participation on substance use outcomes over 3 years among outpatient youth (Chi et al. 2009) and over 8 years for a sample of inpatient youth (Kelly et al. 2008a). In the latter study, for every AA or NA meeting a youth attended, youth were found to gain an additional 2 days of abstinence over and above all other factors associated with good outcomes.

Although participation in 12-step meetings is commonly recommended for youth leaving treatment, and variants of 12-step-oriented treatment are quite common among youth providers (Drug Strategies 2003; Knudsen et al. 2008), limited interest has been demonstrated by the research community. Possible reasons for this lack of interest may include 1) an ambiguous emphasis on spirituality, which has been difficult to define and measure (Kelly et al. 2009); 2) the fact that these programs are a community intervention directed by laypersons and therefore are not under direct researcher control; and 3) its basis in the disease model of addiction, with abstinence as its goal. However, given the programs' widespread use, common 12-step meeting referrals, and promising results, more clinical research is warranted.

Twelve-Step Facilitation Strategies for Youth

Passetti and Godley (2008) studied the referral practice of 28 clinicians at eight different treatment programs, which had follow-up interviews of 1,600 adolescents. Clinicians indicated that referral to 12-step meetings was significantly based on the severity of the substance use and related problems and on whether the adolescents were at a developmental level to grasp 12-step concepts such as "powerlessness." Referral to specific meetings was influenced by the age composition and availability. Attendance rates for different programs varied greatly, from 1% up to 67%. The highest rates of attendance were in those programs that were 12-step based. These programs actively linked adolescents to meetings, sponsors, and sober social activities within the recovery community and monitored their participation.

Passetti and White (2008) discussed specific issues for clinicians to consider in referring adolescents to 12-step groups. To the following summary of their discussion, we have added some further specific recommendations. The paucity of research leaves us to balance recommendations with the successes and failures of frontline clinicians.

1. *Potential negative effects from 12-step meeting attendance.* Although studies support the safety of professionally led adolescent substance abuse group therapy (Burleson et al. 2006), this is not true for unscreened, open, peer-led 12-step meetings. Often adults and adolescents attend meetings to fulfill parole requirements, with no interest in sobriety or working a program,

which, in some instances, could result in some individuals undermining serious attempts at sobriety. Thus, time before and after meetings needs to be structured and contacts with other members need to be monitored. This is especially true for adolescents in early recovery. The so-called 13th step of AA or NA relates to a member flirting with a new member.

2. *Age composition.* Research indicates that meetings with a significant number of other adolescents improve attendance and outcome (Kelly et al. 2005). Professionals should explore which available groups have at least some other adolescents, but this consideration should be balanced with making sure that a significant number are experiencing good recovery.

3. *Ability to understand program concepts.* Recommendations are for professionals to discuss the language and concepts of the program and to correct any misconceptions. The assumption is that the professionals involved are knowledgeable about 12-step recovery. Ideally, professionals need to be familiar with 12-step literature, have attended open meetings, and have spoken to members in good recovery to learn and understand fundamental aspects and more subtle nuances of 12-step recovery. Jaffe's (2000) workbook for the first five steps (as previously described) makes the steps meaningful for adolescents. Twelve-step mutual-help groups are sometimes criticized for being "too abstract" for adolescents. However, the emphasis on sharing experiences and positive relationships, with the goal of sobriety, does not require cognitive formal operations. The concrete higher power conveyed by good feelings (love) and good direction from 12-step program members does not involve an abstract thinking level. In fact, most adolescent attendees report that the feeling of not being alone and of gaining positive attention and support is most important to them (Kelly et al. 2008b).

The spirituality aspects of 12-step programs are important because in the development of addiction, the adolescent has essentially established a negative higher power (the alcohol or drugs). The addicted adolescent devotes all of his or her thoughts, feelings, and actions to acquiring and using alcohol or drugs. The positive, nonreligious higher power of 12-step programs replaces the negative spirituality of addiction. Prayer, meditation, positive affirmations, and altruistic helping of others enhance positive spiritual experiences. In keeping with AA philosophy, the general idea is that adolescents can choose any conception of a "higher power" that they want (e.g., the AA group/fellowship) as long as it is not themselves.

4. *Severity of substance use and related problems.* Adolescents with more severe substance involvement are referred more often and are more likely to attend 12-step meetings (Kelly et al. 2002). Twelve-step recovery was developed as a treatment for addiction. Although some less severely substance-involved youth may benefit from a deterrent effect from some exposure to AA or NA, it does not make good sense to prescribe AA or NA participation for adolescents at the recreational or early abuse level of alcohol or drug involvement. Family therapy treatments are usually more appropriate for early adolescents, with their developmental lack of introspection and less serious alcohol or drug involvement.

5. *Differences in local recovery groups.* Because 12-step program meetings are led by nonprofessionals and are open to anyone with a desire to stop using alcohol or drugs, meetings may vary in their focus, composition, and cultural orientation. Adolescents may need to attend a variety of meetings to find the ones with which they feel the best connection.

6. *Assertive versus passive linkage.* Assertive, monitored linkage is needed for the success and safety of adolescents attending 12-step programs. Sponsors should be screened by the referring clinicians to assess the sponsors' recovery, stability, and appropriateness to work with adolescents.

Conclusion

Twelve-step mutual-help organizations, such as AA and NA, are commonly prescribed as a cost-effective continuing care resource for youth. These free community resources are widely available, are easily accessible, and can be attended for free as intensively and for as long as an individual desires. Because they provide a widely available network of recovery-specific support, particularly at times of high relapse risk when professional support is often not available (e.g., evenings, weekends), these organizations can offer an adaptive community-based system responsive to undulating relapse risk (Kelly and Yeterian, in press). We have presented and suggested some clinical recommendations and strategies to maximize the potential benefits from these community resources. However, given the range of substance involvement and other heterogeneity in youth clinical presentations, more research in general and more rigorous experimental research in particular are needed to understand which youth may benefit from these resources and to what extent.

Key Clinical Concepts

- Clinicians who wish to facilitate 12-step participation among youth would benefit from greater familiarity with 12-step mutual-help organizational concepts and terms.

- The first step of AA, modified for adolescents, emphasizes empowerment; the idea is that one's power is increased if usage of alcohol or drugs is stopped.

- The positive higher power of 12-step programs is nonreligious and involves separating what is in one's control (one's actions) from what is not in one's control (what others say or do), which needs to be turned over to a higher power.

- A significant research base supports the efficacy of 12-step programs, but these studies lack random assignment and are limited mostly to adolescents following discharge from hospital or residential programs.

- Monitored, assertive linking of substance-involved adolescents to 12-step programs (meetings, sponsors, and recovering peers) provides the needed safety and best opportunity for success.

References

Alcoholics Anonymous: Twelve Steps and Twelve Traditions. New York, Alcoholics Anonymous World Services, 1952

Alcoholics Anonymous: 2007 Membership Survey: A Snapshot of AA Membership. New York, Alcoholics Anonymous World Services, 2008

Alford GS, Koehler RA, Leonard J: Alcoholics Anonymous–Narcotics Anonymous model inpatient treatment of chemically dependent adolescents: a 2-year outcome study. J Stud Alcohol 52:118–126, 1991

Brown SA: Recovery patterns in adolescent substance abuse, in Addictive Behaviors Across the Life Span: Prevention, Treatment, and Policy Issues. Edited by Marlatt GA, Baer JS. Newbury Park, CA, Sage, 1993, pp 161–183

Burleson JA, Kaminer Y, Dennis ML: Absence of iatrogenic or contagion effects in adolescent group therapy: findings from the Cannabis Youth Treatment (CYT) study. Am J Addict 15 (suppl 1):4–15, 2006

Chi T, Felicia W, Kaskutas LA, et al: Twelve-step affiliation and 3-year substance use outcomes among adolescents: social support and religious service attendance as potential mediators. Addiction 104:927–939, 2009

Dennis M, Godley S, Diamond G, et al: The Cannabis Youth Treatment (CYT) study: main findings from two randomized trials. J Subst Abuse Treat 27:197–213, 2004

Drug Strategies: Treating Teens: A Guide to Adolescent Programs. Washington, DC, Drug Strategies, 2003

Harrison PA, Hoffman NN: CATOR Report: Adolescent Treatment Completers One Year Later, St Paul, MN, Chemical Abuse/Addiction Treatment Outcome Registry, 1989

Hsieh S, Hoffmann NG, Hollister CD: The relationship between pre-, during-, and post-treatment factors, and adolescent substance abuse behaviors. Addict Behav 23:477–488, 1998

Jaffe SL: Step Workbook for Adolescent Chemical Dependency Recovery: A Guide to the First Five Steps. Washington, DC, American Psychiatric Press, 1990

Jaffe SL: Adolescent Substance Abuse Intervention Workbook: Working a First Step. Washington, DC, American Psychiatric Press, 2000

Jaffe SL, Allen S, Fernandez M, et al: Pilot study of a two-hour workbook intervention for juvenile delinquents with substance abuse. Am J Addict 17:39, 2008

Kelly JF, McCrady BS: Twelve-step facilitation in non-specialty settings, in Research on Alcoholism: Alcoholics Anonymous and Spiritual Aspects of Recovery. Edited by Galanter M. New York, Springer, 2009, pp 797–836

Kelly JF, Myers MG: Adolescents' participation in Alcoholics Anonymous and Narcotics Anonymous: review, implications, and future directions. J Psychoactive Drugs 39:259–269, 2007

Kelly JF, Yeterian J: Mutual-help groups, in Evidence-Based Adjunctive Treatments. Edited by O'Donohue W, Cunningham JR. New York, Elsevier, 2008, pp 61–106

Kelly JF, Yeterian JD: The role of mutual-help groups in extending the framework of treatment. Alcohol Res Health (in press)

Kelly JF, Myers MG, Brown SA: A multivariative process model of adolescent 12-step attendance and substance use outcome following inpatient treatment. Psychol Addict Behav 14:376–389, 2000

Kelly JF, Myers MG, Brown SA: Do adolescents affiliate with 12 step groups? A multivariate process model of effects. J Stud Alcohol 63:293–304, 2002

Kelly JF, Myers MG, Brown SA: The effects of age composition of 12-step groups on adolescent 12-step participation and substance use outcome. J Child Adolesc Subst Abuse 15:63–72, 2005

Kelly JF, Brown SA, Abrantes A, et al: Social recovery model: an 8-year investigation of youth treatment outcome in relation to 12-step group involvement. Alcohol Clin Exp Res 32:1468–1478, 2008a

Kelly JF, Myers MG, Rodolico J: What do adolescents think about 12-step groups? Perceptions and experiences of two AA-exposed clinical samples. J Subst Abuse 29:53–62, 2008b

Kelly JF, Yeterian JD, Myers MG: Treatment staff referrals, participation expectations, and perceived benefits and barriers to adolescent involvement in twelve-step groups. Alcohol Treat Q 26:427–449, 2008c

Kelly JF, Magill M, Stout RL: How do people recover from alcohol dependence? A systematic review of the research on mechanisms of behavior change in Alcoholics Anonymous. Addict Res Theory 17:236–259, 2009

Kennedy BP, Minami M: The Beech Hill Hospital/Outward Bound Adolescent Chemical Dependency Treatment Program. J Subst Abuse Treat 10:395–406, 1993

Knudsen HK, Ducharme LJ, Roman PM, et al: Service Delivery and Use of Evidence-based Treatment Practices in Adolescent Substance Abuse Treatment Settings: Project Report. Athens, University of Georgia, 2008

McCrady BS: Alcoholics Anonymous and behavior therapy: can habits be treated as diseases? Can diseases be treated as habits? J Consult Clin Psychol 62:1159–1166, 1994

Oxford Group: What is the Oxford Group? London, Oxford University Press, 1933

Passetti LL, Godley SH: Adolescent substance abuse treatment clinicians' self-help meeting referral practices and adolescent attendance rates. J Psychoactive Drugs 40:30–40, 2008

Passetti LL, White WL: Recovery support meetings for youths: considerations when referring young people to 12-step and alternative groups. J Groups Addict Recover 2:97–121, 2008

Prochaska JO, DiClemente CC: Transtheoretical therapy: toward a more integrative model of change. Psychotherapy: Theory, Research and Practice 19(3):276-288, 1982

Substance Abuse and Mental Health Services Administration: Results from the 2007 National Survey on Drug Use and Health: National Findings (NSDUH Series H-34; DHHS Publ No SMA 08-4343). Rockville, MD, Office of Applied Studies, 2008

Vaughn MG, Howard MO: Adolescent substance abuse treatment: a synthesis of controlled evaluations. Res Soc Work Pract 14:325–335, 2004

Winters KC, Stinchfield RD, Opland E, et al: The effectiveness of the Minnesota model approach in the treatment of adolescent drug abusers. Addiction 95:601–612, 2000

Winters KC, Stinchfield R, Latimer WW, et al: Long-term outcome of substance-dependent youth following 12 step treatment. J Subst Abuse Treat 33:61–69, 2007

Winters KC, Botzet AM, Fahnhorst T, et al: Adolescent substance abuse treatment: a review of evidence-based research, in Handbook on the Prevention and Treatment of Substance Abuse in Adolescence. Edited by Leukefeld C, Gullotta T, Staton Tindall M. New York, Springer, 2009

Suggested Readings

Humphreys K: Circles of Recovery: Self-Help Organizations for Addictions. Cambridge, UK, Cambridge University Press, 2004

Jaffe SL: The Adolescent Substance Abuse Intervention Workbook: Working a First Step. Washington, DC, American Psychiatric Press, 2000

Jaffe SL: Staff Manual for the Adolescent Substance Abuse Intervention Workbook. Washington, DC, American Psychiatric Press, 2000

Kelly JF, McCrady BS: Twelve-step facilitation in non-specialty settings, in Research on Alcoholism: Alcoholics Anonymous and Spiritual Aspects of Recovery. Edited by Galanter M. New York, Springer, 2008, pp 325–350

Kelly JF, Yeterian J: Mutual-help groups, in Evidence-Based Adjunctive Treatments. Edited by O'Donohue W, Cunningham JR. New York, Elsevier, 2008, pp 61–106

Nowinski J, Baker S, Carroll KM: Twelve-Step Facilitation Therapy Manual: A Clinical Research Guide for Therapists Treating Individuals With Alcohol Abuse and Dependence. NIAAA Project MATCH Monograph Series Vol 1 (DHHS Publ No ADM-92-1893). Rockville, MD, National Institute on Alcohol Abuse and Alcoholism, 1992

White WL: Peer-Based Addiction Recovery Support: History, Theory, Practice, and Scientific Evaluation. Chicago, IL, Great Lakes Addiction Technology Transfer Center and the Philadelphia Department of Behavioral Health and Mental Retardation Services, 2009

Relevant Websites

Alcoholics Anonymous: http://www.aa.org

The Cool Spot (the young teen's place for info on alcohol and resisting peer pressure): http://www.thecoolspot.gov

Narcotics Anonymous: http://www.na.org

12

Attention Deficit–Disruptive Behavior Disorders and Substance Use Disorders in Adolescents

K.A.H. Mirza, M.B., F.R.C.P.C.

Oscar G. Bukstein, M.D., M.P.H.

D isruptive behavior disorders of childhood and adolescence —that is, oppositional defiant disorder, conduct disorder, and attention-deficit/hyperactivity disorder (ADHD)—are the most common comorbid psychiatric disorders diagnosed in youth with substance use disorders (SUDs) (Bukstein et al. 2005). In addition to being highly prevalent in both clinical and community populations of adolescents with SUDs, these disorders, which will be addressed in this chapter as externalizing disorders, have a substantial role in the development of SUDs and influence the course and prognosis.

Epidemiology

In community studies, comorbidity of externalizing disorders in adolescents with substance abuse is high, with a median prevalence of 46% across studies, whereas in the absence of any substance use, reported rates of externalizing disorders range between 0.0% and 12.0% (median between 7.0% and 8.0%) (Armstrong and Costello 2002). There does not appear to be any gradient of comorbidity with increasing severity of substance use.

Oppositional defiant disorder is often associated with substance use. In a comparison of alcohol-dependent and community-control adolescents, those with alcohol dependence were twice as likely as community controls to have oppositional defiant disorder (Clark et al. 1997). Similarly, in a review of 15 community studies of adolescent substance use or SUD, oppositional defiant disorder was one of the most frequently observed comorbid conditions, along with conduct disorder (Armstrong and Costello 2002).

Chan et al. (2008) measured the rates of externalizing problems in a clinical population of adolescents and adults in treatment for SUDs. They reported that the rates of externalizing problems generally decreased with age, going from two-thirds of adolescent groups to one-third of the oldest group. Approximately one-half of adolescents under age 15 and about one-third of adults met criteria for ADHD, and about one-half of adolescents and one-third of adults met criteria for conduct disorder. Among adolescents under age 15 with diagnoses of substance dependence, about 90% had at least one mental health problem in the past year; the most prevalent co-occurring problems were conduct disorder (74.2%), ADHD (63.6%), depression (52.7%), and traumatic distress (50.6%). The estimated odds ratios of comorbidity were 3.4 for conduct disorder and 3.0 for ADHD. From a study of adolescents recruited from clinical treatment programs for alcohol use disorder, Molina et al. (2002) reported that 30% of the adolescents had high ADHD symptom counts and 73% had three or more conduct disorder symptoms.

Relationship Between Conduct Disorder/ Oppositional Defiant Disorder and SUDs

A review of adolescent community surveys found that childhood mental disorders, particularly conduct disorder, generally predicted earlier initiation of substance use and SUD onset (Armstrong and Costello 2002). A robust body of evidence has accumulated over the past few decades to show a strong association between conduct disorder and substance use (Whitmore et al. 1997). This relationship is likely reciprocal, with each exacerbating the expression of the other (Hovens et al. 1994; Le Blanc and Loeber 1998). The onset of conduct disorder almost always precedes or coincides with the onset of SUDs (Clark et al. 1997; Huizinga et al. 1989). In a study by Sung et al. (2004), a history of early conduct disorder doubled the risk for SUD, but oppositional defiant disorder did not increase the risk for SUD. Similarly, a history of conduct disorder independent of substance involvement predicted later alcohol involvement and later antisocial personality disorder (Brown et al. 1996), although it is uncertain whether a decrease in antisocial acts is related to a decrease in substance involvement (Burke et al. 2003). Conduct disorder severity has been found to predict SUD severity (Lynsky and Fergusson 1995; Young et al. 1995).

As with many forms of psychopathology, the etiology of comorbid conduct disorder and SUD is likely to be a combination of genetic predisposition and exposure to environmental risk factors. Findings from genetic studies are consistent with the theoretical formulation proposed by Kendler et al. (2003) that an underlying common genetic basis increases an individual's propensity for behavioral disinhibition leading to conduct disorder, antisocial personality disorder, alcohol dependence, and/or other drug dependence. However, the influence of both specific and common environmental effects, working in concert with these genetic susceptibilities, determines the form and severity of the externalizing disorders (Rutter et al. 2006). Environmental effects emerge from maladaptive interactions with family, school, and peers (Oetting et al. 1998). These environmental risk factors are quite similar for both conduct disorder and SUD. Substance use may result in additional problems with poor judgment and association with delinquent peers, which lead to illegal acts and aggression (Clark and Scheid 2001).

Among treated adolescents, comorbid psychopathology, particularly conduct problems, generally predicted poorer outcomes, including an early return to substance use (Brown et al. 1996; Clark and Scheid 2001) and a more persistent course of substance involvement over 1-year follow-up (Grella et al. 2001). Kaminer et al. (1992) found that among adolescents with SUD, those with only comorbid conduct disorder had a significantly higher treatment dropout rate than did those with both conduct disorder and depression. The authors suggested that youth with comorbid conduct disorder and depression are more amenable to treatment than those with conduct disorder only. A history of conduct disorder, independent of substance use, has been related to greater posttreatment alcohol use and later antisocial personality disorder (Brown et al. 1996; Myers et al. 1995). The same team of researchers reported the results of a 4-year follow-up study of treated youth. The majority (61%) of adolescents with conduct disorder at the time of treatment met criteria for antisocial personality disorder at follow-up, and these individuals had higher levels of drug involvement over follow-up than did those without antisocial personality disorder (Myers et al. 1998).

Relationship Between ADHD and SUDs

Longitudinal studies conducted in community and clinic samples show that children with ADHD are at high risk of developing SUDs (Barkley et al. 2004; Fergusson et al. 1993; Manuzza et al. 1993; Molina and Pelham 2003). The relationship between ADHD and substance abuse is rather complex and relatively understudied. A debate exists in the literature as to whether ADHD in itself poses a significant risk for later substance abuse or whether the substance abuse can be accounted for by the overlap between ADHD and conduct disorder. Some authors suggest that ADHD and conduct disorder interact to increase the risk for substance abuse, so that individuals with both ADHD and conduct disorder are at greater risk for later substance use problems than are those with either disorder alone (Chilcoat and Breslau 1999; Molina et al. 2002). However, some studies have found ADHD to be prospectively associated with cigarette smoking and nicotine dependence, even after controlling for conduct disorder (Biederman et al. 2006; Milberger et al. 1997). A recent review of cross-sectional and longitudinal studies from community and clinical samples by Flory and Lynam (2003) indicated generally consistent results: ADHD appears to confer independent risk only for tobacco use. For all other types of drugs, the relationship with ADHD seems to disappear when controls for comorbid conduct disorder are instituted. A number of other causal pathways or mechanisms may explain the relationship between ADHD and substance abuse. For example, individuals with ADHD may use nicotine, a legal, widely available stimulant drug, to alleviate some of the symptoms of ADHD (Levin et al. 1996). Similarly, in utero exposure to maternal smoking and alcohol abuse may predispose children to develop both ADHD and substance abuse (Milberger et al. 1996; Weissman et al. 1999).

Biological Aspects of Stimulant Medication Abuse

An area of ongoing controversy involves the abuse potential of stimulant medication and the impact of medication treatment on long-term risk of substance abuse. Critics of drug treatment point out that methylphenidate and other stimulants have a strikingly similar pharmacological profile to cocaine, and pharmacotherapy may increase the risk of development of substance abuse through a process of sensitization. Despite suggestive evidence for sensitization from animal models (Kollins et al. 2001), SUDs do not appear to be the result of prior stimulant use for the treatment of ADHD in childhood or early adolescence.

The central role of dopamine and the mesolimbic dopaminergic pathways in addiction has been well substantiated in a large number of studies over several decades. All drugs of abuse act by increasing dopamine in the mesolimbic and mesocortical dopamine pathways. Like cocaine, stimulants exert their pharmacological properties by blocking dopamine reuptake, thereby increasing synaptic dopamine (Volkow et al. 2001). Some studies have shown that methylphenidate is even more potent than cocaine in binding to the dopamine transporter and producing long-lasting neuronal adaptation in the nucleus accumbens (Kim et al. 2009). Studies done in healthy human volunteers showed that subjective effects of intravenous methylphenidate were quite similar to those of cocaine and amphetamine (Kollins 2007). However, Volkow et al. (1995) reported that route of administration and dosages of stimulants are the most important variables that determine abuse potential. When methylphenidate is administered intravenously, it enters the brain like cocaine and peaks rapidly, producing subjective sensations of euphoria. However, when methylphenidate is taken orally, the rate of uptake into striatum is much slower, and subjective sensations of euphoria are significantly reduced or absent. Similarly, regardless of the routes of administration, methylphenidate is cleared from the brain more slowly than cocaine, and this may diminish the reinforcing properties and protect against repeated self-administration and abuse (Volkow et al. 1995). Thus, methylphenidate, when taken orally in therapeutic doses and within a clinical context, appears to be associated with a much lower abuse potential than cocaine.

To date, no long-term randomized controlled studies have directly addressed the question of whether ADHD diagnosed in childhood increases the risk of future substance abuse. Perhaps the best "clinical" evidence may be obtained from longitudinal community studies and naturalistic studies that have followed children diagnosed with ADHD into adolescence or adulthood. In a meta-analysis of prospective and retrospective clinical studies conducted before 2003, Wilens et al. (2003) reported that children treated with stimulant medication were protected against the development of substance-related problems by a factor of two (odds ratio = 1.9) compared with those children who did not receive treatment with stimulant medication for ADHD. However, Lambert and colleagues have shown that childhood ADHD/stimulant treatment is related significantly to rates of tobacco use and dependence and cocaine dependence (Lambert 2002; Lambert and Hartsough 1998). Methodological shortcomings of the above studies included an overrepresentation of children with conduct disorder in the ADHD group and the limited information provided regarding the details of treatment with methylphenidate, including the dosage, age at initiation, and duration of treatment. Therefore, it is difficult to draw any firm conclusions from the study.

More recently, two studies concluded that early stimulant treatment for ADHD does not contribute to substance misuse later in life (Biederman et al. 2008; Manuzza et al. 2008). Similarly, in a naturalistic follow-up study from Germany, Huss et al. (2008) reported that early age at initiation of methylphenidate treatment in children with ADHD does not increase the risk for nicotine dependence and that in fact methylphenidate may delay the onset of continuous nicotine use. Furthermore, observational follow-up of children in the Multimodal Treatment Study of ADHD after 36 months follow-up from assessment has suggested that medication does not contribute significantly to the risk for substance misuse in early adolescence and that behavior therapy is associated with reduction of risk (Molina et al. 2007). In summary, despite the methodological shortcomings of the existing literature, the available data suggest that the net effect of stimulant treatment for ADHD in children and adolescents is to protect against rather than to lead to substance abuse.

Assessment

Clinicians working with adolescents who have comorbid externalizing disorders and SUDs should develop skills in assessing for developmentally appropriate manifestations and impairments associated with adolescent and adult forms of ADHD and should use appropriate instruments, including rating scales, for diagnosing ADHD. The diagnosis of ADHD and/or conduct disorder in adolescents with SUDs is made within a comprehensive evaluation (Bukstein et al. 2005; Pliszka; Work Group on Quality Issues; 1997; Steiner and Remsing; Work Group on Quality Issues 2007) of the multiple needs of the young people affected. The acute status of the patient's SUD may obscure the diagnosis of ADHD, in part because the patient may have difficulty distinguishing drug-induced cognitive status from drug-free cognitive status. Similarly, conduct disorder behaviors may be the result of drug-seeking behaviors, such as stealing and/or lying to maintain a drug use habit. Hyperactivity, agitation, impulsivity, attentional difficulties, aggression, and other antisocial behaviors may also be the result of intoxication or withdrawal from various substances. Features associated with ADHD and conduct disorder include low frustration tolerance; lack of task persistence; conflictual relations with peers, adults, and authorities; contact with the legal system; and increased rates of mood and anxiety disorders.

In the overwhelming majority of cases, both conduct disorder and ADHD will precede the development of SUD; therefore, a premorbid history will often indicate the diagnosis. Review of past records (i.e., psychological or psychiatric evaluations and/or report cards and school records), as well as information from other informants (e.g., parents and teachers), is often critical because both adolescents and adults with ADHD may have poor insight into their level of ADHD symptoms and resulting impairments. Youth should be seen separately from parents for a confidential interview. The clinician should be flexible, empathic, and nonjudgmental to engage the young person in the assessment process and to obtain a valid estimate of substance abuse. The clinician should also be watchful for drug-seeking adolescents with SUDs who may feign ADHD symptoms or history and insist on stimulant treatment; responsible adult informants can be helpful in this detection. Accurate youth self-reports may be challenging to obtain, especially when there are strong incentives to underreport deviant behaviors (e.g., in forensic settings) or to respond in a socially desirable manner (e.g., in clinical settings). The presence of externalizing disorders should prompt special consideration in the inquiry and assessment of substance use behavior, because extremely antisocial adolescents have much higher responses of "faking good" than do clinical samples (Winters 2001).

Given the high prevalence of ADHD and conduct disorder in patients undergoing addiction treatment, all adolescents in treatment for SUDs should be screened and, if needed, evaluated for a diagnosis of ADHD and conduct disorder. A number of well-validated rating scales are available for use with adolescents with ADHD (Collett et al. 2003). Although rating scales are often used for antisocial behaviors, more common is the use of broad-spectrum measures, such as the Child Behavior Checklist (Achenbach 2001a), Youth Self-Report (Achenbach 2001c), and Teacher's Report Form (Achenbach 2001b), or the Strengths and Difficulties Questionnaire (Goodman 2001). Composed of DSM-III-R diagnostic criteria (American Psychiatric Association 1987), the Disruptive Behavior Disorders Rating Scale (Pelham et al. 1992) can be used to obtain parent and teacher ratings of children's symptoms of ADHD, oppositional defiant disorder, and conduct disorder.

The assessment of biological markers indicative of substances of abuse is reviewed in Chapter 4, "Biomarker Testing for Substance Use in Adolescents."

Treatment

Consensus guidelines have been provided for the assessment and treatment of adolescents with SUDs and externalizing disorders (Bukstein et al. 2005; National Institute for Health and Clinical Excellence 2006; Pliszka; AACAP Work Group on Quality Issues 2007; Steiner and Remsing; Work Group on Quality Issues 2007). Integrated, multimodal treatment of both substance misuse and externalizing disorders has been found to be useful in clinical practice. Specific treatment for substance-related problems may often be needed before initiation of treatment for ADHD, especially when evidence indicates substance dependence or extremely chaotic substance misuse. Once some level of stabilization has been reached, further assessment and treatment for ADHD and/or conduct disorder should proceed. Despite the impact of comorbid ADHD and/or conduct disorder on the course and outcome of SUD, limited empirical data are available to guide treatment. Medication should never be provided in isolation from psychosocial treatment directed at a patient's SUD.

Psychosocial Treatments

Treatment for conduct disorder often takes the form of targeting risk factors for the development and maintenance of conduct disorder. This includes targeting social and problem-solving skills, as well as parental supervision and monitoring. Although adolescents with externalizing disorders and SUDs should receive many of the modalities deemed efficacious for adolescents with SUDs in general, several psychosocial treatment modalities deserve special consideration. A specific case has been made for intervention with youth diagnosed with conduct disorder such as multisystemic therapy, other family therapies, and motivational interviewing.

Multisystemic therapy addresses the multidimensional nature of behavior problems in youth with delinquency and/or SUDs (Henggeler et al. 2002). Treatment focuses on those factors in each youth's social network that are contributing to his or her antisocial behavior. The ultimate goal of multisystemic therapy is to empower families to build a healthier environment through the mobilization of existing child, family, and community resources. Multisystemic therapy is delivered in the natural environment (home, school, or community). The typical duration of home-based multisystemic therapy services is approximately 4 months, with multiple, weekly therapist-family contacts. Multisystemic therapy targets risk factors in an individualized, comprehensive, and integrated fashion, allowing families to enhance protective factors. Multisystemic therapy uses specific, empirically supported treatment techniques, including behavioral, cognitive-behavioral, and pragmatic family therapies. It is noteworthy that Henggeler et al. (2002) suggested that the modest effects of multisystemic therapy with substance-abusing and dependent juvenile offenders, when therapy was transported to a community setting, were more dependent on the quality of the research design, including treatment fidelity and supervision oversight, than on other factors. Littell et al. (2005), however, noted that this hypothesis cannot be tested with available data. They noted that although the treatment adherence measure used for multisystemic therapy has some predictive validity, it is not clear whether this is due to fidelity, engagement, treatment participation, alliance, or other constructs.

Although motivation to engage in treatment is a general problem for adolescents with SUDs, this is exacerbated with comorbid disruptive behavior disorders (Kaminer et al. 1992, 2002). Preliminary evidence supports the use of motivational interviewing with incarcerated adolescents (86% with conduct disorder); Stein et al. (2006) reported that adolescents who received motivational interviewing early in treatment evidenced significantly less negative treatment engagement (i.e., poor attitude, dislike for counselor, off-task behavior with peers) during milieu and group-based social skills treatments that focused on substance use. The use of motivational interviewing in more deviant samples of youth with SUDs awaits study.

Development of a prosocial lifestyle is perhaps one of the more difficult goals for SUD treatment in adolescents with externalizing disorders (Bukstein et al. 2005). A supportive environment, especially parents and peers who do not use substances, is important for optimal outcomes (Myers et al. 1995). Use of family therapy specific for youth offenders has been found helpful (Alexander et al. 1999, 2000). A controversial element of traditional treatment programs is the widespread use of group treatment. The consistent empirical support of group cognitive-behavioral therapy for substance-abusing adolescents (Burleson et al. 2006; Kaminer 2005) stands in contrast to the iatrogenic "deviant" peer-group effects reported for group interventions (Dishion et al. 1999, 2002). Neither the Cannabis Youth Treatment study group interventions (Dennis et al. 2004) nor Waldron et al.'s (2001) and Kaminer et al.'s (2002) studies in outpatient settings, which included a significant percentage of adolescents with conduct disorders, demonstrated any severe or unmanageable problems in conducting group therapy (e.g., need to eject subjects, need to discontinue a session, physical abuse). Diverse referral sources apparently allow for a mix of adolescents who are manageable in a group setting once a clearly communicated and signed behavioral contract for ground rules is introduced. Experienced therapists can competently address inappropriate behavior and other "troubleshooting," particularly in a manual-driven treatment.

For a comprehensive review of family therapies, cognitive-behavioral therapy, and motivational interviewing for youth with SUD, the reader is referred to Chapters 9 ("Brief Motivational Interventions, Cognitive-Behavioral Therapy, and Contingency Management for Youth Substance Use Disorders") and 10 ("Multidimensional Family Therapy and the Adolescent Community Reinforcement Approach") in this book.

Pharmacotherapy

In addition to the individual and family treatments for comorbid conduct disorder and SUD, the clinician can consider psychopharmacology as one component of an integrated treatment package. The pharmacological treatment of conduct disorder largely involves the treatment of comorbid conditions, such as ADHD (discussed below), and treatment of aggression and other extreme manifestations of mood dysregulation. Pappadopulos et al. (2003) and Schur et al. (2003) provided 14 recommendations on using antipsychotics to treat acute and chronic aggression in youth, as well as an algorithm on how the clinician can make choices when using these medications. Research indicates that anticonvulsants (Khanzode et al. 2006; Steiner et al. 2003) and atypical antipsychotics (Pappadopulos et al. 2003; Schur et al. 2003) show early efficacy and potential for treating aggressive adolescents. Unfortunately, no studies have been published of using these agents for the treatment of adolescents with SUDs and aggression or conduct disorder comorbidity.

The evidence base for pharmacological treatment of ADHD with comorbid SUD is extremely limited and based primarily on open trials (Szobot et al. 2008; Wilens et al. 2008b), with few empirical studies to help guide the process of choosing the most efficacious treatment approaches for this group. A systematic review of the available evidence in adolescents and adults indicated that stimulants, when given to people with ADHD and drug misuse, led to improvement in ADHD symptoms with no worsening of substance misuse (Wilens et al. 2005).

Treatment may include pharmacotherapy with one of the empirically proven first-line stimulant treatments, such as methylphenidate, amphetamines, or atomoxetine, which are approved by the U.S. Food and Drug Administration (Kollins 2007). Tertiary agents, such as bupropion and venlafaxine, should be reserved for those not responding adequately to the first-line medications. Stimulants remain the most effective treatments for ADHD in all ages. Avoidance of stimulants should be strongly considered in patients with ADHD who have active SUD, especially those with a stimulant or cocaine dependence and those not receiving psychosocial treatment for their SUDs. Individuals with a prior history of SUD or with a reasonable interval of remission of use or symptoms (6–12 months) may benefit from first-line stimulant treatment. Use of longer-acting or extended-release formulations of stimulants is strongly recommended.

If an adequate response to nonstimulants is noted, and especially if uncontrolled ADHD symptoms appear to contribute to relapse or instability of the SUD, stimulant treatment may proceed with careful and frequent monitoring. In addition to being aware of possible abuse of medications by the patients with SUD and ADHD themselves, the clinician should be watchful for possible diversion by either the patient, family members, or peers in every case. Prescription of medications should be carefully monitored, with high suspicion directed toward frequent early requests for refills or "lost" prescriptions.

Pharmacological Strategies to Reduce the Abuse Potential of Medications

Compared with long-acting preparations, short-acting methylphenidate has reinforcing effects, characterized by a rapid rise in serum concentrations and concomitant increases in central nervous system (CNS) dopamine levels. The pharmacokinetic properties of immediate-release stimulant formulations more closely match those of drugs that can induce euphoria. The practice parameters for treatment of ADHD from the American Academy of Child and Adolescent Psychiatry indicate that extended-release stimulants are less likely to be misused or diverted than immediate-release agents (Greenhill et al. 2002). There are several possible reasons that long-acting stimulant medications have a lower risk of abuse. Compared with patients receiving osmotic-release oral system (OROS) methylphenidate, those receiving immediate-release methylphenidate endorsed higher euphoria scores and higher visual analogue drug-liking scales. A neuroimaging study conducted in 12 healthy adults randomly assigned to receive single doses of either immediate-release methylphenidate or OROS methylphenidate indicated that despite similar maximum plasma concentrations, OROS methylphenidate had a prolonged time to maximum concentration and maximum CNS dopamine transporter occupancy, compared with immediate-release methylphenidate (Spencer et al. 2006). The lower risk for abuse of extended-release formulations of methylphenidate or amphetamine may also be related to the fact that active components cannot be readily extracted from the beaded or osmotic extended-release preparations of these stimulants (Wilens et al. 2005). The active compound contained in the OROS methylphenidate preparation is very difficult to obtain by crushing, thus diminishing the abuse potential of methylphenidate, whereas the other long-acting stimulant formulations comprise long-acting beads that are not conducive to abuse by snorting, sniffing, or injecting. These findings are consistent with a report on a group of adolescents with ADHD and SUD who were unable to achieve a high when attempting to inhale a preparation made from OROS methylphenidate (Jaffe 2002).

A methylphenidate transdermal patch that is available in the United States releases 10–30 mg of methylphenidate over a 9-hour period, with peak plasma concentration being achieved after 8 hours (Anderson and Scott 2006). Short-term clinical trials have attested to the safety and efficacy of this transdermal patch, although it has not been studied in patients with comorbid substance misuse. Lisdexamfetamine dimesylate (LDX) is a promising new "prodrug" that could potentially reduce the risk of misuse of dexamphetamine by intra-nasal or intravenous routes (Biederman et al. 2007). In its intact form, LDX is pharmacologically inactive. When LDX is taken orally, the amide linkage is hydrolyzed in the gastrointestinal tract, gradually releasing active D-amphet-amine. Limited biotransformation of LDX occurs when the drug is adminis-tered via parenteral routes. Two double-blind crossover studies in healthy adults with a history of stimulant abuse suggested that LDX had a delayed mean peak effect compared with D-amphetamine, consistent with delayed and less intense pharmacodynamic effects (Jasinski et al. 2006). The relative abuse potential of LDX was less than that for D-amphetamine. However, LDX has not been studied in clinical populations with ADHD and comorbid SUD. It is not yet available in the United Kingdom.

Atomoxetine, a selective norepinephrine reuptake inhibitor, has been re-ported to have little abuse potential, as evidenced by animal studies and small-scale studies in human volunteers (Heil et al. 2002; Lile et al. 2006; Wee and Woolverton 2004). Early clinical experience is encouraging, although no large-scale studies have been undertaken as yet to demonstrate the safety and efficacy of atomoxetine in patients with ADHD and SUD. Meta-analyses have shown that the effect size of atomoxetine is somewhat lower than that of stimulants (Faraone et al. 2006). Some evidence, both from adult literature and from open-label trials in adolescents, supports the use of bupropion. The use of nonstimulant drugs to treat ADHD could potentially reduce the risk of substance abuse, but this should not be at the expense of treatment efficacy. The risk-benefit ratio is generally lower with regard to the use of tricyclic antide-pressants or bupropion.

Diversion and Abuse of Stimulant Medication

Stimulant medications are controlled drugs and have the potential for abuse and diversion, either for subjective euphoric effects or for effects on performance. Methylphenidate can be abused intranasally by crushing the tablets and snorting the powder or intravenously by dissolving the powder in water and injecting it. People who take the drug to induce euphoria prefer intranasal and intravenous routes, and there have been a few case reports of intravenous abuse of methylphenidate in adolescents and young adults (Teter et al. 2006). Extended-release preparations of stimulants are probably less easy to misuse in this way than immediate-release tablets. More commonly, oral stimulants have been misused to enhance performance in sports or some kinds of cognitive tasks and examinations by U.S. (Wilens et al. 2006, 2008a) and Canadian (Barrett et al. 2005) students.

According to a national survey of 10,904 U.S. college students, 4.1% of the students had used stimulants for nonmedical purposes in the previous year, and 54% of students taking medication for ADHD had been approached to divert (sell, trade, or give away) their medication in the past year (McCabe et al. 2005). A report by the Drug Abuse Warning Network indicated that in 2004 in the United States, 48% of the presentations to accident and emergency departments that involved methylphenidate or amphetamines resulted from nonmedical use of prescribed drugs (Drug Abuse Warning Network 2006). A systematic review by Wilens et al. (2008a) indicated that diversion of stimulant medications is rife in North America, and although the extent of diversion in the United Kingdom is not known, the risk is present and possibly growing in view of the increased rates of prescribing stimulant medications. There have been reports of parents with substance abuse histories misusing their children's methylphenidate; in one instance, the son was coached by his mother on symptoms of ADHD to persuade physicians to prescribe methylphenidate (Fulton and Yates 1988). Physicians prescribing stimulants should be vigilant to any phenomenon indicative of medication misuse or diversion. History of familial drug abuse should be a reason for caution when prescribing stimulants. Physicians might need to count pills and meet one-on-one with the youth and the parent(s) to inquire about discrepancies.

Conclusion

Conduct disorder and ADHD are significant risk factors for the development of substance abuse through a number of causal pathways. In adolescents with SUDs, conduct disorder and ADHD are among the most common comorbid disorders. Because of the potential influence of conduct disorder and ADHD on the course of SUDs, these problems should be identified and treated with a combination of psychosocial and pharmacological interventions. Active treatment of ADHD is likely to reduce the development of conduct disorder and SUD, and many adolescents with SUD can take stimulants safely and appropriately. However, in view of the potential misuse of stimulants and diversion of stimulant medication, clinicians, teachers, and other professionals should be made aware of the scope and context of the problem and closely monitor adolescents being treated with these agents.

The choice of medication is dependent on the personal and family history of substance abuse, including the potential risk of abuse and diversion. In treating adolescents with ADHD and active SUD symptoms and behaviors, nonstimulant agents (atomoxetine) or antidepressants (bupropion) may be preferable to stimulants, given the absence of more substantial evidence of stimulant efficacy in this population. For those with poor response to these agents, those whose SUD has been stabilized, or those with merely a prior history of SUD (assuming nonamphetamine SUD), the use of extended-release or longer-acting stimulants with lower abuse liability and diversion potential is a reasonable option. The role of optimal treatment of ADHD and conduct disorder on the course of SUD has yet to be fully studied.

Key Clinical Concepts

- Persistent conduct disorder in children and adolescents is among the most robust predictors of adolescent SUDs.
- Children with ADHD and conduct disorder are at increased risk of developing substance abuse in adolescence and adulthood, and the risk is higher for those with coexistent social adversity and other environmental risk factors.
- The existing literature suggests that treatment of ADHD with medication does not increase the risk of development of substance abuse. In

fact, it may protect against the development of substance abuse in children with ADHD.

- Abuse of stimulants employed for the treatment of ADHD is not uncommon. Stimulant medications are diverted or abused either for subjective euphoric effects or for effects on performance.

- Treatment of ADHD or conduct disorder alone will not improve the outcome for people with disruptive behavior disorder and comorbid SUD. Integrated, multimodal treatment packages incorporating specific psychosocial and pharmacological treatments for SUD and other comorbidities, such as conduct disorder, should be provided along with optimal treatment of ADHD.

- Careful selection of agents for the treatment of patients with ADHD has the potential to limit drug diversion and abuse, particularly in high-risk groups, such as those with a comorbid SUD or conduct disorder. Extended-release stimulants, nonstimulants, or "prodrugs" are preferred to short-acting stimulants, because they are less likely to be misused or diverted.

References

Achenbach TM: Child Behavior Checklist for Ages 6–18. Burlington, VT, ASEBA Research Center for Children, Youth, and Families, 2001a

Achenbach TM: Teacher's Report Form. Burlington, VT, ASEBA Research Center for Children, Youth, and Families, 2001b

Achenbach TM: Youth Self-Report. Burlington, VT, ASEBA Research Center for Children, Youth, and Families, 2001c

Alexander JF, Robbins MS, Sexton TL: Family therapy with older, indicated youth: from promise to proof to practice, in Center for Substance Abuse Prevention Science Symposium: Bridging the Gap Between Research and Practice. Edited by Kumpfer K. Washington, DC, Center for Substance Abuse and Prevention, 1999, pp 1–164

Alexander JF, Pugh C, Parsons BV, et al: Functional family therapy, in Blueprints for Violence Prevention (Book 3), 2nd Edition. Edited by Elliott DS. Boulder, CO, Center for the Study and Prevention of Violence, Institute of Behavioral Science, University of Colorado, 2000

American Psychiatric Association: Diagnostic and Statistical Manual of Mental Disorders, 3rd Edition, Revised. Washington, DC, American Psychiatric Association, 1987

Anderson VR, Scott LJ: Methylphenidate transdermal system: in attention-deficit hyperactivity disorder in children. Drugs 66:1117–1126, 2006

Armstrong TD, Costello EJ: Community studies on adolescent substance use, abuse, or dependence and psychiatric comorbidity. J Consult Clin Psychol 70:1224–1239, 2002

Barkley RA, Fischer M, Smallish L, et al: Young adult follow-up of hyperactive children: antisocial activities and drug use. J Child Psychol Psychiatry 45:195–211, 2004

Barrett SP, Darredeau C, Lana E, et al: Characteristics of methylphenidate misuse in a university student sample. Can J Psychiatry 50:457–461, 2005

Biederman J, Monuteaux MC, Mick E, et al: Young adult outcome of attention deficit hyperactivity disorder: a controlled 10-year follow-up study. Psychol Med 36:167–179, 2006

Biederman J, Krishnan S, Zhang Y, et al: Efficacy and tolerability of lisdexamfetamine dimesylate (NRP-104) in children with attention-deficit/hyperactivity disorder: a phase III, multicenter, randomized, double-blind, forced-dose, parallel-group study. Clin Ther 29:450–463, 2007

Biederman J, Monuteaux MC, Spencer T, et al: Stimulant therapy and risk for subsequent substance use disorders in male adults with ADHD: a naturalistic controlled 10-year follow-up study. Am J Psychiatry 165:597–603, 2008

Brown SA, Gleghorn A, Schuckit MA, et al: Conduct disorder among adolescent alcohol and drug abusers. J Stud Alcohol 57:314–324, 1996

Bukstein OG, Bernet W, Arnold V, et al: Practice parameter for the assessment and treatment of children and adolescents with substance use disorders. J Am Acad Child Adolesc Psychiatry 44:609–621, 2005

Burke JD, Loeber R, Lahey BB: Course and outcomes, in Conduct and Oppositional Defiant Disorders. Edited by Essau CA. Mahwah, NJ, Erlbaum, 2003, pp 61–95

Burleson JA, Kaminer Y, Dennis M: Absence of iatrogenic or contagion effects in adolescent group therapy: findings from the Cannabis Youth Treatment (CYT) study. Am J Addict 15 (suppl 1):4–15, 2006

Chan YF, Dennis ML, Funk RR: Prevalence and comorbidity of major internalizing and externalizing problems among adolescents and adults presenting to substance abuse treatment. J Subst Abuse Treat 34:14–24, 2008

Chilcoat HD, Breslau N: Pathways from ADHD to early drug use. J Am Acad Child Adolesc Psychiatry 38:1347–1354, 1999

Clark DB, Scheid J: Comorbid mental disorders in adolescents with substance use disorders, in Substance Abuse in the Mentally and Physically Disabled. Edited by Hubbard JR, Martin PR. New York, Marcel Dekker, 2001, pp 133–167

Clark DB, Pollock NK, Bukstein OG, et al: Gender and comorbid psychopathology in adolescents with alcohol dependence. J Am Acad Child Adolesc Psychiatry 36:1195–1203, 1997

Collett BR, Ohan JL, Myers KM: Ten-year review of rating scales, VI: scales assessing externalizing behaviors. J Am Acad Child Adolesc Psychiatry 42:1143–1170, 2003

Dennis ML, Godley SH, Diamond G, et al: The Cannabis Youth Treatment (CYT) study: main findings from two randomized trials. J Subst Abuse Treat 27:197–213, 2004

Dishion TJ, McCord J, Poulin F: When interventions harm: peer groups and problem behavior. Am Psychol 54:755–764, 1999

Dishion TJ, Poulin F, Barraston B: Peer group dynamics associated with iatrogenic effects in group interventions with high-risk young adolescents. New Dir Child Adolesc Dev 91:79–92, 2002

Drug Abuse Warning Network: Emergency department visits involving ADHD stimulant medications, 2006. Available at: https://dawninfo.samhsa.gov/files/TNDR09ADHDmedsForHtml.pdf. Accessed January 2, 2010.

Faraone SV, Biederman J, Spencer TJ, et al: Comparing the efficacy of medications for ADHD using meta-analysis. MedGenMed 8:4, 2006

Fergusson DM, Lynskey MT, Horwood LJ: Conduct problems and attention deficit behaviour in middle childhood and cannabis use by age 15. Aust N Z J Psychiatry 27:673–682, 1993

Flory K, Lynam DR: The relationship between attention deficit hyperactivity disorder and substance abuse: what role does conduct disorder play? Clin Child Fam Psychol Rev 6:1–16, 2003

Fulton AI, Yates WR: Family abuse of methylphenidate. Am Fam Physician 38:143–145, 1988

Goodman R: Psychometric properties of the Strengths and Difficulties Questionnaire (SDQ). J Am Acad Child Adolesc Psychiatry 40:1337–1345, 2001

Greenhill LL, Pliszka S, Dulcan MK, et al: Practice parameter for the use of stimulant medications in the treatment of children, adolescents, and adults. J Am Acad Child Adolesc Psychiatry 41 (2 suppl):26S–49S, 2002

Grella CE, Hser Y, Joshi V, et al: Drug treatment outcomes for adolescents with comorbid mental and substance use disorders. J Nerv Ment Dis 189:384–392, 2001

Heil SH, Holmes HW, Bickel WK, et al: Comparison of the subjective, physiological, and psychomotor effects of atomoxetine and methylphenidate in light drug users. Drug Alcohol Depend 67:149–156, 2002

Henggeler SW, Clingempeel WG, Brondino MJ, et al: Four-year follow up of multisystemic therapy with substance abusing and substance-dependent juvenile offenders. J Am Acad Child Adolesc Psychiatry 41:868–874, 2002

Hovens JG, Cantwell DP, Kiriakos R: Psychiatric comorbidity in hospitalized adolescent substance abusers. J Am Acad Child Adolesc Psychiatry 33:476–483, 1994

Huizinga DH, Menard S, Elliot DS: Delinquency and drug use: temporal and developmental patterns. Justice Q 6:419–455, 1989

Huss M, Poustka F, Lehmkuhl G, et al: No increase in long-term risk for nicotine use disorders after treatment with methylphenidate in children with attention-deficit/hyperactivity disorder (ADHD): evidence from a non-randomised retrospective study. J Neural Transm 115:335–339, 2008

Jaffe SL: Failed attempts at intranasal abuse of Concerta (letter). J Am Acad Child Adolesc Psychiatry 41:5, 2002

Jasinski D, Krishnan S, Kehner G: Abuse liability of intravenous lisdexamfetamine (LDX; NRP 104). Program and Abstracts of the 2006 Annual Meeting of the Society for Developmental and Behavioral Pediatrics. Philadelphia, PA, September 16–18, 2006

Kaminer Y: Challenges and opportunities of group therapy for adolescent substance abuse: a critical review. Addict Behav 30:1765–1774, 2005

Kaminer Y, Tarter RE, Bukstein OG, et al: Comparison between treatment completers and noncompleters among dually diagnosed substance-abusing adolescents. J Am Acad Child Adolesc Psychiatry 31:1046–1049, 1992

Kaminer Y, Burleson JA, Goldberger R: Cognitive-behavioral coping skills and psychoeducation therapies for adolescent substance abuse. J Nerv Ment Dis 190:737–745, 2002

Kendler KS, Prescott CA, Myers J, et al: The structure of genetic and environmental risk factors for common psychiatric and substance use disorders in men and women. Arch Gen Psychiatry 60:929–937, 2003

Khanzode LA, Saxena K, Kraemer H, et al: Efficacy profiles of psychopharmacology: divalproex sodium in conduct disorder. Child Psychiatry Hum Dev 37:55–64, 2006

Kim Y, Teylan MA, Baron M, et al: Methylphenidate-induced dendritic spine formation and DeltaFosB expression in nucleus accumbens. Proc Natl Acad Sci U S A 106:2915–2920, 2009

Kollins SH: Abuse liability of medications used to treat attention-deficit/hyperactivity disorder (ADHD). Am J Addict 16 (suppl 1):35–42; quiz 43–44, 2007

Kollins SH, MacDonald EK, Rush CR: Assessing the abuse potential of methylphenidate in nonhuman and human subjects: a review. Pharmacol Biochem Behav 68:611–627, 2001

Lambert NM: Stimulant treatment as a risk factor for nicotine use and substance abuse, in Diagnosis and Treatment of Attention-Deficit Hyperactivity Disorder: An Evidence-Based Approach. Edited by Jensen PS, Cooper JR. Kingston, NJ, Civic Research Institute, 2002, pp 1811–1820

Lambert NM, Hartsough CS: Prospective study of tobacco smoking and substance dependencies among samples of ADHD and non-ADHD participants. J Learn Disabil 6:533–544, 1998

Le Blanc M, Loeber R: Developmental criminology updated, in Crime and Justice: A Review of Research. Edited by Ohlin L, Tonry M. Chicago, IL, University of Chicago Press, 1998, pp 245–265

Levin ED, Connors CK, Sparrow E, et al: Nicotine effects on adults with attention-deficit/hyperactivity disorder. Psychopharmacology (Berl) 123:55–63, 1996

Lile JA, Stoops WW, Durell TM, et al: Discriminative-stimulus, self-reported, performance, and cardiovascular effects of atomoxetine in methylphenidate-treated humans. Exp Clin Psychopharmacol 14:136–147, 2006

Littell JH, Popa M, Forsythe B: Multisystemic therapy for social, emotional, and behavioral problems in youth aged 10–17. Cochrane Database Syst Rev CD004797, 2005

Lynsky MT, Fergusson DM: Childhood conduct problems, attention deficit behaviors, and adolescent alcohol, tobacco, and illicit drug use. J Abnorm Child Psychol 23:281–302, 1995

Mannuzza S, Klein RG, Bessler A, et al: Adult outcome of hyperactive boys: educational achievement, occupational rank, and psychiatric status. Arch Gen Psychiatry 50:565–576, 1993

Mannuzza S, Klein RG, Truong NL, et al: Age of methylphenidate treatment initiation in children with ADHD and later substance abuse: prospective follow-up into adulthood. Am J Psychiatry 165:604–609, 2008

McCabe SE, Knight JR, Teter CJ, et al: Non-medical use of prescription stimulants among U.S. college students: prevalence and correlates from a national survey. Addiction 100:96–106, 2005

Milberger S, Biederman J, Faraone S, et al: Is maternal smoking during pregnancy a risk factor for attention-deficit/hyperactivity disorder in children. Am J Psychiatry 153:1138–1142, 1996

Milberger S, Biederman J, Faraone S, et al: ADHD is associated with early initiation of cigarette smoking in children and adolescents. J Am Acad Child Adolesc Psychiatry 36:37–44, 1997

Molina BS, Pelham WE: Childhood predictors of adolescent substance use in a longitudinal study of children with ADHD. J Abnorm Psychol 112:497–507, 2003

Molina BS, Bukstein OG, Lynch K: Attention-deficit/hyperactivity disorder and conduct disorder symptomatology in adolescents with alcohol use disorder. Psychol Addict Behav 16:161–164, 2002

Molina BS, Flory K, Hinshaw SP, et al: Delinquent behavior and emerging substance use in the MTA at 36 months: prevalence, course, and treatment effects. J Am Acad Child Adolesc Psychiatry 46:1028–1040, 2007

Myers MG, Brown SA, Mott MA: Preadolescent conduct disorder behaviors predict relapse and progression of addiction for adolescent alcohol and drug abusers. Alcohol Clin Exp Res 19:1528–1536, 1995

Myers MG, Stewart DG, Brown SA: Progression from conduct disorder to antisocial personality disorder following treatment for adolescent substance abuse. Am J Psychiatry 155:479–485, 1998

National Institute for Health and Clinical Excellence: Methylphenidate, atomoxetine and dexamfetamine for the treatment of attention deficit hyperactivity disorder in children and adolescents (Technology Appraisal 98). 2006. Available at: www.nice.org.uk/TA98. Accessed January 2, 2010.

Oetting ER, Deffenbacher JL, Donnermeyer JF: Primary socialization theory: the role played by personal traits in the etiology of drug use and deviance, II. Subst Use Misuse 33:1337–1366, 1998

Pappadopulos E, Macintyre JC II, Crismon ML, et al: Treatment recommendations for the use of antipsychotics for aggressive youth (TRAAY), part II. J Am Acad Child Adolesc Psychiatry 42:145–161, 2003

Pelham WE, Gnagy EM, Greenslade KE, et al: Teacher ratings of the DSM-III-R symptoms of the disruptive behavior disorders. J Am Acad Child Adolesc Psychiatry 31:210–218, 1992

Pliszka S; Work Group on Quality Issues: Practice parameter for the assessment and treatment of children and adolescents with attention-deficit/hyperactivity disorder. J Am Acad Child Adolesc Psychiatry 46:894–921, 2007

Rutter M, Moffitt TE, Caspi A: Gene-environment interplay and psychopathology: multiple varieties but real effects. J Child Psychiatry 47:226–261, 2006

Schur SB, Sikich L, Findling RL, et al: Treatment recommendations for the use of antipsychotics for aggressive youth (TRAAY), part I: a review. J Am Acad Child Adolesc Psychiatry 42:132–144, 2003

Spencer TJ, Biederman J, Ciccone PE, et al: PET study examining pharmacokinetics, detection and likeability, and dopamine transporter receptor occupancy of short- and long-acting oral methylphenidate. Am J Psychiatry 163:387–395, 2006

Stein LAR, Colby SM, Barnett NP, et al: Effects of motivational interviewing for incarcerated adolescents on driving under the influence after release. Am J Addict
15 (suppl 1):50–57, 2006

Steiner H, Petersen ML, Saxena K, et al: Divalproex sodium for the treatment of conduct disorder: a randomized controlled clinical trial. J Clin Psychiatry 64:1183–1191,
2003

Steiner H, Remsing L; Work Group on Quality Issues: Practice parameter for the assessment and treatment of children and adolescents with oppositional defiant disorder. J Am Acad Child Adolesc Psychiatry 46:126–141, 2007

Sung M, Erkanli A, Angold A, et al: Effects of age at first substance use and psychiatric
comorbidity on the development of substance use disorders. Drug Alcohol Depend 75:287–299, 2004

Szobot CM, Rohde LA, Katz B, et al: A randomized crossover clinical study showing
that methylphenidate-SODAS improves attention-deficit/hyperactivity disorder
symptoms in adolescents with substance use disorder. Braz J Med Biol Res
41:250–257, 2008

Teter CJ, McCabe SE, LaGrange K, et al: Illicit use of specific prescription stimulants
among college students: prevalence, motives, and routes of administration. Pharmacotherapy 26:1501–1510, 2006

Volkow ND, Ding YS, Fowler JS, et al: Is methylphenidate like cocaine? Studies on
their pharmacokinetics and distribution in the human brain. Arch Gen Psychiatry 52:456–463, 1995

Volkow ND, Wang GK, Fowler JS, et al: Therapeutic doses of oral methylphenidate
significantly increase extracellular dopamine in the human brain. J Neurosci
21:1–5, 2001

Waldron HB, Slesnick N, Brody JL, et al: Treatment outcomes for adolescent substance
abuse at 4- and 7-month assessments. J Consult Clin Psychol 69:802–813, 2001

Wee S, Woolverton WL: Evaluation of the reinforcing effects of atomoxetine in mon-
keys: comparison to methylphenidate and desipramine. Drug Alcohol Depend
75:271-276, 2004

Weissman MM, Warner V, Wickramaratne PJ, et al: Maternal smoking during pregnancy and psychopathology in offspring followed to adulthood. J Am Acad Child
Adolesc Psychiatry 38:892–899, 1999

Whitmore EA, Mikulich SK, Thompson LL, et al: Influences on adolescent substance
dependence: conduct disorder, depression, attention deficit hyperactivity disorder, and gender. Drug Alcohol Depend 47:87–97, 1997

Wilens TE, Faraone SV, Biederman J, et al: Does stimulant therapy of attention-
deficit/hyperactivity disorder beget later substance abuse? A meta-analytic review
of the literature. Pediatrics 111:179–185, 2003

Wilens TE, McBurnett K, Stein M, et al: ADHD treatment with once-daily OROS methylphenidate: final results from a long-term open label study. J Am Acad Child Adolesc Psychiatry 44:1015–1023, 2005

Wilens TE, Gignac M, Swezey A, et al: Characteristics of adolescents and young adults with ADHD who divert or misuse their prescribed medications. J Am Acad Child Adolesc Psychiatry 45:408–414, 2006

Wilens TE, Adler LA, Adams J, et al: Misuse and diversion of stimulants prescribed for ADHD: a systematic review of the literature. J Am Acad Child Adolesc Psychiatry 47:21–31, 2008a

Wilens TE, Adler LA, Weiss MD, et al: Atomoxetine treatment of adults with ADHD and comorbid alcohol use disorders. Drug Alcohol Depend 96:145–154, 2008b

Winters KC: Assessing adolescent substance use problems and other areas of functioning: state of the art, in Adolescents, Alcohol, and Substance Abuse: Reaching Teens Through Brief Interventions. Edited by Monti PM, Colby SM, O'Leary TA. New York, Guilford, 2001, pp 80–108

Young SE, Mikulich SK, Goodwin MB, et al: Treated delinquent boys' substance use: onset, pattern, relationship to conduct and mood disorders. Drug Alcohol Depend 37:149–162, 1995

13

Assessment and Treatment of Internalizing Disorders

Depression, Anxiety Disorders, and Posttraumatic Stress Disorder

Yifrah Kaminer, M.D., M.B.A.

Julian D. Ford, Ph.D.

Duncan Clark, M.D., Ph.D.

The population of adolescents with substance use disorders (SUDs) is heterogeneous. One of the largest subgroups is composed of those with one or more comorbid psychiatric disorders, also known as dual diagnosis. Dual diagnosis is the rule rather than the exception and amounts to 70%–80% in clinical samples (Kaminer and Bukstein 2008). Comorbid psychiatric disorders influence the development, course, treatment, and outcomes of SUDs in adolescents (Clark and Kirisci 1996).

Clinical consensus is growing for a coordinated intervention toward both SUDs and comorbid psychiatric disorders. Piecemeal treatments targeting depression in the absence of treatment for SUD, or vice versa, have a higher risk of failure than treatments that simultaneously target both disorders (Bukstein et al. 2005). Barriers for integrating treatment services for patients with dual diagnoses include 1) the historical separation of substance abuse and mental health services, 2) a limited number of clinicians and researchers who focus on youth with dual diagnoses, and 3) the tendency to exclude youth with SUDs from medication clinical trials for psychiatric disorders (Libby and Riggs 2005).

Our first objective in this chapter is to enhance practitioners' understanding of the relationship between concomitant SUD and comorbid internalizing disorders, including unipolar depression, anxiety disorders, and posttraumatic stress disorder (PTSD). Second, we aim to increase the knowledge regarding assessment and coordinated treatment of adolescents with these comorbid disorders. Each section addresses the characteristics, epidemiology, assessment, and treatment of the specific disorder among youth with SUDs.

Association Between Internalizing Disorders and SUDs

Psychiatric disorders in childhood confer an increased risk for the development of SUDs (Kaminer and Bukstein 2008); however, the etiological mechanisms have not been systematically researched. A number of possible relationships exist between SUD and psychopathology. Psychiatric disorders may precede SUDs, may develop as a consequence of preexisting SUDs, may moderate the severity of SUDs, or may originate from a common vulnerability (Hovens et al. 1994).

A pivotal source of knowledge about the relationship between psychiatric disorders and substance abuse in the general population is the Epidemiologic Catchment Area study (Regier et al. 1990). Almost three of every four participants with psychiatric comorbidity indicated that the substance abuse started later than other psychiatric disorders (Christie et al. 1988). Indeed, many clinicians believe that substance abuse is the result of the need to self-medicate emotional stress and affective symptomatology (Khantzian 1997). Limited evidence supports the popular self-medication theory (Degenhardt et al. 2003; Fergusson et al. 2009). However, there is empirical support for the rebound effects (i.e., symptom exacerbation) of substance use on psychiatric symptom severity in youth with dual diagnoses (Tomlinson et al. 2005). These rebound effects carry added risk for physical and psychological adverse effects.

Depression

Characteristics and Epidemiology

The comorbidity of SUD with unipolar depression in adolescents is well established. Developmentally, adolescence is a time when the prevalence of both depression and substance use increases in nonreferred community samples. The median age for the onset of unipolar depression is 19 years (Christie et al. 1988). Moreover, a secular trend of a shift to an earlier age at onset for major depression has been reported (Helzer and Pryzbeck 1988). Up to 8.3% of adolescents (Birmaher et al. 1996) are affected by the unipolar depressive disorders spectrum in the *Diagnostic and Statistical Manual of Mental Disorders*, 4th Edition, Text Revision (DSM-IV-TR; American Psychiatric Association 2000), which includes major depressive disorder, dysthymia, and depressive disorder not otherwise specified.

The odds ratio between alcohol use disorders and both depression and dysthymia is between 1.7 and 1.8 (Helzer and Pryzbeck 1988). Thus, it is not surprising that adolescents may have both a depressive disorder and an SUD. The prevalence of comorbid unipolar depressive disorders in clinical samples of adolescents with SUD ranges from 24% to 50% (Kaminer and Bukstein 2008).

The etiological mechanisms for dual diagnosis of SUD and depression have not been extensively studied. However, they may have important therapeutic and prognostic implications, including increased risk of treatment dropout, poorer treatment response, and earlier relapse (Curry et al. 2003). SUDs among depressed youths are a risk factor for suicidal behaviors, including ideation, attempts, and completed suicide. (For further information on suicidal behavior, see Chapter 14, "Assessment and Treatment of Suicidal Behavior.")

Assessment of Depression in Youth With SUD

The psychiatric assessment of adolescents with SUD should routinely include screening questions about depressive symptoms, including depressive or sad mood, irritability, anhedonia, and suicidality. Symptoms should be considered clinically significant if they are present most of the time, affect the teenager's daily psychosocial or academic functioning, and are above and beyond what is expectable for the adolescent's chronological and psychological age. Validated rating scales that screen for depression using either a parent report or self-report are used to quantify depressive symptoms. If screening suggests significant depressive symptoms, a thorough clinical evaluation should be completed to determine the presence of a depressive disorder and other comorbid psychiatric and medical conditions. Table 13–1 presents some of these rating scales.

Treatment of SUD and Comorbid Depression

Adolescents with combined depression and SUD have higher rates of perceived service needs and receive more treatment services than adolescents with depression and no comorbid disorder (Grella et al. 2001). However, adolescents with SUD have been excluded from all adolescent treatment studies for depression, thus making it impossible to develop a rational, empirically based clinical treatment for these youths with dual diagnosis. Similarly, although depressed youths have been included in some samples in treatment studies for SUD, results generally have not been analyzed separately for this dual-diagnosis group. Therefore, a great need exists to scientifically develop and test interventions for youths with SUD and depression.

Evidence-based research of the treatment of SUD and depression in adolescents includes either psychosocial interventions or psychosocial interventions integrated with selective serotonin reuptake inhibitor (SSRI) pharmacotherapy when indicated (Brent et al. 1997; March et al. 2004). In terms of individual antidepressants, there have been reports of three positive trials of fluoxetine, one trial of citalopram, one trial of escitalopram (the therapeutically active enantiomer of racemic citalopram), and a positive pooling of two trials of sertraline (Emslie et al. 2009).

The guidelines for the treatment of depression in adolescents with dual diagnosis are the same as the guidelines for the treatment of depression not com-

Table 13–1. Rating scales that are used to screen for depression in adolescents

Measure	Age appropriateness (approximate years)	Reading level (grade)	Number of items	Time to complete (approximate minutes)
Beck Depression Inventory (Beck et al. 1996)	14 and older	6th	21	5–10
Center for Epidemiologic Studies— Depression Scale (Radloff 1977)	14 and older	6th		5–10
Center for Epidemiologic Studies— Depression Scale for Children (Fendrich et al. 1990)	12–18	6th	20	5–10
Children's Depression Inventory (Kovacs 1992)	7–17	1st	27	10–15
Reynolds Adolescent Depression Scale (Reynolds 1986)	13–18	3rd	30	10–15
Reynolds Child Depression Scale (Reynolds 1989)	8–12	2nd	30	10–15

plicated by alcohol or substance abuse. However, because substance abuse may impair judgment and increase impulsivity, close and frequent monitoring of the depressed teenager with dual diagnosis is mandatory. Because depression in adolescents is often a chronic and intermittently recurring illness that predicts increased risk for depression in the adult years, and because comorbid SUDs may increase depression severity, the treatment of depression should always include acute and continuation phases. The main goals of the acute phase are to develop a treatment plan that is acceptable to the adolescent and parents and that addresses the substance abuse issues; to provide education about the nature of depression, including how ongoing substance abuse can worsen depressive symptoms, and about the risks and benefits of various treatments, including the risk accruing from a decision not to seek treatment; to introduce an intervention or interventions; and to achieve a response to treatment. The acute phase generally takes from several weeks to 3 months. Continuation treatment is required for all depressed youth to consolidate the response during the acute phase and to avoid depressive relapse. The consolidation phase generally lasts 6–12 months. Thus, the total length of time to treat a single episode of adolescent depression, including the acute and continuation phases, may be 9–15 months.

Maintenance treatment is used to avoid depressive episode recurrences in adolescents who have had a more recurrent, severe, and chronic disorder. Maintenance treatment may last several years or more (Birmaher et al. 2007).

Psychosocial Treatment

An important question is whether psychosocial treatment that targets both SUD and depression is more efficacious than treatment targeting only SUD for substance use outcomes in teens with depression and SUD. Studies have demonstrated that treatments sometimes have beneficial effects for nontargeted yet comorbid conditions. Youth with depression have been included in some studies of psychotherapy for SUDs, but analyses have not always investigated comparative efficacy for this subgroup. In some studies, comorbidity, including depression, has been associated with poorer outcome of SUD treatment (Grella et al. 2001).

Another important question is whether psychosocial treatment that targets both SUD and depression is more efficacious in terms of depression outcomes in teens than similar treatment targeting only SUD. Although successful treatment of SUD could hypothetically reduce secondary depression, two studies did not find this outcome, suggesting a need to target depression even in secondary depression cases (Kaminer et al. 2002; Riggs et al. 1995).

Psychosocial treatment for adolescents with SUD and depression ideally should arise from a theoretical model with demonstrated efficacy in the treatment of both disorders. Cognitive-behavioral therapy (CBT), broadly construed, provides such a foundation. Family systems, behavioral, and cognitive-behavioral therapy models have all shown promise in treating adolescent SUDs. Only one study utilizing a psychosocial approach to the treatment of SUD and depression in youth has been reported. Curry et al. (2003) developed family and coping skills therapy as an integrated family and peer group CBT intervention for adolescents with SUD and depression. Family and coping skills therapy combines adolescent group skills training with cognitive-behavioral family therapy, using modalities and components from effective interventions for both problems. Adolescents also complete periodic urine drug screens. Adolescents attend one family and two group therapy sessions per week. Thus, the treatment approximates an intensive outpatient intervention. Pilot testing indicates considerable promise. A larger-scale randomized controlled study is necessary to replicate and expand on this preliminary study.

Pharmacotherapy

Given the high placebo response rates (35%–60%) in clinical antidepressant trials for youth depression, an advisable practice would be to initiate treatment for youth depression with psychotherapy for mild to moderate depression, and to assess outcome over 4–8 weeks before consideration of adding antidepressant medication (Hughes et al. 2007). It is recommended that depressed youth be seen every week for the first 4 weeks and biweekly thereafter. Determining whether and when to add an antidepressant to the treatment plan for a dually diagnosed adolescent can be difficult. Psychosocial interventions may be sufficient for patients with SUD and uncomplicated and mild depression. However, in adolescents with more severe depression, chronic or recurrent depressive episodes, functional impairment, suicidality, and/or agitation, the addition of antidepressant therapy and specific types of empirically supported psychotherapy (see subsection "Psychosocial Treatment" above) may be necessary. The adolescent with dual diagnosis requires close clinical evaluation and monitoring of treatment. For depressed adolescents with complications such as those noted above, the clinician should consider prescribing an antidepressant as well as psychosocial treatment. Extant psychopharmacological research supports using an algorithmic approach to adolescent antidepressant treatment, beginning with an SSRI (fluoxetine, citalopram, or sertraline). Fluoxetine has the most empirical support, with three large, positive studies indicating superiority to placebo in the treatment of depression (March et al. 2004). Venlafaxine has shown more side effects. The reported remission rates were from 23% at 12 weeks posttreatment to 55% at 36 weeks (Kennard et al. 2009; March et al. 2004). Only five studies have evaluated the efficacy of SSRI antidepressants in depressed adolescents with SUDs (see Table 13–2).

The clinician needs to be aware of potential side effects of antidepressants. An ongoing debate involves whether—and, if so, to what degree—the use or lack of use of SSRIs for the treatment of depression in youth may contribute to increased suicidality (Gibbons et al. 2007; Leckman and King 2007). Concerns about the risk of suicide in youth have led not only to fewer SSRI prescriptions without substitution of alternative medications or psychotherapies, but also to a decrease in predicted rates of diagnosis of mood disorders (Libby et al. 2007). Since the decrease in prescription rates for adolescents in 2004 and 2005 (Gibbons et al. 2007), the suicide rate has increased in that age group (Bridge et al. 2008).

Integrative Treatment

Two recent reports addressed integrative treatment for youth with comorbid major depression using double-blind placebo-controlled trials of fluoxetine. In the first study, by Riggs et al. (2007), all 126 subjects received CBT for SUD concurrent with the medication trial. Fluoxetine had superior efficacy to placebo for remission of depression at and after 13 weeks of treatment. Those adolescents whose depression remitted, regardless of medication group assignment, significantly reduced their drug use, whereas those whose depression did not remit showed no change in drug use. This might be attributed to the CBT effects. It is notable that the separation of effects from fluoxetine versus placebo occurred further along in treatment of these dually diagnosed youths than in studies of children and adolescents without SUDs, suggesting that a longer treatment period may be necessary for substance-abusing adolescents with major depressive disorder (Emslie et al. 1997; March et al. 2004). In the second study, Cornelius et al. (2009) reported the lack of a significant differ-

Table 13–2. Adolescent treatment trials for dually diagnosed depressed adolescents

Substance/study	Study design	N	Intervention/medication	Response
Alcohol use disorder				
Deas et al. 2000	Placebo controlled	10	Sertraline	Improvement in depressive symptoms and drinking in both groups
Cornelius et al. 2001	Open label	13	Fluoxetine	Within-group significant improvement in depression and drinking
Cornelius et al. 2009	Double blind, placebo controlled	50	Fluoxetine	Improvement in depressive symptoms and drinking in both groups; no difference between conditions
Substance use disorder				
Riggs et al. 1997	Open label	8	Fluoxetine	Improvement in depressive symptoms in 7 of 8 subjects
Curry et al. 2003	Pilot	13	Integrated family and cognitive-behavioral therapy	Feasibility demonstrated, and trial associated with improvements in both disorders
Riggs et al. 2007	Double blind, placebo controlled	126	Fluoxetine	Significant improvement in depression in fluoxetine vs. placebo group; no difference between groups in substance abuse outcomes

ence between fluoxetine and placebo groups. Subjects in both groups showed significant improvement in both depressive symptoms and level of alcohol consumption. These findings may be the result of a limited sample size ($N=$ 50) or due to the noteworthy efficacy of the CBT/motivational enhancement therapy provided to all participants.

Case Vignette

Jim, age 15 years 11 months, is a white male who, following an arrest for drug dealing, was referred by a juvenile drug court social worker for psychiatric and substance abuse evaluation and treatment. Jim started smoking marijuana at age 13 after his older brother introduced the drug to him. Jim gradually escalated his use of marijuana over the next 3 years and presently smokes one to two joints daily. He reports a calming effect from the marijuana and frequently goes to school "high." Beginning this year, Jim has occasionally worked for a drug dealer distributing marijuana to students on the grounds of his high school. He started smoking cigarettes at age 11 and is now smoking one-half pack per day. He started drinking alcohol at age 13, and in the last year he has been consuming one six-pack of beer per night on Friday and Saturday to intoxication. All of Jim's friends are drug and/or alcohol users. Jim was an average student, but his grades have gradually deteriorated since seventh grade. Despite a Full Scale IQ of 106, he must make a considerable effort to complete his work in school. He currently has a C– average, and his attendance has been compromised. He is now repeating ninth grade.

When Jim was 11 years old, his mother died in a car accident. She had been in treatment for unipolar depression. When he was 14 years old, Jim was diagnosed with depression after he reported intense symptoms, dating to the loss of his mother, which consisted of daily anhedonia and boredom, irritability, and uncontrollable anger, especially when he perceived himself as being provoked. He was referred to an anger management group but did not attend. The clinician prescribed sertraline, but Jim took it only briefly. He did not disclose his substance use.

Jim lives with his biological father, who works as an electrician; a 13-year-old sister; and his 19-year-old brother, who is an unemployed high school dropout and heavy cannabis user. Upon evaluation, Jim reported feeling depressed and irritable, and reported anhedonia. Jim completed the Beck Depression Inventory and obtained a total score of 26 (moderate depression). He said he believes marijuana "worked better" for calming himself. Upon evaluation, Jim was not yet motivated to abstain from drug use, but was willing to discuss a treatment option in order to avoid legal consequences and to have his pending charges dropped. No suicidal ideation was evident, and no symptoms of bipolar illness were present on mental status examination.

Case Discussion

Treatment goals: The goals for Jim's treatment should be realistic and attainable. Realistic expectancies, including that treatment is a process and not an event, should be conveyed to both Jim and his father. Although the ultimate goal is abstinence, recovery often involves periods of improvement, followed by relapse, and changes in symptom severity.

Treatment setting: Because Jim is not suicidal or dangerous, treatment can occur in an outpatient setting. After 3 years of continuous abuse, he is at risk of withdrawal once he stops using cannabis (Vandrey et al. 2005). A duration of 12 weeks is recommended for a first treatment episode for cannabis use disorders.

Treatment for SUD: Psychosocial treatment strategies that have shown promise in reducing SUD among adolescents are reviewed in Chapters 9–11.

Because Jim demonstrates little motivation for change and the status of his coping skills to resist substance use in high-risk situations is unknown, the clinician recommended an integrated intervention of motivational enhancement therapy and CBT. In this context, *motivational* refers to addressing readiness to change behavior toward abstinence.

A therapeutic contract is recommended. Periodic urinalyses to monitor abstinence, with consequences for negative or positive urine tests, are recommended. A contract negotiated early in treatment between Jim, his father, and the clinician included changes in curfew times, allowance, or other incentives, such as entertainment items (e.g., CDs, DVDs, movie tickets) and clothing. Adjustments to the contract may follow during treatment, based on Jim's progress. An effort to engage Jim's father as an ally in treatment is important to encourage Jim to achieve and maintain abstinence as well as to contain the drug-using activities of Jim's older brother at home.

Psychosocial and pharmacological treatment for comorbid depression: On clinical assessment, Jim met criteria for major depressive disorder. CBT was recommended for Jim's depression and focused on increasing positive activities, improving problem-solving skills, and learning how to restructure unrealistic negative thoughts. Given his lack of suicidal ideation and the moderate severity of his depressive symptoms, beginning antidepressant medication immediately is not mandatory. Because evidence suggests that depression in adolescents is influenced by psychosocial variables and given the high placebo response rates in clinical trials for youth depression, a period of watchful waiting, with ongoing monitoring of Jim's clinical status, is indicated. Suggestions for lifestyle management, including increased engagement with non-drug-involved peers, daily exercise, and the creation of a daily activity schedule to increase pleasurable activities were encouraged.

Two weeks after the onset of treatment for SUD and with the prompting of his father, Jim agreed to an antidepressant trial "to see if it would help." After a risk-benefit discussion with Jim and his father, fluoxetine was initiated at 10 mg/day and increased to 20 mg/day after 1 week. Three weeks after initiating medication, Jim scored 18 on the Beck Depression Inventory (a 30% improvement over baseline). He requested to continue his combined medication and psychosocial treatment. Jim adhered to his recommended treatment for 2 months, with significant improvement in SUD and depression. He then became noncompliant with his scheduled visits and medication. Six months later, his father reported that Jim had relapsed and was smoking marijuana daily, although he was not depressed. Jim refused to return to treatment. The clinician is maintaining contact with his father in order to enable access to treatment.

Conclusion

In the "Practice Parameter for the Assessment and Treatment of Children and Adolescents With Substance Use Disorders," the American Academy of Child and Adolescent Psychiatry (AACAP) Work Group on Quality Issues (Bukstein et al. 2005) concluded that it is essential to treat psychiatric disorders that are comorbid with SUDs among adolescents, and that integration of psychotherapy and medication therapy is currently the best treatment for that population. The Work Group also suggests that SSRI antidepressants are a promising form of therapy for depressive disorders in combination with SUDs among adolescents. Nevertheless, the advice to the savvy clinician is to "proceed with caution" until additional studies clarify the status of the alleged increased probability of suicidality associated with SSRIs in youth (Gibbons and Mann 2009).

Heavy, sustained substance use or poor compliance or refusal of medication may preclude pharmacotherapy. Once abstinence or a reduction in use has occurred, physicians may proceed with a trial of antidepressant medications. For example, in a study of treatment of adolescents with depression, continuation and maintenance treatment out to 36 weeks was included, and continued response and improved rates of remission were noted over this period (Kennard et al. 2009).

Finally, given the relapsing and remitting nature of both SUD and depression (Hawke et al. 2008), treatment may need to be long-term. Continuity of care should already be considered at the onset rather than at the end of treatment, given the potential for dropout.

Anxiety Disorders

Anxiety disorders influence the development, course, treatment, and outcomes of SUDs in adolescents. Anxiety disorders are among the most common mental disorders in adolescents, and are prevalent among adolescents with SUDs (Clark et al. 1994b). The diverse range of problems represented by anxiety disorders complicates the relationships of these disorders with substance use and SUDs (Clark and Sayette 1993). For some anxiety disorders, an association with adolescent SUD has been demonstrated, and plausible models with some empirical support may be presented as a framework for understanding their comorbidity. For other anxiety disorders, there is little or no evidence indicating a clinically meaningful relationship between the specific anxiety disorder and adolescent SUD (Clark et al. 2008).

Characteristics and Epidemiology

The median age at onset of anxiety disorders is 15 years (Christie et al. 1988). DSM-IV-TR includes the following anxiety disorders: social phobia, separation anxiety disorder, specific phobias, panic disorder, agoraphobia, obsessive-compulsive disorder, generalized anxiety disorder, acute stress disorder, and PTSD. *Social phobia* (social anxiety disorder) is characterized by the persistent fear of embarrassment in situations involving social scrutiny. In the most limited form, the fear may be specific to a particular performance situation, such as public speaking. In the most severe and generalized form, social anxiety may include virtually all social situations and be associated with disabling avoidance. *Separation anxiety disorder* is defined by excessive anxiety about separation from parents or other attachment figures. *Specific phobias* include persistent fear of other well-defined objects or situations, with the most common foci including animals or insects, heights or flying, blood or injury, and dental or medical procedures. *Panic disorder* is defined by relatively short periods of intense fear that are not the result of exposure to a feared situation. Panic disorder is often accompanied by *agoraphobia*, a fear of being in situations from which it may be difficult to escape in the event of incapacitating symptoms. In *obsessive-compulsive disorder*, obsessions are persistent thoughts that are experienced as intrusive, and compulsions are repetitive, intentional, and purposeful behaviors performed in response to obsessions. *Generalized anxiety disorder* involves excessive, unrealistic, and persistent worry about two or more life circumstances.

The rates of specific anxiety disorders in community samples (Clark et al. 1994b) provide a context for examining their comorbidity with SUD. Social phobia has been found to be about as common in adolescence as in adulthood. Social phobia has been found to occur in about 1.5% of adolescents, although this figure excludes those with milder forms of performance anxiety. Separation anxiety disorder occurs in about 4% of preadolescent children, and the rate declines during the course of adolescence. Specific phobias occur in about 5% of community adolescent samples, although clinically significant impairment is present in a small proportion of these cases. Although subclinical panic attacks are relatively common, panic disorder occurs in less than 1% of community adolescent samples, and agoraphobia is also uncommon. Obsessive-compulsive disorder occurs in 1% of adolescents. Generalized anxiety disorder also occurs in about 1% of adolescents. Approximately 25% of adolescents with anxiety disorder have multiple anxiety disorders (Clark et al. 1994b). The overlap of social phobia, separation anxiety disorder, and generalized anxiety disorder has been noted to be common in clinical samples (Clark et al. 2005). Depression also commonly accompanies anxiety disorders (Clark et al. 1994b; Kilpatrick et al. 2003). The odds ratios between alcohol use disorders and panic disorder, phobic disorders, and obsessive-compulsive disorders are 2.4, 2.1, and 1.4, respectively (Helzer and Pryzbeck 1988).

Anxiety Disorders and SUD

Demonstrated anxiolytic effects of a substance would to some extent provide supportive evidence for a model proposing that anxiety disorders cause substance involvement. Benzodiazepines, for example, have proven anxiolytic effects and produce a dependence syndrome. Benzodiazepine abuse and dependence are, however, uncommon among adolescents. The evidence for anxiolytic effects of other more commonly abused substances is less clear. The effects of alcohol on anxiety are complex and depend on dose, individual differences, anxiety type, and use circumstances (Clark and Sayette 1993). Stimulants, on the other hand, can lead to or exacerbate anxiety disorders. The theory that adolescents with anxiety disorders consume abused substances for their anxiolytic effects and thereby develop SUD is not consistent with data from adolescent samples.

The influences of anxiety disorders on substance use and related problems likely vary by developmental stage, substance type, stage of substance involvement, and anxiety symptom characteristics. For example, children with anxiety disorders may be risk averse and may therefore show a delay in early adolescent drug and alcohol experimentation. Anxiety disorders have been found to inhibit tobacco use initiation (Clark and Cornelius 2004; Costello et al. 1999) but to be associated with higher rates of daily smoking and nicotine dependence (Breslau et al. 2004). After a substance is tried and adverse consequences do not occur, individuals with anxiety disorders may have an acceleration of the development of substance-related problems. More complex and comprehensive models need to be developed that take into consideration the mechanisms of interactions among different anxiety disorders, specific substances, and developmental stage.

The age at onset of SUD and the relationship of anxiety disorder to SUD onset depend on the specific anxiety disorder. W. M. Compton et al. (2000) found that among adults with substance dependence, phobic disorders predated SUD onset by an average of over 10 years, whereas generalized anxiety disorder and SUD have similar onset ages, with SUD typically preceding generalized anxiety disorder. The specificity of social anxiety disorder as a risk factor for alcohol or other SUDs has been established after depression and other anxiety disorders are controlled for (Buckner et al. 2008). Other anxiety and mood disorders were not associated with subsequent alcohol or other SUDs. However, little published information is available on the sequences of disorders for adolescents with SUD and comorbid anxiety disorders. Several studies have noted that anxiety disorders occur more often in adolescent females than in adolescent males (Clark et al. 1997b).

Anxiety symptoms and disorders have been found to predict substance use and related disorders in adolescents. In a prospective study of community adolescents, baseline social phobia predicted the onset of hazardous alcohol use, and panic disorder predicted persistent alcohol abuse and dependence (Zimmermann et al. 2003). In a large New Zealand birth cohort, adolescents with anxiety disorders were shown to have increased odds of developing substance dependence (Goodwin et al. 2004). Rather than indicating a direct causal link, however, the association observed was thought to be largely attributable to covariates, including childhood, family, and peer factors; prior substance use; and comorbid depression. Anxiety disorders were also shown to predict substance dependence in a community sample of young adults (ages 18–23 years). In these young adults (Lopez et al. 2005), anxiety disorders generally predated SUD, and the increased risk for SUD was attributable to PTSD; anxiety disorders other than PTSD were not predictive of SUD. Although the relationship was not as strong as that for PTSD and major depressive episode, there was some comorbidity, as described in more detail later in this chapter (see section "Adolescent Posttraumatic Stress Disorder and SUD").

To complicate the matter, it is important to note that some anxiety disorders have been shown to be associated with a delay of substance use initiation, diminished substance use overall, or less SUD severity (Clark and Sayette 1993; Myers et al. 2003). Taken together, these studies suggest that anxiety disorders such as separation anxiety may delay experimentation with substance use, whereas adolescent PTSD, social phobia, and panic disorder may contribute to the development of SUD.

Assessment of Anxiety Disorders in Youth With SUD

The assessment of anxiety and anxiety disorders is a recommended component of the psychiatric evaluation of adolescents (Connolly et al. 2007) and is often clinically useful in evaluating adolescents with SUDs. Assessment instruments designed for adolescents are available to identify and evaluate anxiety disorders (Clark et al. 1997a). Tools to screen for anxiety disorders may be particularly useful in the context of the multiple demands placed on the initial assessment for addictions treatment. For example, the Screen for Child Anxiety Related Emotional Disorders (SCARED) is a psychometrically sound 41-item instrument used for child or parent report of a child's DSM-IV anxiety disorder symptoms (Birmaher et al. 1997, 2003; Clark et al. 2005). For adolescents likely to have anxiety disorders, reliance on systematic methods for determining diagnoses is preferred. Although often difficult to achieve, a period of abstinence from alcohol and drugs is very useful in evaluating anxiety disorders in adolescents with SUD, because substantial improvement may occur early in the course of treatment without specific interventions.

Interview methods appropriate for adolescents, such as the Schedule for Affective Disorders and Schizophrenia for School-Age Children—Present and Lifetime Version (K-SADS-PL; Kaufman et al. 1997), typically include the relevant anxiety disorders. This and other semistructured interviews are intended to be administered by clinically experienced and thoroughly trained interviewers. A computer-assisted structured diagnostic interview has been developed for the National Survey on Drug Use and Health (NSDUH) for determining DSM-IV mental disorder diagnoses, including anxiety disorders and SUDs. The NSDUH approach has been extensively evaluated (Caspar and Penne 2002).

Instruments providing graded severity ratings are often more sensitive change indicators than are diagnostic assessments. SCARED scores may be used as a broad change indicator (e.g., Clark et al. 2005). The assessment of global anxiety provides a useful guide for severity and change with treatment that applies across anxiety disorders. Global anxiety may be assessed through interview and questionnaire approaches. The Hamilton Anxiety Rating Scale is an interview method that has been demonstrated to have good psychometric properties in adolescents with SUDs (Clark and Donovan 1994). The clinician-rated Pediatric Anxiety Rating Scale includes a 7-item anxiety severity rating scale that has been shown to have good psychometric properties and sensitivity to treatment effects (Birmaher et al. 2003; Clark et al. 2005). The State-Trait Anxiety Inventory for Children may also be used to determine global anxiety (Kirisci et al. 1996). Focusing on specific anxiety dimensions may also be useful. For example, several scales have been demonstrated to be appropriate for the assessment of social anxiety in adolescents (Clark et al. 1994a, 1997a).

The presence of comorbid anxiety disorders and SUD in adolescents has been found to be associated with decrements in multiple psychosocial and health dimensions (Clark and Kirisci 1996). Consultation with the primary care physician may be helpful in determining whether medical conditions or medication side effects may be contributing to symptoms.

Treatment of SUD and Comorbid Anxiety Disorders

Treatment for anxiety disorders ideally includes all treatment modalities that may improve outcomes (Connolly et al. 2007). Intervention modalities that may be considered in planning treatment for anxiety disorders include education of the adolescent and parents, family therapy, individual psychosocial interventions, and pharmacotherapy. The potential contribution of SUD to exacerbating anxiety symptoms also needs to be addressed in treatment planning.

Although anxiety disorders in some adolescents may be fully responsive to a period of alcohol and drug abstinence, most adolescents with comorbid anxiety disorders and SUDs continue to experience anxiety symptoms despite successful addictions treatment. Furthermore, anxiety disorders may alter response to addictions treatment. Adolescents with social phobia may be less willing to participate in group interventions. When anxiety symptoms persist after a period of abstinence, targeting these symptoms with specific interventions is appropriate. Simultaneous treatment for SUDs and anxiety disorders may be challenging and is largely empirically untested in this population, but it is clinically necessary.

Psychosocial Treatment

Although educational activities and effective communication with parents are a standard and necessary element of treatment with adolescents, the extent and focus of family interventions may vary. In the treatment of youth SUDs, adequate parental supervision contributes to fostering an environment wherein other interventions may lead to successful outcomes (Clark et al. 2005). Family interventions for anxiety disorders in children and adolescents, on the other hand, often focus on fostering independence (Connolly et al. 2007). The appropriate balance between parental involvement and adolescent autonomy at a given time in the course of treatment depends on the adolescent's self-regulation capabilities, peer characteristics, developmental considerations, and parental strengths and limitations.

Psychosocial treatments advocated for anxiety disorders run the gamut, but relatively few approaches have been consistently demonstrated to be effective in controlled trials. Although there are adherents to the practice of psychodynamic psychotherapy for anxiety disorders in adolescents, no large, well-controlled studies have yet been done to demonstrate clinically significant benefits in this population. Furthermore, observational studies have indicated that psychodynamic approaches tend to be more successful in preadolescent children than in adolescents (Target and Fonagy 1994). Empirically demonstrated approaches for anxiety disorders have generally utilized CBT approaches (Connolly et al. 2007).

In a comprehensive review, CBT has been shown to be effective for a range of anxiety and depressive disorders (S. N. Compton et al. 2004), and outcome studies indicate that CBT confers long-term benefit (Kendall et al. 2004). Individual and group CBT approaches have proven successful (Manassis et al. 2002). The elements of CBT thought to be important include exposure to feared stimuli, cognitive restructuring, and relaxation training, with specific features emphasized for particular anxiety disorders (Connolly et al. 2007). For example, individual sessions with graded exposure to feared external stimuli have been emphasized for specific phobias, exposure to interoceptive cues is a unique focus for panic disorder, and group exposure exercises may be useful for social phobia. These approaches may be applicable to adolescents with comorbid anxiety disorders and SUDs. For most adolescents with SUDs, psychosocial interventions are preferred over pharmacological interventions for initial treatment. In patients with SUDs, treatments targeted to anxiety disorders have long been advocated as an approach to diminishing the probability of relapse (Clark et al. 2002).

Pharmacotherapy

Pharmacological approaches to adolescent anxiety disorders include SSRIs, tricyclic antidepressants, benzodiazepines, and buspirone (Birmaher et al. 1998). SSRIs have been demonstrated to be helpful for children and adolescents with common clinical presentations of separate or overlapping anxiety disorders (Birmaher et al. 2003). The effects of SSRIs on anxiety disorders in children and adolescents have also been shown to continue over an extended period (Clark et al. 2005; Walkup et al. 2008). The combination of CBT and sertraline reduced the severity of anxiety disorders in children and adolescents and was superior to each intervention alone (Walkup et al. 2008). For adults, paroxetine has been shown to be helpful for the treatment of comorbid social phobias and SUD, with decreased symptoms of social anxiety and reduced reliance on alcohol to engage in social situations (Thomas et al. 2008). However, these relationships are rather complex: although paroxetine reduced symptoms of social anxiety, it did not reduce drinking in individuals who were not seeking treatment for alcohol problems.

Compared with SSRIs, the other medication classes have disadvantages. Tricyclic antidepressants can have adverse cardiac effects in children and adolescents, and close monitoring is clinically prudent. In addition, the evidence for the effectiveness of tricyclic antidepressant medications for anxiety disorders in children and adolescents is not compelling (Connolly et al. 2007). Due to the risk of abuse and dependence, benzodiazepines are contraindicated in adolescents with SUDs (Clark et al. 2002). Finally, buspirone hydrochloride is an anxiolytic drug that is pharmacologically different from the benzodiazepines. This agent has been marketed as a less sedative anxiolytic that does not potentiate alcohol effects and has a low abuse potential. Buspirone has been used to successfully treat an adolescent with overanxious disorder who did not tolerate treatment with desipramine, and compared with placebo, buspirone therapy was associated with reduced anxiety among adults with anxiety disorder and alcoholism. In conclusion, SSRIs are the mainstay of adolescent anxiety disorder pharmacotherapy.

Integrative Interventions

At this time, recommendations for treating comorbid anxiety disorders and SUDs in adolescents are based on little empirical study and therefore tend to follow the recommendations that would be suggested for adolescents with anxiety disorders without SUDs (Myrick and Brady 2003). For adolescents with comorbid anxiety disorders and SUDs, the integration of treatment options relies on clinical judgment. Prolonged abstinence, however, is achieved by only the minority of treated adolescents. The treatment of anxiety disorders may therefore need to proceed under less than ideal circumstances. Psychosocial treatments are available for adolescents with anxiety disorders, and their integration into addictions treatment does not pose undue problems. Pharmacological treatments for anxiety disorders are also available and need to be considered, especially in more severe and treatment-resistant cases. Benzodiazepines should be avoided due to their potential for abuse or diversion in adolescents with SUDs and have been found to be rarely used in clinical practice with these adolescents (Clark et al. 2002, 2003). Comprehensive treatment guidelines for adolescents with comorbid anxiety disorders and SUDs, however apparent their components, are unfortunately not supported by an empirical literature, and therefore treatment needs to be guided by clinical judgment.

Conclusion

Anxiety disorders vary in their prevalence in adolescence, features, relevance to adolescent SUDs, and treatment implications. Some anxiety disorders overlap in their symptoms, and combinations of disorders represent commonly observed syndromes. Similarly, the overlap between some anxiety disorders and depression may indicate a syndrome rather than independent conditions. The heterogeneity among anxiety disorders is important to acknowledge and to take into consideration in clinical and research applications.

There are many unanswered questions in the area of comorbid anxiety disorders and adolescent SUDs. Additional research needs to be done to determine the extent to which anxiety disorders are relevant for adolescent SUD etiology and treatment. Clinical and community studies have suggested that some anxiety syndromes lead to SUDs, but the role of child maltreatment and PTSD reviewed in the next section is often not considered as an alternative explanation. Some substances cause anxiety in some adolescents, but whether substance-induced anxiety induces long-term changes remains unclear.

Multifaceted models of the comorbidity between SUDs and anxiety disorders need to be developed, tested, and refined. For example, the pharmacological effects of some substances may lead to neurobiological changes that exacerbate anxiety disorders, such as downregulation of the gamma-aminobutyric acid (GABA)–benzodiazepine receptor complex (Clark et al. 2000).

Treatment needs to proceed under less than ideal conditions with an unsatisfactory knowledge base. For adolescents with comorbid anxiety disorders and SUDs, approaches gleaned from other populations, including adolescents and adults with anxiety disorders but not SUDs, need to be applied based on clinical judgment.

Adolescent Posttraumatic Stress Disorder and SUD

Characteristics and Epidemiology

PTSD is the only anxiety disorder that requires not only a pattern of symptoms and psychosocial impairment but also a history of exposure to a stressor. To qualify for PTSD, an adolescent must have "experienced, witnessed, or [been] confronted with an event or events that involved actual or threatened death or serious injury, or a threat to the physical integrity of self or others" (Criterion A1) *and also* have had a response during or soon after the event that "involved intense fear, helplessness, or horror…[which] in children…may be expressed instead by disorganized or agitated behavior" (Criterion A2) (American Psychiatric Association 2000, p. 467). In addition, the adolescent must have experienced three types of symptoms for more than a month. Intrusive reexperiencing symptoms are unwanted memories or distress when reminded of the traumatic event(s) (Criterion B). Avoidance and emotional numbing symptoms are attempts to avoid recalling or being faced with reminders of the event(s), feelings of anhedonia, feelings of detachment from one's own emotions or from relationships, psychogenic amnesia for "an important part" of the traumatic event, and a sense that life will be cut short (distinct from suicidality) (Criterion C). Symptoms of increased arousal include sleep difficulty, irritability or anger outbursts, difficulty concentrating, hypervigilance, and exaggerated startle responses (Criterion D). Most persons with PTSD do not have all of these symptoms; a diagnosis of PTSD requires at least one of reexperiencing symptoms, three of the avoidance or numbing symptoms, and two of the arousal symptoms. Notably, substance use may be directly involved in PTSD avoidance symptoms, and several PTSD symptoms (e.g., anger, poor concentration, emotional numbing) are also symptoms or impairments often involved in SUDs. PTSD also may include several complex "associated features" that are more common when the traumatic event(s) include childhood maltreatment or family violence (e.g., dissociation).

As many as two in three adolescents report having been exposed to traumatic stressors at some point in their lives (Copeland et al. 2007), including directly experiencing or witnessing intentional or accidental violence, abuse, injury, or loss (Kilpatrick et al. 2000); war and terrorism (Pat-Horenczyk et al. 2007); and life-threatening disasters (Anthony et al. 2005). Trauma-exposed adolescents are at risk for PTSD, major depressive disorder, and substance abuse, and those who develop PTSD are at further risk for drug abuse or dependence (Ford et al. 2008; Kilpatrick et al. 2000) and related serious behavioral and psychosocial problems (e.g., depression, suicidality, and oppositionality, as well as SUD; Ford et al. 2000).

Although the prevalence of PTSD in adolescent community populations has been estimated to be as low as 1% (Copeland et al. 2007), estimates from an epidemiological sample of adolescents (Kilpatrick et al. 2003) and from a community-based clinical sample of youth with alcohol use disorders (Hawke et al. 2009) were approximately 5% (five times the prevalence of current or past-year PTSD in an adult community sample) (Kessler et al. 1995). Prevalence estimates among troubled adolescents range from more than twice as high as in community samples (11% among youth in juvenile justice detention programs; Abram et al. 2004) to three to five times as high as in a psychiatric sample (Deykin and Buka 1997) or SUD clinical sample (Lubman et al. 2007) compared with community samples of adolescents. PTSD involves severe impairment across multiple biopsychosocial domains and often is treatment refractory when it becomes chronic (i.e., more than 6 months' duration; American Psychiatric Association 2000).

SUD is a common comorbidity of PTSD among persons of all ages (Mills et al. 2006), but particularly for adolescents and young adults (Kessler et al. 1996). In the National Survey of Adolescents in the United States (Kilpatrick et al. 2003), 24% of girls and 30% of boys who had PTSD also had a SUD, and 25% of girls and 14% of boys who had an SUD also had comorbid PTSD. Although these comorbidity levels were only one-half to one-third of those for PTSD and major depression (especially for girls), they nevertheless suggest that a substantial subgroup of adolescents (approximately 1.5% in the community population) have comorbid SUD and PTSD. Youths at greatest risk for comorbid SUD and PTSD were those who reported having witnessed violence, had been sexually or physically assaulted, had a parent with substance use problems, or were older (Kilpatrick et al. 2003).

In clinical samples receiving treatment for PTSD (Cook et al. 2005) or SUD (Clark et al. 1997b; Jaycox et al. 2004; Lubman et al. 2007), co-occurring PTSD and SUD problems consistently are associated with more severe symptoms and poorer functioning, and prevalence estimates of comorbid SUD and PTSD are higher but consistent with the approximately 20%–25% comorbidity estimate for youth with one or the other disorder reported by Kilpatrick et al. (2003). Compared with SUD treatment clients without PTSD, adolescents in SUD treatment with comorbid PTSD were found to have approximately four times as many additional comorbid psychiatric disorders (on average, two other psychiatric diagnoses in addition to SUD and PTSD), more severe depression symptoms, twice as many SUD diagnoses (on average, two SUDs), more frequent use of and dependence on multiple types of substances (on average, 7.5 types of substances), more relationship problems, more unprotected sex, and more self-harm (Lubman et al. 2007). Further evidence suggesting a risk relationship between SUD and PTSD is provided by results of a study with juvenile justice–involved adolescents, which showed that a combination of substance use problems, past exposure to potentially traumatic stressors, and PTSD symptoms was associated with particularly serious risk of suicidal ideation (Chapman and Ford 2008).

PTSD often has onset among (pre)adolescents prior to SUD. Two community studies with older adolescents and adults found that approximately two-thirds of persons with comorbid PTSD and SUD had an onset of PTSD prior to that of SUD (Epstein et al. 1998; Kessler et al. 1995, 1996). Another study of adolescents and young adults found that several anxiety disorders often preceded SUD but that PTSD was the only anxiety disorder that was predictive of subsequent SUD (Lopez et al. 2005). PTSD has been shown to independently increase the risk among adolescents of marijuana or hard drug abuse (Kilpatrick et al. 2000). The epidemiological research on PTSD and SUDs in adolescents is limited but indicates that PTSD is associated with a 3–14 times greater risk of SUDs (Chilcoat and Menard 2003; Giaconia et al. 2003) and that PTSD more often (i.e., in 53%–85% of cases) predates SUDs than vice versa, with only one exception: 18-year-olds were slightly more likely (54%) to report that alcohol dependence preceded PTSD than vice versa (46%). A prospective study of primarily white middle-class adults in a health maintenance organization (ages 21–35 years) found that PTSD led to a fourfold increased risk of developing SUD independent of the influence of prior conduct problems or depression, but SUD did not increase the risk of either exposure to trauma or developing PTSD (Chilcoat and Menard 2003). The strongest relationship between PTSD and SUD was with abuse of or dependence on prescription drugs but not street drugs, consistent with the higher levels of use of prescription drugs versus street drugs by this particular subgroup of young adults. Thus, SUD may predate PTSD, but it is more likely that SUDs will develop or worsen as a result of attempts to cope with PTSD.

Assessment of PTSD in Youth With SUD

The first step in assessment is screening to identify whether an adolescent with SUD is likely to have comorbid PTSD. Although no validated brief screening measure for PTSD has yet been reported, a four-item Primary Care PTSD (PC-PTSD) questionnaire has been validated for the identification of adults with undetected PTSD in primary care and SUD treatment (Kimerling et al. 2006) populations. The screener asks a single question for each of the four factor–analytically derived categories of PTSD symptoms: intrusive reexperiencing, avoidance of trauma reminders, emotional numbing, and hyperarousal. The PC-PTSD questionnaire has been shown to be reliable and (with a cut score of three items endorsed) to predict PTSD cases in primary care and SUD treatment (Kimerling et al. 2006) samples. The PC-PTSD questionnaire showed evidence of temporal stability, internal consistency, predictive efficiency (0.91), sensitivity (0.91), and specificity (0.87) in identifying SUD treatment patients with PTSD (Kimerling et al. 2006). Validation with adolescent SUD treatment recipients is necessary before the PC-PTSD questionnaire can be used on more than a provisional basis, but it shows promise for quickly identifying youth who otherwise may not be recognized as having comorbid PTSD.

When PTSD is identified as potentially present in a youth with SUD, the second step is to assess the individual's history of (and current) exposure to traumatic stressors. A number of trauma history measures have been developed specifically to assess whether children or adolescents have experienced event(s) that qualify as DSM-IV-TR Criterion A traumatic stressors. A widely used trauma history interview (for parent or youth) that also has a self-report version for adolescents, the Traumatic Events Screening Instrument (TESI; Ford et al. 2000), asks behaviorally anchored questions about 12 distinct domains of potentially traumatic events (e.g., sexual abuse: "Has someone ever made you see or do something sexual against your wishes or when you were helpless?" "Have you seen or heard someone else being forced to do sex acts?"). Following each lead question, probes inquire as to the severity of the event(s) ("Who did this?" "Did anyone die?")—PTSD Criterion A1—and the youth's immediate subjective reactions ("Did you feel really bad, upset, scared, sad, or mixed up the worst time this happened?")—PTSD Criterion A2. The TESI is available at no charge from the National Center for PTSD (http://www.ncptsd.va.gov). Other trauma history measures and specific assessment tools for particular types of traumatic stressor exposure (e.g., childhood physical or sexual abuse; interpersonal violence; disasters; traumatic loss) are described by Nader (2008).

Assessment of PTSD symptom severity and diagnosis is the third step in addressing PTSD in a youth with SUD. Standardized questionnaires and structured interviews have been developed to assess PTSD symptom severity and PTSD diagnosis, respectively (see Nader 2008 for a detailed review). Although a number of validated questionnaires and interviews can be used to efficiently and accurately assess PTSD with children and adolescents, the gold standard for PTSD symptom assessment is the UCLA PTSD Reaction Index; for PTSD diagnostic assessment, the most detailed and widely used is the Clinician-Administered PTSD Scale for Children and Adolescents (CAPS-CA; Nader et al. 1996; see also Nader 2008). The UCLA measure provides a brief but thorough assessment of trauma history and 22 items on which the youth (or a parent) can numerically rate how troubling each of the PTSD symptoms has been. It is brief enough to be suitable for use periodically during treatment as a check on progress in reducing the severity of PTSD symptoms. To make a clinical (or research) diagnosis of PTSD, a structured interview is necessary, in order to probe sufficiently to accurately determine the presence and severity of each symptom and the degree to which the symptoms are causing impairment.

A critical fourth step is to assess comorbid psychiatric disorders and risk behaviors or vulnerability factors, because adolescents with comorbid SUD and PTSD have been shown to be more likely than those with SUD alone to have these additional impairments. Hawke et al. (2009) empirically determined that sexual abuse history, comorbid psychiatric symptom severity, and suicidal ideation were particularly strongly associated with the presence of PTSD among youth receiving psychosocial treatment for SUD in a research study.

Assessment of potential protective factors is an important but often overlooked step in developing a complete clinical formulation and treatment plan for youths with comorbid SUD and PTSD. Protective factors that may reduce the severity of SUD and PTSD and enhance sustained recovery by adolescents from the disorders include positive (nonconflictual) social support, developmentally appropriate parental monitoring, self-efficacy, development, and adherence to regular healthy routines and activities, and emotion regulation skills (Pat-Horenczyk et al. 2006; Saxe et al. 2007).

Treatment of SUD and Comorbid PTSD

The scientific evidence base for treatment of comorbid SUD and PTSD with adolescents is very limited. Although the AACAP's practice guidelines for both SUD (Bukstein et al. 2005) and PTSD (Cohen et al. 2010) note that the disorders often co-occur, they do not provide any treatment recommendations for comorbid SUD and PTSD. Treatment for adolescents with co-occurring SUD and PTSD therefore must be guided by approaches developed for adults, with adaptations to fit the developmental needs and challenges of adolescents.

Among adults with SUD, having PTSD (Najavits et al. 2007) and complex PTSD (Ford et al. 2007a) at baseline, as well as unremitted PTSD (Read et al. 2004), has been found to be associated with poorer SUD treatment outcomes. Improvements in PTSD symptoms (particularly reduced hyperarousal) have been found to be more strongly associated with improvement in alcohol use disorder symptoms than vice versa. Alcohol-related symptoms tended to begin improving slightly before PTSD symptoms did (Back et al.

2006). Concurrent PTSD treatment has been shown to reduce not only immediate but also long-term risk of SUD relapse if provided during the transitional period beginning soon after discharge from inpatient SUD treatment and during the long-term recovery period (Ouimette et al. 2003). Concurrent treatment also was associated with reduced PTSD symptom severity and improved overall functioning 1 year after initiation of treatment (Amaro et al. 2007). Consistent with these research findings, adult patients with comorbid SUD and PTSD tend to express a preference for treatment that simultaneously or concurrently addresses both disorders in an integrated rather than compartmentalized or sequential way (Read et al. 2004).

Virtually no research has been done with adolescents concerning whether PTSD influences retention or outcome in SUD treatment, or SUD influences retention or outcome in PTSD treatment. Jaycox et al. (2004) reported that adolescents in inpatient SUD treatment were more likely to end treatment earlier if they had a history of experiencing traumatic stressors but did not endorse sufficient symptoms to qualify for a diagnosis of PTSD (compared with those having no reported traumatic stressor history or those with PTSD). Unfortunately, it was not clear if PTSD is beneficial as a motivator for retention in treatment, or if the adolescents who did not have PTSD underreported their PTSD symptoms. Also, it was not clear whether earlier departure from treatment reflected a positive or negative outcome. Thus, the role of PTSD in SUD treatment and SUD in PTSD treatment, with adolescents and young adults, remains in need of empirical study.

Psychosocial Treatment

Seeking Safety, a psychosocial intervention originally designed for women with comorbid SUD and PTSD, has been adapted for adolescent girls and found to be associated with reduced sexual concerns/distress and reduced problems with anorexia, somatization, and depression, as well as sustained sense of control in relation to substance use (Najavits et al. 2006). Seeking Safety provides 25 sessions of psychoeducation about PTSD and SUD and their interrelationship; training in skills for changing cognitions, behaviors, and relationships that enhance recovery from both PTSD and SUD; and case management to help recipients address current stressors and access resources. Attendance was problematic (on average, fewer than half of the sessions were attended), and benefits have not been shown with regard to PTSD or SUD per se, but the intervention demonstrated that integrated PTSD-SUD psychosocial treatment can be accomplished and may yield substantial benefits for girls with comorbid PTSD and SUD.

Although one intervention, trauma-focused cognitive-behavioral therapy (TF-CBT), has extensive validation for children who have PTSD following sexual abuse (Cohen et al. 2006), treatments for adolescents who have experienced sexual abuse or other forms of traumatic stressors have not received sufficient clinical and scientific testing to be considered validated (Saxe et al. 2007). TF-CBT requires involvement in treatment by a stable supportive parent and no ongoing traumatic exposure, which are problematic if substance abuse and conflict are chronic and family based, in which case traumatic exposure is likely to be complex for the adolescent as well as for the parent(s) (e.g., domestic violence, child maltreatment, sexual and physical assault, and community violence; Hanson et al. 2006).

Independent of the functionality of the family system and parents, when community violence is an ongoing threat, the relative degree of safety required by both Seeking Safety and TF-CBT is not likely to be possible. Under those conditions, such as when children are living under the constant threat of harm due to terrorism or war, helping the adolescent to develop or maintain a regular healthy routine of activities has been found to be associated with psychological resilience (i.e., lower self-reported levels of impairment in school, family, peer group, extracurricular, and personal safety domains; Pat-Horenczyk et al. 2006). A cognitive-behavioral psychoeducation program for groups of children in school settings in which violence often is ongoing has been shown to be effective in reducing PTSD symptom severity (Stein et al. 2003), but adaptations for adolescents with SUD have not been reported or tested as yet.

Pharmacotherapy

Pharmacotherapy for children and adolescents with PTSD is in the early stages of development, with no FDA-approved indications (unlike pharmacotherapy for adult PTSD, for which two SSRI antidepressants, paroxetine and sertraline, have been approved by the FDA) (Connor and Fraleigh 2008). Numerous classes of medications have been found effective in some children and adolescents with PTSD (e.g., alpha- and beta-adrenergic agents, antipsychotics, anticonvulsants/mood stabilizers, antidepressants), but only in open-label trials and not specifically with youth with SUD. One randomized controlled trial found that sertraline did not enhance the efficacy of TF-CBT, so the best approach to pharmacotherapy with youth with comorbid PTSD and SUD is to follow guidelines formulated by Connor and Fraleigh (2008), who recommend

> to tailor the decision to use medications to individual patient needs, safety, preferences, and concerns. Medication therapy is considered adjunctive to other psychosocial treatments in childhood PTSD,...to: 1) Target disabling PTSD symptoms so that daily impairment is diminished and the child may pursue a healthier developmental and psychosocial trajectory; and 2) Help traumatized children tolerate emotionally painful material in order to participate in rehabilitative psychosocial therapy. (p. 423)

In addition to seeking to reduce PTSD symptoms of intrusive memories and nightmares, avoidance, and hyperarousal, when SUD is comorbid with PTSD, pharmacotherapy should be prescribed only if it is not likely to result in cross-tolerance with or adverse effects on problematic substance use or cravings, and only in the presence of an ongoing psychosocial therapy that addresses both PTSD and SUD.

Case Vignette

Leshonda is a 16-year-old black female who was court-mandated to receive an evaluation and treatment for PTSD after her fifth confinement in juvenile detention with legal charges, including felony assault, destruction of property, possession of illegal substances and alcohol, and repeated violations of probation. Leshonda was placed on house arrest and ordered to resume attendance at the alternative school from which she had been truant or suspended for more than two-thirds of the past 18 months. She had been placed in residential treatment for polysubstance abuse three times, and each time she was sent back to detention prior to completing the program, because of assaultive behavior toward peers and staff. Leshonda and her family, including her mother and father and four younger siblings, had received three types of in-home family intervention for substance abuse, which she and her parents agreed had led to some improvement in Leshonda's willingness to abide by family rules but only temporary reductions in or abstention from drinking and smoking marijuana, heroin, and methamphetamine.

In court-ordered evaluations, the clinician had noted that from age 5 to 7, Leshonda experienced sexual abuse by an uncle and adult neighbor, which she did not disclose until a child protective services investigation was initiated by her false accusation of rape by her father at age 13. Leshonda subsequently was raped at age 14 by a young adult male whom she had met while she was associating exclusively with adults rather than peers her own age. She was in supportive counseling for a few months after each of those incidents, stopping when, by her own account, "I had nothing more to say, and the counselor thought I was doing fine."

Leshonda answered all four screening questions affirmatively, although she said that she had gotten so used to living with "shut-down" feelings, episodes of rage, and bad memories and "using whatever I can to avoid them" that "it really doesn't bother me." On the TESI, she disclosed the sexual molestation and rape, as well as traumatic losses (of a friend who overdosed and a grandmother who died of a heart attack at age 50) and gang-related physical assaults. On the CAPS-CA, Leshonda initially said that she did not have any bad memories or reminders of even the worst of these experiences (which she identified as the rape) and that she didn't have to avoid them anymore because she just never let them bother her. Upon further inquiry, she said that the memories of that (and other) traumatic event(s) actually are "always just in the back of my mind, I just tell myself they're gone away," and that she avoided going to school because that was where the physical assaults had occurred "and I have to see those same fools every day, looking at me like they're laughing and about to jump me again if I'm not careful." Leshonda described nightmares of being attacked, anger, jumpiness, "my mind going blank" when preparing to go to school as well as at school, always having to keep her guard up (hypervigilance), and not being able to let anyone get close to her or to really enjoy activities she used to find rewarding. Although she did not report having flashbacks or memory gaps regarding the traumatic events, Leshonda was diagnosed with PTSD with severe impairment in school and social functioning.

Leshonda noted that the PTSD symptoms were much worse since she had not been able to drink or use drugs because of the court-ordered random urinalyses and escalating legal sanctions. She said she really did not miss the "high" associated with using as much as the relief that drugs and alcohol temporarily offered from the PTSD symptoms. She had tried to use the coping and substance refusal skills she had learned in SUD treatment, "but they just don't cut it when I get to feeling really bad, sad, or mad." She believed she could not stop using unless there was a way to reduce the frequency and intensity of what she now understood were symptoms of PTSD.

Case Discussion

Treatment goals: The PTSD assessment indicates that Leshonda will be most likely to actually commit to a goal of abstinence if treatment enables her to cope successfully with and diminish the severity of her PTSD symptoms. She may then be motivated to consider sober choices both for dealing with stressors without using or reacting with anger and aggression, and for seeking out and engaging in relationships and activities that are prosocial and that provide her with greater safety, social support, and opportunities for achievement and self-efficacy.

Treatment setting: Although Leshonda is in very serious trouble legally and at school, the legal sanctions and supervision have increased her safety, and she has parents who are invested in supporting her recovery. Outpatient treatment is a reasonable least restrictive option, with close coordination with the probation officer and school social worker who also are working with her.

Psychosocial and pharmacological treatment for PTSD and SUD: In individual, group, and family therapy, Leshonda (and her parents) was provided with psychoeducation explaining how PTSD, SUD, and problems with anger and aggressive behavior share the common feature of biologically based stress reactivity, which begins as a healthy adaptation to traumatic stressors but can become a serious emotional and behavioral problem (Ford et al. 2007a). Leshonda was taught skills for managing reactivity to reminders of traumatic past events, such as being at school or encountering hostile peers, by regulating her emotions (Ford et al. 2007b). The SUD recovery skills she had learned previously (e.g., drug refusal, cognitive reappraisal, assertiveness) were reinforced as she learned how to maintain sufficient emotional equilibrium to use those skills in a timely and effective manner. In individual and family therapy, Leshonda was helped to gradually create a personal narrative ("tell the story") of the rape and the worst physical assault, in writing (poetry as well as prose) and through drawings and collage, and to share this with her parents in a therapeutic manner that enabled them to feel a stronger bond and genuine hope for the future.

Concurrently, Leshonda was evaluated by a child psychiatrist, who recommended to her and her parents that she receive a trial of an SSRI to reduce her underlying dysphoria and irritability, and a mildly sedating antidepressant medication at bedtime to help her regain a more normal sleep cycle. Stimulant medication was considered for her difficulty with sustaining focused attention, but was withheld pending evaluation of her progress in reducing stress reactivity (which might be the source of concentration problems). Leshonda was reluctant to take medications at first, and particularly did not want anything that would cause weight gain (e.g., atypical antipsychotic medications that may be prescribed for the agitation associated with severe PTSD). She and her parents agreed to a trial of the antidepressants, which were associated with reductions in "moodiness" that helped Leshonda to engage in psychosocial therapy. The combined benefit enabled Leshonda to feel able to go to school and deal with peer and other stressors without becoming "too angry to think straight." Although she continued to have periodic spikes in anger and cravings for alcohol or drugs, Leshonda felt increasingly confident that she could cope with those reactions ("it's just my stress alarm—no one's gonna die").

Conclusion

Treatment for youth with comorbid SUD and PTSD involves the challenge of addressing two mutually exacerbating conditions. PTSD symptoms are likely to be precipitated or intensified by substance use, particularly by the patterns of problematic use in substance abuse or dependence, despite the youth intending to use alcohol or other substances to reduce awareness or the severity of intrusive memories and hyperarousal (i.e., as a form of PTSD avoidance symptoms, which in turn is likely to lead over time to increased dysphoria, emotional numbing, and social detachment, which are further symptoms of PTSD). SUD is likely to be intensified by PTSD symptoms, in the form of increased cravings, impulsive use or overuse of substances, or association with peers who use substances to cope with distress. SUD also may lead to additional exposure to traumatic stressors in the form of severe accidents or violence.

Assessment, therefore, should systematically include a careful review of the adolescent's history of substance use, abuse, and dependency, as well as of exposure to traumatic stressors and the onset of PTSD symptoms, which often develop sequentially rather than simultaneously (e.g., first a generalized sense of hyperarousal, followed by nightmares and daytime hypervigilance, and then by progressive impairment as avoidance coping and emotional numbing become pronounced). Treatment is best done with an integrative approach addressing PTSD and SUD as literally co-occurring sets of symptoms on a moment-to-moment as well as day-to-day basis (Ford et al. 2007b). Promising models of integrative PTSD-SUD and SUD-PTSD treatment have been adapted for youth (e.g., Seeking Safety) and offer the practicing clinician a starting point for developing an evidence-based approach in real-world practice.

Developing clinician knowledge and "buy-in" for integrated PTSD-SUD treatment is a key challenge and should begin with preprofessional training in the use of empirically validated interventions that are readily replicated in clinical practice with fidelity. Research on the neurobiology of PTSD and SUD has identified a number of potential targets for biological interventions (e.g., opiate and GABA-benzodiazepine receptors) that may lead to additional advances in pharmacotherapy for comorbid SUD and PTSD. In the meantime, the treatment of comorbid SUD and PTSD depends largely on careful clinical testing of specific hypotheses about the interplay of the specific symptoms of the two disorders with each individual youth, and the application of promising combined psychosocial and biological approaches to treatment.

Key Clinical Concepts

- The treatment of SUD and comorbid depression and/or anxiety disorders in youth should be conducted simultaneously.
- Mild depression accompanying SUD responds to CBT. Moderate to severe depression requires an integrative approach including pharmacotherapy.
- Treatment of SUD accompanied by social phobia should be conducted individually and not in a group setting, until significant improvement of this anxiety disorder has been reached.
- Identifying cues that trigger PTSD-related hyperarousal or avoidance reactions can enhance treatment of substance use problems with adolescents by providing a basis for helping the youth to understand and replace substance-seeking behavior or craving for substances with stress-coping skills (e.g., relaxation skills to reduce arousal, assertive rather than avoidant responses).
- Although it once was believed that PTSD could not be treated unless substance use problems had been successfully treated, conducting CBT for PTSD concurrently with therapy for substance abuse can enhance the latter treatment. CBT for PTSD involves helping develop emotion, and behavior-regulation skills in relation to traumatic stress that are complementary with the coping skills taught in addictions treatment.

References

Abram KM, Teplin LA, Charles DR, et al: Posttraumatic stress disorder and trauma in youth in juvenile detention. Arch Gen Psychiatry 61:403–410, 2004

Amaro H, Dai J, Arevalo S, et al: Effects of integrated trauma treatment on outcomes in a racially/ethnically diverse sample of women in urban community-based substance abuse treatment. J Urban Health 84:508–522, 2007

American Psychiatric Association: Diagnostic and Statistical Manual of Mental Disorders, 4th Edition, Text Revision. Washington, DC, American Psychiatric Association, 2000

Anthony JL, Lonigan CJ, Vernberg E, et al: Multisample cross-validation of a model of childhood posttraumatic stress disorder symptomatology. J Trauma Stress 18:667–676, 2005

Back SE, Brady KT, Sonne S, et al: Symptom improvement in co-occurring PTSD and alcohol dependence. J Nerv Ment Dis 194:690–696, 2006

Beck AT: Beck Depression Inventory. Philadelphia, PA, Center for Cognitive Therapy, 1961

Beck AT, Steer RA, Brown GK: Beck Depression Inventory: Manual, 2nd Edition. Boston, MA, Harcourt Brace, 1996

Birmaher B, Ryan ND, Williamson DE, et al: Childhood and adolescent depression: a review of the past 10 years, Part II. J Am Acad Child Adolesc Psychiatry 35:1575–1583, 1996

Birmaher B, Khetarpal S, Brent D, et al: The Screen for Child Anxiety Related Emotional Disorders (SCARED): scale construction and psychometric characteristics. J Am Acad Child Adolesc Psychiatry 36:545–553, 1997

Birmaher B, Yelovich AK, Renaud J: Pharmacologic treatment for children and adolescents with anxiety disorders. Pediatr Clin North Am 45:1187–1204, 1998

Birmaher B, Axelson DA, Monk K, et al: Fluoxetine for the treatment of childhood anxiety disorders. J Am Acad Child Adolesc Psychiatry 42:415–423, 2003

Birmaher B, Brent D; Work Group on Quality Issues: Practice parameter for the assessment and treatment of children and adolescents with depressive disorders. J Am Acad Child Adolesc Psychiatry 46:1503–1526, 2007

Brent DA, Holder D, Kolko, D, et al: A clinical psychotherapy trial for adolescent depression comparing cognitive, family, and supportive therapy. Arch Gen Psychiatry 54:877–885, 1997

Breslau N, Novak SP, Kessler RC: Psychiatric disorders and stages of smoking. Biol Psychiatry 55:69–76, 2004

Bridge JA, Greenhouse JB, Weldon AH, et al: Suicide trends among youths aged 10 to 19 years in the United States, 1996–2005. JAMA 300:1025–1026, 2008

Buckner JD, Schmidt NB, Lang AR, et al: Specificity of social anxiety disorder as a risk factor for alcohol and cannabis dependence. Psychiatry Res 42:230–239, 2008

Bukstein OG, Bernet W, Beitchman J, et al; Work Group on Quality Issues: Practice parameter for the assessment and treatment of children and adolescents with substance use disorders. J Am Acad Child Adolesc Psychiatry 44:609–621, 2005

Caspar RA, Penne M: Assessment of the computer-assisted instrument, in Redesigning an Ongoing National Household Survey: Methodological Issues (DHHS Publ No 03-3768). Edited by Gfroerer J, Eyerman J, Chromy JR. Rockville, MD, Substance Abuse and Mental Health Services Administration, Office of Applied Statistics, 2002, pp 53–84

Chapman JF, Ford JD: Relationships between suicide risk, traumatic experiences, and substance use among juvenile detainees screened with the MAYSI-2 and Suicide Ideation Questionnaire. Arch Suicide Res 12:50–61, 2008

Chilcoat HD, Menard C: Epidemiological investigations: comorbidity of posttraumatic stress disorder and substance use disorder, in Trauma and Substance Abuse. Edited by Ouimette P, Brown PJ. Washington, DC, American Psychological Association 2003, pp 9–28

Christie KA, Burke JD, Regier DA, et al: Epidemiologic evidence for early onset of mental disorders and higher risk of drug abuse in young adults. Am J Psychiatry 145:971–975, 1988

Clark DB, Cornelius J: Childhood psychopathology and adolescent cigarette smoking: a prospective survival analysis in children at high risk for substance use disorders. Addict Behav 29:837–841, 2004

Clark DB, Donovan JE: Reliability and validity of the Hamilton Anxiety Rating Scale in an adolescent sample. J Am Acad Child Adolesc Psychiatry 33:354–360, 1994

Clark DB, Kirisci L: Posttraumatic stress disorder, depression, alcohol use disorders and quality of life in adolescents. Anxiety 2:226–233, 1996

Clark DB, Sayette MA: Anxiety and the development of alcoholism: clinical and scientific issues. Am J Addict 2:59–76, 1993

Clark DB, Beidel DC, Turner SM, et al: Reliability and validity of the Social Phobia and Anxiety Inventory for adolescents. Psychol Assess 6:135–140, 1994a

Clark DB, Hirsche BE, Smith MG, et al: Anxiety disorders in adolescents: characteristics, prevalence, and comorbidities. Clin Psychol Rev 14:113–137, 1994b

Clark DB, Feske U, Masia CL, et al: Systematic assessment of social phobia in clinical practice. Depress Anxiety 6:47–61, 1997a

Clark DB, Lesnick L, Hegedus AM: Trauma and other stressors in adolescent alcohol dependence and abuse. J Am Acad Child Adolesc Psychiatry 36:1744–1751, 1997b

Clark DB, Rao A, Greer P, et al: A pilot study of anterior cingulate cortex benzodiazepine receptor binding in adolescent onset alcohol use disorders. Alcoholism Clinical and Experimental Research 24:713A, 2000

Clark DB, Bukstein OG, Cornelius J: Alcohol use disorders in adolescents: epidemiology, diagnosis, psychosocial interventions, and pharmacological treatment. Paediatr Drugs 4:493–502, 2002

Clark DB, Cornelius JR, Wood DS, et al: Clinical practices in the pharmacological treatment of comorbid psychopathology in adolescents with alcohol use disorders. J Subst Abuse Treat 25:293–295, 2003

Clark DB, Birmaher B, Axelson D, et al: Fluoxetine for the treatment of childhood anxiety disorders: open-label, long-term extension to a controlled trial. J Am Acad Child Adolesc Psychiatry 44:1263–1270, 2005

Clark DB, Thatcher DL, Cornelius JR: Anxiety disorders and adolescent substance use disorders, in Adolescent Substance Abuse: Psychiatric Comorbidity and High-Risk Behaviors. Edited by Kaminer Y, Bukstein O. New York, Routledge/Taylor & Francis, 2008

Cohen JA, Mannarino AP, Deblinger E: Treating Trauma and Traumatic Grief in Children and Adolescents. New York, Guilford, 2006

Cohen JA, Bukstein O, Walter H, et al; AACAP Work Group on Quality Issues: Practice parameter for the assessment and treatment of children and adolescents with posttraumatic stress disorder. J Am Acad Child Adolesc Psychiatry 49(4):414–430, 2010

Compton SN, March JS, Brent D, et al: Cognitive-behavioral psychotherapy for anxiety and depressive disorders in children and adolescents: an evidence-based medicine review. J Am Acad Child Adolesc Psychiatry 43:930–959, 2004

Compton WM, Cottler LB, Phelps DL, et al: Psychiatric disorders among drug dependent subjects: are they primary or secondary? Am J Addict 9:126–134, 2000

Connolly SD, Bernstein GA; Work Group on Quality Issues: Practice parameter for the assessment and treatment of children and adolescents with anxiety disorders. J Am Acad Child Adolesc Psychiatry 46:267–283, 2007

Connor DF, Fraleigh L: Pharmacotherapy, child, in The Encyclopedia of Psychological Trauma. Edited by Reyes G, Elhai JD, Ford J. New York, Wiley, 2008, pp 471–474

Cook A, Spinazzola J, Ford JD, et al: Complex trauma in children and adolescents. Psychiatr Ann 35:390–398, 2005

Copeland WE, Keeler G, Angold A, et al: Traumatic events and posttraumatic stress in childhood. Arch Gen Psychiatry 64:577–584, 2007

Cornelius JR, Bukstein OG, Birmaher B, et al: Fluoxetine in adolescents with major depression and alcohol use disorder: an open-label trial. Addict Behav 26:735–739, 2001

Cornelius JR, Bukstein OG, Wood DS, et al: Double-blind placebo-controlled trial of fluoxetine in adolescents with comorbid major depression and an alcohol use disorder. Addict Behav 34:905–909, 2009

Costello EJ, Erkanli A, Federman E, et al: Development of psychiatric comorbidity with substance abuse in adolescents: effects of timing and sex. J Clin Child Psychol 28:298–311, 1999

Curry JF, Wells KC, Lochman JE, et al: Cognitive-behavioral intervention for depressed, substance-abusing adolescents: development and pilot testing. J Am Acad Child Adolesc Psychiatry 42:656–665, 2003

Deas D, Randall CL, Roberts JS, et al: A double-blind placebo-controlled trial of sertraline in depressed adolescent alcoholics: a pilot study. Hum Psychopharmacol 15:461–469, 2000

Degenhardt L, Hall W, Lyskey M: Exploring the association between cannabis use and dependence. Addiction 98:1493–1504, 2003

Deykin EY, Buka SL: Prevalence and risk factors for posttraumatic stress disorder among chemically dependent adolescents. Am J Psychiatry 154:752–757, 1997

Emslie GJ, Rush AJ, Weinberg WA, et al: A double-blind, randomized, placebo-controlled trial of fluoxetine in children and adolescents with depression. Arch Gen Psychiatry 54:1031–1037, 1997

Emslie GJ, Ventura D, Korotzer A, et al: Escitalopram in the treatment of adolescent depression: a randomized placebo-controlled multisite trial. J Am Acad Child Adolesc Psychiatry 48:721–729, 2009

Epstein JN, Saunders BE, Kilpatrick DG, et al: PTSD as a mediator between childhood rape and alcohol use in adult women. Child Abuse Neglect 22:223–234, 1998

Fendrich M, Weissman MM, Warner V: Screening for depressive disorder in children and adolescents: validating the Center for Epidemiologic Studies Depression Scale for Children. Am J Epidemiol 131:538–551, 1990

Fergusson DM, Boden JM, Horwood LJ: Tests of causal links between alcohol abuse or dependence and major depression. Arch Gen Psychiatry 66:260–266, 2009

Ford JD, Racusin R, Ellis C, et al: Child maltreatment, other trauma exposure and posttraumatic symptomatology among children with oppositional defiant and attention deficit hyperactivity disorders. Child Maltreat 5:205–217, 2000

Ford JD, Hawke J, Alessi S, et al: Psychological trauma and PTSD symptoms as predictors of substance dependence treatment outcomes. Behav Res Ther 45:2417–2431, 2007a

Ford JD, Russo EM, Mallon S: Integrating treatment of posttraumatic stress disorder (PTSD) and substance use disorder. J Couns Dev 85:475–489, 2007b

Ford JD, Hartman JK, Hawke J, et al: Traumatic victimization, posttraumatic stress disorder, suicidal ideation, and substance abuse risk among juvenile justice–involved youths. J Child Adolesc Trauma 1:75–92, 2008

Giaconia RM, Reinherz HZ, Paradis A, et al: Comorbidity of substance use disorders and posttraumatic stress disorder in adolescents, in Trauma and Substance Abuse. Edited by Ouimette P, Brown PJ. Washington, DC, American Psychological Association, 2003, pp 227–242

Gibbons R, Mann JJ: Proper studies of selective serotonin reuptake inhibitors are needed for youth with depression. CMAJ 180:270–271, 2009

Gibbons RD, Brown CH, Hur K, et al: Early evidence on the effects of regulators' suicidality warnings on SSRI prescriptions and suicide in children and adolescents. Am J Psychiatry 164:1356–1363, 2007

Goodwin RD, Fergusson DM, Horwood LJ: Association between anxiety disorders and substance use disorders among young persons: results of a 21-year longitudinal study. J Psychiatr Res 38:295–304, 2004

Grella CE, Hser YI, Joshi V, et al: Drug treatment outcomes for adolescents with comorbid mental and substance use disorders. J Nerv Ment Dis 189:384–392, 2001

Hanson RF, Self-Brown S, Fricker-Elhai A, et al: The relations between family environment and violence exposure among youth: findings from the National Survey of Adolescents. Child Maltreat 11:3–15, 2006

Hawke JM, Kaminer Y, Burke R, et al: Stability of comorbid psychiatric diagnosis among youths in treatment and aftercare for alcohol use disorders. Subst Abus 29:33–42, 2008

Hawke J, Ford JD, Kaminer Y, et al: Trauma and PTSD among youths in outpatient treatment for alcohol and other substance use disorders. J Child Adolesc Trauma 2:1–14, 2009

Helzer JE, Pryzbeck TR: The co-occurrence of alcoholism with other psychiatric disorders in the general population and its impact on treatment. J Stud Alcohol 49:219–224, 1988

Hovens JG, Cantwell DP, Kiriakos R: Psychiatric comorbidity in hospitalized adolescent substance abusers. J Am Acad Child Adolesc Psychiatry 33:476–483, 1994

Hughes CW, Emslie GJ, Crismon ML, et al: Texas Children's Medication Algorithm Project: update from Texas Consensus Conference Panel on Medication Treatment of Childhood Major Depressive Disorder. J Am Acad Child Adolesc Psychiatry 46:667–686, 2007

Jaycox LH, Ebener P, Damesek L, et al: Trauma exposure and retention in adolescent substance abuse treatment. J Trauma Stress 17:113–121, 2004

Kaminer Y, Bukstein O (eds): Adolescent Substance Abuse: Psychiatric Comorbidity and High-Risk Behaviors. New York, Routledge/Taylor & Francis, 2008

Kaminer Y, Burleson JA, Goldberger R: Cognitive-behavioral coping skills and psychoeducation therapies for adolescent substance abuse. J Nerv Ment Dis 190:737–745, 2002

Kaufman J, Birmaher B, Brent D, et al: Schedule for Affective Disorders and Schizophrenia for School-Age Children—Present and Lifetime Version (K-SADS-PL): initial reliability and validity data. J Am Acad Child Adolesc Psychiatry 36:980–988, 1997

Kendall PC, Safford S, Flannery-Schroeder E, et al: Child anxiety treatment: outcomes in adolescence and impact on substance use and depression at 7.4-year follow-up. J Consult Clin Psychol 72:276–287, 2004

Kennard BD, Silva SG, Tonev S, et al: Remission and recovery in the Treatment of Adolescents with Depression Study (TADS): acute and long-term outcomes. J Am Acad Child Adolesc Psychiatry 48:186–195, 2009

Kessler RC, Sonnega A, Bromet E, et al: Posttraumatic stress disorder in the National Comorbidity Survey. Arch Gen Psychiatry 52:1048–1060, 1995

Kessler RC, Nelson CB, McGonagle KA, et al: The epidemiology of co-occurring addictive and mental disorders: implications for prevention and service utilization. Am J Orthopsychiatry 66:17–31, 1996

Khantzian EJ: The self-medication hypothesis of substance use disorders: a reconsideration and recent applications. Harv Rev Psychiatry 4:231–244, 1997

Kilpatrick DG, Acierno R, Saunders B, et al: Risk factors for adolescent substance abuse and dependence: data from a national sample. J Consult Clin Psychol 68:19–30, 2000

Kilpatrick DG, Ruggiero KJ, Acierno R, et al: Violence and risk of PTSD, major depression, substance abuse/dependence, and comorbidity: results from the National Survey of Adolescents. J Consult Clin Psychol 71:692–700, 2003

Kimerling R, Trafton JA, Ngyuen B: Validation of a brief screen for posttraumatic stress disorder with substance use disorder patients. Addict Behav 31:2074–2079, 2006

Kirisci L, Clark DB, Moss HB: Reliability and validity of the State-Trait Anxiety Inventory for Children in adolescent substance abusers: confirmatory factor analysis and item response theory. J Child Adolesc Subst Abuse 5:57–69, 1996

Kovacs M: Children's Depression Inventory. North Tonawanda, NY, Multi-Health Systems, 1992

Leckman JF, King RA: A developmental perspective on the controversy surrounding the use of SSRIs to treat pediatric depression. Am J Psychiatry 164:1304–1306, 2007

Libby AM, Riggs PD: Integrated substance use and mental health treatment for adolescents: aligning organizational and financial incentives. J Child Adolesc Psychopharmacol 15:826–834, 2005

Libby AM, Brent DA, Morrato EH, et al: Decline in treatment of pediatric depression after FDA advisory on risk of suicidality with SSRIs. Am J Psychiatry 164:884–891, 2007

Lopez B, Turner RJ, Saavedra LM: Anxiety and risk for substance dependence among late adolescents/young adults. J Anxiety Disord 19:275–294, 2005

Lubman DI, Allen NB, Rogers N, et al: The impact of co-occurring mood and anxiety disorders among substance-abusing youth. J Affect Disord 103:105–112, 2007

Manassis K, Mendlowitz SL, Scapillato D, et al: Group and individual cognitive-behavioral therapy for childhood anxiety disorders: a randomized trial. J Am Acad Child Adolesc Psychiatry 41:1423–1430, 2002

March J, Silva S, Petrycki S, et al: Fluoxetine, cognitive-behavioral therapy, and their combination for adolescents with depression. JAMA 292:807–820, 2004

Mills KL, Teesson M, Ross J, et al: Trauma, PTSD, and substance use disorders: findings from the Australian National Survey of Mental Health and Well-Being. Am J Psychiatry 163:652–658, 2006

Myers MG, Aarons GA, Tomlinson K, et al: Social anxiety, negative affectivity, and substance use among high school students. Psychol Addict Behav 17:277–283, 2003

Myrick H, Brady K: Current review of the comorbidity of affective, anxiety, and substance use disorders. Curr Opin Psychiatry 16:261–270, 2003

Nader K: Understanding and Assessing Trauma in Children and Adolescents: Measures, Methods, and Youth in Context. New York, Routledge, 2008

Nader K, Kriegler JA, Blake DD, et al: Clinician Administered PTSD Scale, Child and Adolescent Version. White River Junction, VT, National Center for PTSD, 1996

Najavits LM, Gallop RJ, Weiss RD: Seeking safety therapy for adolescent girls with PTSD and substance use disorder: a randomized controlled trial. J Behav Health Serv Res 33:453–463, 2006

Najavits LM, Harned MS, Gallop RJ, et al: Six-month treatment outcomes of cocaine-dependent patients with and without PTSD in a multisite national trial. J Stud Alcohol Drugs 68:353–361, 2007

Ouimette P, Moos RH, Finney JW: PTSD treatment and 5-year remission among patients with substance use and posttraumatic stress disorders. J Consult Clin Psychol 71:410–414, 2003

Pat-Horenczyk R, Schiff M, Doppelt O: Maintaining routine despite ongoing exposure to terrorism: a healthy strategy for adolescents? J Adolesc Health 39:199–205, 2006

Pat-Horenczyk R, Peled O, Miron T, et al: Risk-taking behaviors among Israeli adolescents exposed to recurrent terrorism: provoking danger under continuous threat? Am J Psychiatry 164:66–72, 2007

Radloff LS: The CES-D Scale: a self-report depression scale for research in the general population. Appl Psychol Meas 1:385–401, 1977

Read JP, Brown PJ, Kahler CW: Substance use and posttraumatic stress disorders: symptom interplay and effects on outcome. Addict Behav 29:1665–1672, 2004

Regier DA, Farmer ME, Rae DS, et al: Comorbidity of mental disorders with alcohol and other drug abuse: results from the Epidemiologic Catchment Area (ECA) study. JAMA 264:2511–2518, 1990

Reynolds WM : Reynolds Adolescent Depression Scale. Odessa, FL, Psychological Assessment Resources, 1986

Reynolds WM: Reynolds Child Depression Scale. Odessa, FL, Psychological Assessment Resources, 1989

Riggs PD, Baker S, Mikulich SK, et al: Depression in substance-dependent delinquents. J Am Acad Child Adolesc Psychiatry 34:764–771, 1995

Riggs PD, Mikulich SK, Coffman LM, et al: Fluoxetine in drug-dependent delinquents with major depression: an open trial. J Child Adolesc Psychopharmacol 7:87–95, 1997

Riggs PD, Mikulich-Gilbertson SK, Davies RD, et al: A randomized controlled trial of fluoxetine and cognitive behavioral therapy in adolescents with major depression, behavior problems, and substance use disorders. Arch Pediatr Adolesc Med 161:1026–1034, 2007

Saxe GN, MacDonald HZ, Ellis BH: Psychosocial approaches for children with PTSD, in Handbook of PTSD: Science and Practice. Edited by Friedman MJ, Keane TM, Resick PA. New York, Guilford, 2007, pp 359–375

Stein BD, Jaycox LH, Kataoka SH, et al: A mental health intervention for schoolchildren exposed to violence: a randomized controlled trial. JAMA 290:603–611, 2003

Target M, Fonagy P: The efficacy of psychoanalysis for children: prediction of outcome in a developmental context. J Am Acad Child Adolesc Psychiatry 33:1134–1144, 1994

Thomas SE, Randall PK, Book SW, et al: A complex relationship between co-occurring social anxiety and alcohol use disorders: what effect does treating social anxiety have on drinking? Alcohol Clin Exp Res 32:77–84, 2008

Tomlinson KL, Tate SR, Anderson KG, et al: An examination of self-medication and rebound effects: psychiatric symptomatology before and after alcohol or drug relapse. Addict Behav 31:461–474, 2005

Vandrey R, Budney AJ, Kamon JL, et al: Cannabis withdrawal in adolescent treatment seekers. Drug Alcohol Depend 78:205–210, 2005

Walkup JT, Albano AM, Piacentini J, et al: Cognitive behavioral therapy, sertraline, or a combination in childhood anxiety. N Engl J Med 359:2753–2766, 2008

Zimmermann P, Wittchen HU, Höfler M, et al: Primary anxiety disorders and the development of subsequent alcohol use disorders: a 4-year community study of adolescents and young adults. Psychol Med 33:1211–1222, 2003

Relevant Websites

National Center for PTSD: www.ncptsd.va.gov

The National Child Traumatic Stress Network: http://www.nctsnet.org/nccts/nav.do?pid=hom_main

14

Assessment and Treatment
of Suicidal Behavior

David B. Goldston, Ph.D.

John F. Curry, Ph.D.

Karen C. Wells, Ph.D.

Michelle Roley, B.A.

Adolescents who use substances and are suicidal are a diverse and high-risk group, with multiple comorbidities, life stresses, and developmental trajectories. This group of adolescents also can be especially challenging for clinicians because of their multiple treatment needs; comorbid psychiatric problems; legal, academic, and family difficulties; impulsivity; and ambivalence about participating in treatment and changing maladaptive behavior patterns. Careful assessment, safety monitoring, and integrated treatment for this population are important in clinical care, but treatment research in this area is lacking, and only indirect evidence is available regarding the most promising targets for intervention with this group.

The objectives of this chapter are threefold. First, we review for the practitioner the problem of suicidal behaviors among youths with substance abuse problems, and the interrelationship between risk for suicidal behaviors and substance abuse. Second, we discuss issues in the assessment and treatment of suicidal behaviors among youths with substance abuse problems, along with practical considerations regarding integrated treatment. Last, we present a clinical vignette for illustrative purposes, with discussion of the treatment approach.

Definitions of Suicidal Behaviors

Suicide-related terms have been used inconsistently in the literature, a situation that has impeded progress in research and created difficulties in communication for practitioners (O'Carroll et al. 1996). In this chapter, we operationally define *suicide* as a fatality that is the result of a self-injurious behavior that was associated with at least some evidence of intent to die (O'Carroll et al. 1996; Posner et al. 2007). The term *suicide attempt* is used to refer to potentially self-injurious behaviors associated with at least some (i.e., nonzero) intent to end one's life (O'Carroll et al. 1996; Posner et al. 2007). Our references to "at least some" or "nonzero" intent are made in acknowledgment of the reality that suicidal behavior is often associated with multiple motives and ambivalence (Goldston 2003; Shneidman 1996). *Suicidal ideation*, in this chapter, refers to thoughts about killing oneself, regardless of whether a specific plan is envisioned and regardless of intent to act on these thoughts. Suicidal ideation can be differentiated from thoughts of wishing one were dead or wanting to be dead that are not accompanied by thoughts about killing oneself. The term *suicidality* is used in this chapter when referring globally to all of the aspects of suicidal behavior (i.e., suicidal ideation, attempts, deaths by suicide). *Nonsuicidal self-injurious behavior* refers to self-harm that is not associated with any intent to kill oneself. For example, cutting of oneself to relieve tension or an accidental overdose of drugs in an effort to get high would not be considered suicidal.

The definitions of *suicide, suicide attempt,* and *suicidal ideation* are largely consistent with those referenced in the "Practice Guideline for the Assessment and Treatment of Patients With Suicidal Behaviors" published by the American

Psychiatric Association (Jacobs; APA Work Group on Suicidal Behaviors 2003) and with operational definitions proposed in collaborative work groups sponsored by the National Institute of Mental Health and the Center for Mental Health Services (O'Carroll et al. 1996). With the exception of the term *suicidal ideation*, these terms are also consistent with the operational definitions used by the U.S. Food and Drug Administration in classifying self-harm adverse events associated with pharmacotherapy (Posner et al. 2007).

These operational definitions notwithstanding, the classification of suicidal behaviors among individuals who are intoxicated or have substance use problems can sometimes be difficult. For example, substance abuse can be related to memory difficulties (Millsaps et al. 1994), and respondents sometimes find it difficult to remember the intent or motives associated with behaviors in which they engaged while under the influence of substances. In addition, death via ingestion of substances or injection drug use can be very difficult to classify accurately, particularly in cases where there is no communication of intent (e.g., a "suicide note") and/or when the decedent is known to have a history of depression or suicidal behavior in addition to substance use (Cantor et al. 2001).

Characteristics and Epidemiology

According to data from the self-report Youth Risk Behavior Surveillance, administered anonymously during the year 2007 to high school students in selected schools throughout the United States, a surprisingly high percentage of adolescents (14.5%; 18.7% of girls, 10.3% of boys) reported that they had "seriously considered" killing themselves (i.e., had suicidal ideation) in the last year (Eaton et al. 2008). Moreover, 11.3% of high school students (13.4% of girls, 9.2% of boys) reported that they had made a specific suicide plan in the preceding year. A total of 6.9% of the students (9.3% of girls, 4.6% of boys) responding to the survey said that they had made suicide attempts in the last year. In addition, 2.0% of students (2.4% of girls, 1.5% of boys) reported that they had made suicide attempts in the last year that required treatment by a doctor or a nurse.

Data from both community and clinical samples suggest that the rate of suicide attempts increases as youths enter adolescence, particularly for girls, but then declines again during the transition from adolescence to young adulthood

(Angle et al. 1983; Kovacs et al. 1993; Lewinsohn et al. 2001). The primary methods of attempted suicide among young people are overdose and cutting (Brent 1987; Lewinsohn et al. 1996; Spirito et al. 1987). The majority of suicide attempts, however, do not result in a high degree of medical lethality (Goldston et al. 2009; Lewinsohn et al. 1996).

Rates of death by suicide are considerably lower than rates of nonlethal suicidal behavior, with an average of 5.5 per 100,000 youth ages 12–19 dying by suicide per year from 1999 to 2006 in the United States (Centers for Disease Control and Prevention 2010). Nonetheless, suicide is the third leading cause of death in this age group, surpassed only by accidents and homicide (Centers for Disease Control and Prevention 2010). The main methods of death by suicide in the United States in this age group are firearms and hanging or strangulation (Centers for Disease Control and Prevention 2010).

There are marked gender and ethnic differences in rates of suicidal thoughts and behaviors. In general, adolescent girls have suicidal ideation and make suicide attempts more than boys, but adolescent boys have a higher rate of dying by suicide (Centers for Disease Control and Prevention 2010; Eaton et al. 2008). Native Americans appear to have the highest rates of suicidal ideation, suicide attempts, and deaths by suicide of all racial and ethnic groups (Goldston et al. 2008). However, Asian American/Pacific Islander high school girls also have relatively high rates of suicidal ideation, and Latinas have relatively high rates of suicide attempts (Goldston et al. 2008). Although the rates of suicide have generally been lower for African Americans than other racial and ethnic groups, there was a 114% increase in suicides among African Americans ages 10–19 from 1980 to 1995 (Centers for Disease Control and Prevention 1998). This increase was primarily notable for males and was related to increased suicides associated with firearms (Joe and Kaplan 2002). Rates of suicide attempts also increased for African American males from 1991 to 2001 (Joe and Marcus 2003).

Suicidal Ideation and Behaviors and Substance Use Disorders

In population studies and clinical samples of adolescents, substance and/or alcohol use and suicidal behaviors co-occur at rates that exceed what would be expected on the basis of their prevalence rates. For example, in some samples of adolescents presenting for substance abuse treatment, between 18% and 36% reported past suicide attempts (Berman and Schwartz 1990; Cavaiola and Lavender 1999; Deykin and Buka 1993; Kelly et al. 2001). In a longitudinal, repeated assessments study of adolescents who had been psychiatrically hospitalized and then followed through young adulthood, substance use disorders (SUDs) were associated with a threefold increased proximal risk for suicide attempts. SUDs also were associated with 38% of all repeat attempts, although this risk was almost always associated with comorbid depressive or disruptive behavior disorders (Goldston et al. 2009). Moreover, the risk associated with contemporaneous SUDs for suicide attempts tended to increase from adolescence through young adulthood (Goldston et al. 2009); that is, SUDs became a stronger risk factor for suicide attempts as individuals got older.

Across studies, more severe, impairing, or long-lasting alcohol and substance use problems generally are more likely to be associated with suicidal behaviors than are less severe alcohol and substance abuse problems (Goldston 2004). In community-based samples of youths, for example, SUDs were associated with suicide attempts but not with suicidal ideation (Gould et al. 1998). In a longitudinal study of a previously hospitalized sample of adolescents, the risk over time for suicide attempts was higher for participants who had a lifetime history of both alcohol and other SUDs than it was for young people who had a lifetime history of either alone (Goldston et al. 2009). In addition, across studies, more severe suicidal thoughts and behavior tended to have a greater likelihood of being associated with substance abuse problems than less severe suicidality (Goldston 2004). For example, based on Youth Risk Behavior Surveillance data collected anonymously in schools, it appears that there are progressively increased odds of suicidal ideation, suicide attempts without medical consequences, and suicide attempts with medical consequences with binge drinking, drinking frequency, marijuana use, cocaine use, and intravenous drug use (Garrison et al. 1993).

In several studies, between 28% and 33% of youth and young adults who died by suicide were found to have positive evidence of intoxication or recent alcohol use (Brent et al. 1988; Hoberman and Garfinkel 1988; Houston et al. 2001). Among adults, it has been noted that suicide may account for between one-fifth and one-third of the increased mortality rate among alcoholic individuals (Hufford 2001). In a systematic literature review of published studies of suicide deaths and SUDs, Wilcox et al. (2004) found that mixed drug use was associated with the greatest likelihood of suicide, but that opioid use disorder and intravenous drug use were also associated with high risk of suicide deaths. Alcohol use disorder and heavy drinking also were associated with increased risk of suicide.

Nature of Relationship Between Alcohol and Substance Use Disorders and Suicidal Behaviors

Multiple potential reasons may explain why suicidal behaviors and substance abuse are related among young people. First, some of the motives associated with the desire to kill oneself and to abuse substances may be similar. Adolescents, for instance, may try to kill themselves because they find their life circumstances intolerable, and may be having a great deal of difficulty with the depression or psychological pain associated with these difficulties; to this end, they may see suicide as a potential solution or way to escape from these intolerable life circumstances and pain (Boergers et al. 1998; Kienhorst et al. 1995). Similarly, young people may use alcohol or other substances to help them escape from their current difficulties and distress, or because the substances dampen the psychological pain or distract them from their upsetting circumstances. In this way, both substance use and suicidality can be understood as methods of avoidance (Hufford 2001; Khantzian 1997).

Second, common risk factors may increase the likelihood both of suicidal thoughts and behaviors and of substance use. For example, impulsivity and aggressiveness (Moeller et al. 2001; Prevette et al. 2005), sexual abuse (Bailey and McCloskey 2005; Beautrais et al. 1996; Brent et al. 2002; Moeller et al. 2001), family environment and stresses (Gould et al. 1996; Wu et al. 2004), academic and disciplinary problems (Eggert and Herting 1993; Gould et al. 1996), and psychiatric diagnoses of depressive and disruptive disorders (Costello et al. 1999; Foley et al. 1996; Goldston et al. 2009) have all been found to be related to suicidal thoughts or behavior as well as to alcohol and substance use. A variety of risk-taking or health-endangering behaviors, including physical fighting (Centers for Disease Control and Prevention 2004; Rudatsikara et al. 2008) and more frequent or risky sexual behavior (Burge et al. 1995; Crockett et al. 2006; Epstein and Spirito 2009), also have been found to be related to both suicidality and substance use.

Third, substance use can indirectly increase risk for suicidality via its effects on associated risk factors. For example, substance abuse can result in depressed mood (Bovasso 2001), and comorbid substance abuse in adolescent girls has been found to be associated with longer episodes of depression (King et al. 1996). Longer episodes of depression, in turn, have been associated with increased risk of suicidal behaviors (Brent et al. 1990). Relatedly, substance use sometimes may be associated with decreasing motivation to engage in activities other than those associated with substance abuse. This lack of participation in activities may be associated with intoxication and residual effects of substances and/or motivational deficits (e.g., Lane et al. 2005). Less frequent pleasant activities, in turn, have been found to be related to slower recovery from depression in response to cognitive-behavioral group treatment (Clarke et al. 1992). Substance use and related conduct problems also may be the triggers for arguments and conflicts within families, which in turn can be triggers or precipitants for depression and suicidal thoughts and behaviors (see Conner and Goldston 2007). Substance abuse also can increase impulsivity and disinhibition (Schuckit and Schuckit 1989), increasing the likelihood that a young person will act on self-destructive urges.

Fourth, at a biological level, studies of individuals who have died by suicide and of individuals who have had difficulties with substance abuse or dependence have implicated altered serotonergic functioning or the role of serotonin transporter genes (Arango et al. 2001; Boldrini et al. 2008; Pinto et al. 2008). Neuropsychological studies also have found that chronic substance abusers show a pattern of focusing on short-term rewards rather than long-term rewards (Whitlow et al. 2004); a similar pattern of focusing on acute or current distress, rather than focusing on long-term possibilities, is also characteristic of suicidal individuals (Shneidman 1996).

Finally, alcohol and substance use also can provide young people with readily accessible means for attempting suicide, such as by overdose (Goldston 2004). For example, a teenager with alcohol dependence may try to commit suicide by "drinking himself to death," and a girl who is using pills recreationally may try to take multiple pills in an overdose; in both cases, the troubled teenagers have easy access to the methods for attempting suicide.

Clinical Characteristics of Youth With Both Substance Abuse Problems and Suicidal Behaviors

Youths who engage in co-occurring suicidal and substance abuse behaviors can present numerous challenges for clinicians (see Esposito-Smythers and Goldston 2008). They sometimes are reluctant to enter or to continue in treatment; they may lack motivation to work on substance abuse problems, despite clear negative consequences in multiple domains that are associated with the substance abuse; or they may feel that it is not important to continue working on life difficulties once immediate distress has been ameliorated in the initial stages of intervention. Many of these youths also are having school difficulties, including school suspensions and expulsions related to substance abuse or conduct problems associated with substance abuse, lack of attendance in school, and declining grades. Many of these youths socialize in deviant peer groups that use alcohol or other substances, and that engage in other rule-breaking, risk-taking, and self-harmful behaviors. These youths may give up contacts with non-substance-abusing peers, because of perceptions that they have little in common with other youth. Because of higher degrees of substance abuse in their peer groups, these teens often fail to recognize the degree to which their own substance abuse is not normative for other youth their age. Throughout the course of interventions, these youths may express or display a strong degree of ambivalence about substance abuse, treatment involvement, and living versus dying. Families of these youths, who have often experienced multiple adversities or life stresses, are often very concerned, but also frustrated, and sometimes have begun to give up hope regarding attempts to change the behaviors of their adolescent children.

Assessment of Suicidal Behaviors Among Youth With Substance Abuse Problems

With any clinical population, but particularly with a group at higher risk for suicidal behaviors, such as youth with substance abuse problems, it is important for clinicians to assess both previous and current suicidal thoughts, behavior, and risk. Unfortunately, in part because of fragmented care between mental health and substance abuse professionals for youths with comorbid psychiatric disorders and SUDs, assessment of suicidal thoughts and behavior may not always occur. Substance abuse practitioners sometimes avoid asking about suicidal thoughts and behaviors, with the assumption that the mental health professional is assessing for suicide risk and that their own focus should be limited to substance use. Also, mental health professionals do not always assess for suicidal thoughts and behavior when they are not obvious presenting problems. Moreover, assessment of suicidal thoughts and behaviors can be anxiety provoking for even experienced clinicians, who may be uncomfortable working with high-risk clients, or who may be unsure of their ability to intervene effectively with this population.

Unfortunately, without direct assessment, suicidal behavior among adolescents can go undiscovered by adults. For example, comparisons of adolescent and parent reports in response to structured and semistructured diagnostic interviews have revealed that parents are typically unaware of many youths' suicidal thoughts and behaviors (Breton et al. 2002; Foley et al. 2006; Klaus et al. 2009; Klimes-Dougan 1998; Velez and Cohen 1988; Walker et al. 1990). Because of lack of parental knowledge of much adolescent suicidal behavior, assessment of suicidality must include the adolescent, and not simply rely on reports of parents or other adult informants. Assessment is important so that the clinician can ascertain level of risk, implement appropriate safety plans with the adolescents and families, better understand the context of suicidal behaviors for purposes of psychotherapy, and monitor the course of the adolescents' difficulties during treatment.

Self-report measures and interviews can be used as tools to assist in the assessment of suicidal behaviors and risk. However, as suggested by Goldston (2003), these assessments should never be the only considerations in determination of risk and should never supplant clinical judgment. Rather, they should be used as an additional source of information for clinicians, complementing other available information.

Generally, two types of clinical instruments may be of most use to clinicians working with substance use clients in assessing suicidal behaviors and risk. The first set consists of *detection instruments* (Goldston 2003). As indicated by their name, these instruments are used primarily to detect the presence or absence as well as the severity of past and current suicidal thoughts and behaviors. These instruments can be used both during an initial assessment and as a continuing form of assessment for emergent suicidality or the course of suicidality during treatment. Detection assessments comprise both semistructured and structured interviews and standardized questionnaires. In clinical research settings in particular, two semistructured diagnostic interviews, the Schedule for Affective Disorders and Schizophrenia for School-Aged Children—Epidemiologic Version (Orvaschel 1994) and the Present and Lifetime Version (Kaufman et al. 1997), have been used to assess suicidal ideation and suicide attempts. In addition to assessing history of and current suicidality, these two instruments assess the severity of current symptoms, and other childhood and adolescent psychiatric disorders. Two other interviews that can be used in assessment of suicidal behaviors are the Suicidal Behaviors Interview (Reynolds 1990), an instrument with excellent psychometric properties that assesses suicidal thoughts, plans, attempts, and associated distress and life events, and the Lifetime Parasuicide Count (Linehan and Comtois 1997), which assesses both nonsuicidal and suicidal self-harm behaviors.

Among the most widely used standardized questionnaires are the Suicidal Ideation Questionnaire (SIQ; Reynolds 1988) and the Beck Scale for Suicide Ideation (BSI; Beck and Steer 1991). Psychometrically, both measures have excellent test-retest reliability and have been used in clinical trials with adolescents (Goldston 2003). In particular, the SIQ has been used in a pilot randomized controlled trial of a combined motivational interviewing and cognitive-behavioral intervention for alcohol- and substance-abusing suicidal teenagers (Esposito-Smythers et al. 2006, 2008). The SIQ was used in the Treatment for Adolescents with Depression Study and demonstrated significant change with treatment (March et al. 2007). Both the SIQ and the BSI focus primarily on suicidal thoughts, although the BSI has a single item asking about past history of suicide attempts. Hence, questionnaires or other assessments that focus primarily on suicidal thoughts should be supplemented with assessments of recent and past suicidal behaviors; this is important because suicidal ideation can be ephemeral and wax and wane over time, but past suicide attempts in numerous studies have been found to be the best predictor of suicidal ideation and current suicidal behaviors (e.g., Joiner et al. 2005). Regardless of which assessments are used, given the predictive power of past suicide attempts, it is important always to assess at intake not only for recent suicidal behavior but also for history of any past attempts.

The second group of instruments that are potentially useful to clinicians is *risk assessment instruments.* As their name implies, these instruments are used primarily to ascertain level of risk, or to predict future suicidal behaviors. These assessment instruments may focus on adolescent suicidal behavior risk factors, protective factors, or their combination. Two examples of risk assessments are the Beck Hopelessness Scale (Beck and Steer 1988) and the Columbia Suicide Screen (Shaffer et al. 2004). The Beck Hopelessness Scale assesses hopelessness as a risk factor associated with suicide attempts and previously has been shown to have predictive validity (Goldston 2003). The Columbia Suicide Screen is used as an initial assessment for suicidal behaviors, is a good tool for identifying at-risk adolescents in a community or school setting, and has been shown to be reliable and valid (Shaffer et al. 2004). One of the few inventories that has focused on protective factors and that has demonstrated predictive validity in assessing adolescent repeat suicide attempts in a clinical sample is the Reasons for Living Inventory (Linehan et al. 1983). Although risk assessment instruments can provide very useful information about risk for future behaviors and potential targets for treatment, clinicians should be cautious in their use because the great majority of instruments of this type have not been validated in prospective studies. Instead, the validation strategy for many of these instruments has focused on the ability of the instrument to differentiate between suicidal and nonsuicidal youths at a single point in time, rather than on the utility of the instrument in predicting future behavior (Goldston 2003).

Occasionally, clinicians use information about intent or lethality of past suicide attempts to help estimate risk for future suicidal behavior. In this regard, it should be noted that intent and lethality of adolescent suicidal behavior are not always highly correlated across studies (Goldston 2003), and may not even be highly correlated within the same individuals across suicide attempts (D.B. Goldston, unpublished data). In addition, although some data are emerging regarding medical lethality of past suicidal behavior as a possible predictor of future suicide attempts (D.B. Goldston, unpublished data, April 2010), there is little research documenting the predictive validity of clinical characteristics of past attempts. Hence, clinicians should be cautious about relying on clinical characteristics of past suicidal behavior when estimating future risk.

Assessment of Imminent Risk

One primary purpose of clinical assessment is to determine the degree to which an adolescent patient poses imminent risk of harm to self. This determination is important in decisions regarding level of clinical care, and in decisions to implement crisis management procedures to de-escalate level of risk so that the patient can be managed effectively in the least restrictive setting. In determining whether patients are at imminent risk to themselves, the report of adolescents regarding their intent and perceptions of whether they can keep themselves safe (and participate in a safety plan, as described in the later section on treatment) is of primary importance. With that said, there are certain situations when adolescents' reports of suicidality may be influenced by environmental contingencies. For example, an adolescent may deny suicidal intent if she is trying to avoid being hospitalized because of previous bad experiences in the hospital. Other factors that should be considered in the clinical judgment of imminent risk are whether the adolescent's family and social environment can provide close monitoring, whether lethal means for attempting suicide are accessible, and whether the adolescent can articulate alternatives to suicidal behavior if the crisis that precipitated a suicide attempt should recur. Additional considerations in assessing imminent risk include the adolescent's past history of suicidal behavior and associated risk factors, and whether situational factors contributing to acute risk have been reduced. For example, if an adolescent reports that he will try to kill himself the next time his mother yells at him and that he has a gun hidden, but his mother does not believe him and says she fully intends to "give him a piece of her mind" when she gets home, that adolescent would be considered at imminent risk because of intent, availability of method, and the high likelihood that a crisis will occur without intervention.

Functional Assessments

Over and beyond simply determining the presence and severity of suicidal ideation, behavior, or risk for suicidal behavior, a functional analysis of suicidal thoughts and behavior can provide important insight into the context of suicidality and possible targets for intervention to reduce risk for future suicidal behaviors (see Goldston 2004). In describing the functional analysis, we follow the SORC (Stimulus-Organism-Response-Consequence) model described by Goldfried and Sprafkin (1974). In the service of developing integrative and individualized treatment approaches for suicidal and substance-abusing youths, the SORC model can be used to help identify functional commonalities (e.g., common triggers, risk and protective factors, consequences) as well as functional relationships between substance abuse and suicidality. In this model, "S" refers to the antecedent events or circumstances that precipitate or serve as the trigger for substance use and suicidality. "O" refers to the person variables (e.g., feelings, cognitions, history, risk and protective factors) that moderate or mediate relationships between the triggers and the substance use and/or suicidality. For example, an adolescent might not always react to a stressful family interaction (e.g., a trigger) with substance abuse or suicidal behavior; rather, there may be factors, such as preexisting levels of depression, anxiety, and anger, or low perceived social support, that increase the likelihood of the maladaptive behaviors' occurring in the presence of environmental triggers. "R" refers to the behavior or response(s) of interest in the functional analysis (i.e., substance use and suicidality). "C" refers to the consequences that serve to maintain or reinforce or that function to decrease the likelihood of recurrence of the behavior of interest. For example, to the extent that suicidal behavior and substance-abusing behavior are associated with removal or diminution of unpleasant affective states, these behaviors will be negatively reinforced and the likelihood of their recurrence in the presence of similar environmental circumstances (i.e., triggers) will increase. As described previously, there are often common triggers, risk and protective factors, and even consequences for suicidal and substance-abusing behaviors (Goldston 2004). Identification of these functional commonalities can be of assistance in choosing appropriately targeted and integrated interventions that can decrease the likelihood of multiple negative outcomes.

Treatment of SUD and Suicidal Ideation and Suicide Attempts

Psychosocial Interventions

No randomized controlled studies have been published evaluating the efficacy of psychosocial interventions specifically developed for suicidal youths with SUDs. With that said, there are several promising psychosocial approaches. Wood et al. (2001) examined the potential effectiveness of adjunctive group therapy (i.e., an add-on or augmenting therapy in addition to usual care received in the community) in reducing incidents of repeat (both suicidal and nonsuicidal) self-harm. Prior to randomization, 44% of adolescents reported intoxication at least once a week, and 37% reported using drugs at least once a week.

The group therapy in this study was eclectic in orientation, drawing from cognitive-behavioral therapy (CBT), dialectical behavior therapy (DBT), and psychodynamic therapy approaches and focusing on themes relevant to the developmental level of the youths, including peer and family issues. The adjunctive group therapy intervention resulted in reductions in incidents of repeat self-harm behaviors and improvements in behavior problems; effects on drinking or other substance use were not described. This study is one of the very few randomized controlled studies with suicidal adolescents showing greater efficacy for an experimental intervention in reducing self-harm behaviors.

Kaminer et al. (2006) compared two alternative approaches for providing aftercare for adolescents with alcohol use disorders following completion of 9 weeks of group CBT. The effectiveness of aftercare was examined because of the relatively high rate of relapse among alcohol- and substance-abusing youths. The two aftercare conditions included in-person relapse-prevention sessions, and relapse-prevention sessions delivered via telephone. Both aftercare approaches used both CBT and motivational interviewing approaches, and consisted of four sessions over 3 months. Both the initial treatment and the aftercare focused on alcohol and substance use, and did not focus on suicidal behaviors or risk. In addition to beneficial effects on substance use outcomes, the in-person CBT–motivational interviewing aftercare intervention resulted in greater reductions in suicidal ideation relative to the telephone aftercare or no aftercare, although the magnitude of the difference between the groups was small.

Esposito-Smythers et al. (2006, 2008) developed a flexible and integrated CBT–motivational interviewing intervention for suicidal youths with alcohol and/or other substance use problems. With this intervention approach, parents and youths had their own separate therapist in a coordinated approach to treatment because of the severity and multiplicity of the problems of this population. In addition to the integrated intervention, youths and families also received case management assistance, and psychiatric referrals for monitoring of medications. The intervention consisted of 6 months of weekly active treatment, 3 months of biweekly maintenance sessions, and 3 monthly booster sessions. Modules in the CBT–motivational interviewing intervention for the adolescents included safety planning, motivational interviewing, and cognitive-behavioral skills training. Modules for work with parents included, but were not limited to, monitoring, consequences, beliefs regarding adolescents, and communication with adolescents. This intervention was contrasted with enhanced treatment as usual (treatment as usual in the community, in addition to case management and provision of a psychiatrist for medications). Although this was a pilot study, the results with this intervention were very encouraging, with fewer suicide attempts, fewer rehospitalizations, fewer emergency room visits, fewer residential out-of-home placements, fewer arrests, fewer runaway episodes, and greater reductions in suicidal thoughts, depressive symptoms, anxiety symptoms, aggression, number of days using alcohol, and number of days using cannabis by 12 months after study entry.

Brown et al. (2005) described a randomized controlled trial of brief CBT for individuals presenting in an emergency department following attempted suicide. The sample consisted primarily of adults but also included adolescents age 16 and older. In this sample, 68% of participants had SUDs. The augmenting 10-session CBT intervention focused on suicide attempts and, in particular, relapse prevention. The CBT intervention was effective in reducing the rates of suicide attempts by half. Effects of the intervention on substance use were not reported, although this was not the primary focus of the intervention.

Dialectical behavior therapy is a variant of combined individual and group CBT that focuses on acceptance, emotion regulation, distress tolerance, mindfulness meditation and mindful awareness, and interpersonal effectiveness. DBT has been shown in randomized controlled trials with adults to be effective in reducing rates of suicide attempts relative to patients with other forms of treatment (Linehan et al. 2006). DBT also has been shown to reduce drug abuse among adult women with borderline personality disorder (Linehan et al. 1999). DBT has been adapted for use with adolescents, to include involvement of parents and to focus on developmentally appropriate issues, such as the balance between the need for parental monitoring versus the adolescent strivings for autonomy (Rathus and Miller 2000, 2002). Nonetheless, randomized controlled trials of DBT with adolescents have not yet been conducted.

Drawing from these psychosocial studies, as well as our own work in developing an integrated intervention with motivational interviewing and CBT approaches for suicidal dually diagnosed youths, we describe several approaches to intervention with the suicidal and substance-abusing adolescent. Prior to suggesting changes, the clinician should begin gathering information about the context of the suicide attempt or crisis—that is, to hear the "story" (Berk et al.

2004). This information about the context of suicidality, along with information regarding the history of substance abuse, can be used to develop a functional analysis regarding substance use and suicidality, as described earlier in this chapter (see "Functional Assessments"), which in turn can be used to identify treatment targets. Complementing this emphasis on "understanding the story" early in intervention, motivational interviewing approaches are useful in helping the adolescent to consider reasons for living and for quitting substance use, and in highlighting ambivalence and discrepancies between these reasons and current behavioral patterns. Motivational interviewing approaches also can be used with parents, given the importance of parents in monitoring adolescents, reinforcing change, and helping the adolescent continue in treatment (Logan and King 2001).

It is important to develop in a collaborative manner a safety plan of action for when the adolescent is beginning to feel distressed or in danger of hurting himself or herself. The safety plan can refer to coping thoughts and strategies learned in therapy, as well as individuals the adolescent may contact when feeling suicidal or unsafe, generally including the therapist (and after-hours contact information). Safety considerations also should be reviewed with the adolescent's parents, who should be strongly encouraged to remove access to potential means for attempting suicide, including firearms. The therapist should monitor for suicidal ideation and behavior at every treatment session, and should collaborate with the adolescent and family throughout the course of treatment in revising the safety plan as needed.

Increased participation in potentially enjoyable, pleasant activities other than alcohol and drug use is often encouraged with the suicidal, substance-abusing teen. The giving up of previously important social or recreational activities in favor of increased drug use is one symptom of substance dependence in adolescents or adults (American Psychiatric Association 2000). Depressed adolescents engage in more unpleasant activities than do nondepressed adolescents (Carey et al. 1986), and those with comorbid substance abuse engage in few social activities (Becker and Curry 2007). The therapist can work with the adolescent to help discover, or rediscover, and increase participation in pleasant activities, at least some of which can be social.

Another useful approach for the suicidal, substance-abusing adolescent is to focus on enhancing problem-solving skills. Suicidal, depressed adolescents show deficiencies in social problem solving (Speckens and Hawton 2005), and

problem-solving training is often included in treatment programs for substance-abusing adolescents (Latimer et al. 2003; Waldron et al. 2001). With
problem-solving training, the adolescent may learn to relax and try to "step back"
before solving problems, to brainstorm about possible alternatives, to identify
both advantageous and disadvantageous consequences associated with different options, to choose a possible solution, and to give himself or herself credit
for methodically thinking through how to handle the situation.

One therapy goal common to CBT approaches is to increase awareness of
and to challenge patterns of negative thoughts. The suicidal client is especially
likely to have negative thoughts about the future (hopelessness). The therapist
may counter this problem by increasing the adolescent's awareness of this negative pattern of thinking and coaching the adolescent to externalize and challenge these thoughts (e.g., by focusing on reasons for living and future goals).
Teenagers also may have distorted thoughts about substance abuse; for example, they may focus only on the positive consequences of use, and they may
not consider or may minimize the significance of the problems associated with
substance abuse. Similar to the approach with depression-related cognitions,
the therapist can help the adolescent to cultivate greater awareness of distor-
tions in thoughts and to challenge these thoughts.

In working with suicidal, substance-abusing youth, the therapist should involve parents or caregivers in a collaborative treatment approach. Parents can
be provided information about monitoring the adolescent for signs of escalating depression, withdrawal, and/or suicidal ideation and behavior. Although
some teens will tell their parents if they have made a suicide attempt, other
teens will not inform anyone, so parents of teens who have a history of previous suicide attempts should be on the lookout for evidence of another suicide
attempt. If parent monitoring reveals that suicidal thinking or behavior is increasing, then the parents and teen must be encouraged to use the safety plan
developed earlier in the treatment. Because the level of parent monitoring is
strongly related to teen conduct problems, such as substance use, increasing
parent monitoring of substance use and peer group activity, especially early in
treatment, may be an important goal. Likewise, monitoring the whereabouts
of the teen when out of the house and aspects of behavior such as curfew adherence can be very important treatment targets.

As parents monitor their teenager more accurately, it may become necessary to develop a plan for administering consequences. Monitoring may reveal

that the teenager is associating with drug-using peers, is coming home on the weekends drunk or high, or is consistently breaking curfew. Likewise, increased monitoring may show that the teen is becoming more depressed and/or experiencing an increase in suicidal ideation. Treatment sessions can be devoted to collaboratively developing a plan for exactly what consequences will be applied when the teenager comes home drunk or high or breaks curfew. Likewise, if increased monitoring reveals that the teen is becoming more hopeless or suicidal, then parents may need to apply interventions such as checking on the teenager at frequent intervals, looking for evidence of suicidal behavior, and implementing agreed-upon responses if such evidence is obtained (e.g., calling the therapist, taking the teen to the emergency room).

Negative communication is another potentially important treatment target in working with parents of suicidal, substance-using youth. Negative communication behaviors in home interactions may serve as a precipitant of suicidal behavior or substance use, and also may occur in the course of therapy sessions and interfere with the goals and content of these therapy sessions. If parents and teens engage in sarcastic, hostile, accusatory, blaming, or verbally aggressive behaviors during therapy sessions, then these communication behaviors will sidetrack or interfere with proactive, collaborative discussions. Alternatively, hostile family communication can result in family members shutting down, behaviorally and emotionally, and withdrawing from one another. Therapeutic work focusing on negative communication patterns may involve directly labeling the negative communication behaviors, based on the observation by the therapist in actual sessions or based on family reports of what occurs in the home, and teaching and then prompting more effective communication skills, such as active listening and reflecting without necessarily agreeing.

One last common area of intervention with parents and teens together involves family problem solving. Problem solving is an important family skill, because unresolved family problems or conflict can lead to negative "expressed emotion" (anger, hostility, contempt) among family members, and this process is known to be related to depression, suicidality, and recurrence of various mental health problems in adults and teens. In addition, suicidality can result from the hopelessness, helplessness, anxiety, and feelings of low self-esteem that arise from overwhelming unsolved problems. The urge to use substances also can be prompted by an impulse to reduce or escape from the negative feelings that arise from the inability to solve problems effectively and respectfully as a family. The approach to teaching family problem-solving skills is analogous to the process described above for working individually with the adolescent, with the major difference being that the problem-solving steps are collaborative (e.g., the family works together to identify the problem they are having together in concrete, nonpejorative terms, brainstorms and evaluates solutions together, and agrees together on an ultimate solution).

Pharmacotherapy

To our knowledge, no published controlled studies with comparison groups have shown the effectiveness of pharmacotherapy in reducing risk for suicidal behaviors or suicide specifically among individuals with substance abuse problems, or in reducing risk for both suicidal behaviors and substance abuse among adolescents. As described elsewhere in this book (see, e.g., Chapter 13, "Assessment and Treatment of Internalizing Disorders"), pharmacotherapy may be useful in reducing risk factors (e.g., anxiety, depression) that contribute to both suicidal behavior and substance abuse.

Integrative Treatment

No studies have been published describing the efficacy of combined pharmacotherapy and psychosocial treatment approaches for substance-abusing and suicidal adolescents. As described earlier, however, promising results have been obtained with integrated motivational interviewing and CBT approaches.

Case Vignette

Cathy is a 15-year-old female who lives with her biological mother and her younger brother. She presents for treatment after discharge from the hospital following her second suicide attempt by overdose, which was discovered by her mother. Cathy had been drinking when she took the pills in an effort to kill herself because she said she was tired of being depressed and she was upset after an argument with her mother about her skipping school and her declining grades. Cathy said that she had been depressed for approximately 3 years after an incident of sexual abuse. Since the abuse, she had been feeling very poorly about herself. Following this incident, she also began drinking and using cannabis, and experimenting with taking pills. Cathy's mother knew she had been using alcohol and drugs, but she was not fully aware of her daughter's use until the hospitalization.

By the time of this most recent suicide attempt, Cathy had developed a tolerance to both alcohol and cannabis. She said that she liked to drink and use pills to feel better because she did not like to feel depressed, but also acknowledged that "partying" was an important part of her social life, and she liked to "party" because all of her friends used substances at these occasions. Increasingly, Cathy had chosen to give up activities so she could more singularly focus her energies on activities related to alcohol and drug use with the permissive peer group. In the home, Cathy was often punished by her mother (generally by being grounded or with restrictions of privileges) because of the lying associated with substance abuse, breaking of curfew, and sneaking out of the home.

Cathy's history revealed that she tended to have intense suicidal ideation when inebriated, particularly when she was feeling anxious about other issues (e.g., school difficulties, problems with peers, conflict with her mother over her friends and substance abuse). Also when inebriated, she sometimes had intense memories of depression and anxiety from other upsetting experiences, including the sexual abuse. During these times of inebriation, she was sometimes impulsive and had difficulty following her safety plan. Her mother was very frustrated with Cathy and feeling increasingly hopeless, because she felt she was unable to keep her daughter safe. She tried to punish her daughter and lecture her, but her daughter tended to ignore these consequences and to sneak out of the home even more often when angry following arguments.

Case Discussion

Treatment goals: The immediate treatment goal is to ensure safety of the suicidal client. Ultimate treatment goals are reduction in suicidal thoughts and the risk for suicidal behaviors, reduction in depression and anxiety, and reduction in alcohol and substance abuse. Related goals include reduction in problems contributing to these issues, such as family conflict, negative thoughts and low self-esteem, lack of involvement in activities other than those focused on substance abuse, poor problem-solving skills, and lack of effective communication and parental monitoring in the home.

Treatment setting: The preferred choice for treatment setting is outpatient, although it is very likely that Cathy may need more than the usual 1-hour-per-week psychotherapy session (either longer or more frequent sessions, as well as emergency sessions when crises occur). If Cathy cannot be kept safe, cannot agree to a safety plan, or makes another suicide attempt, psychiatric hospitalization is an option. If the substance abuse or dependence problems are recalcitrant or worsen, intensive outpatient therapy or residential treatment may be warranted.

Treatment: Initially, and usually separately in psychotherapy, Cathy and her mother will be invited to "tell their story" regarding the events that led up to the suicidal behaviors and current substance abuse patterns. On the basis of this information, the therapist will begin working with Cathy and her mother to develop a functional analysis of the context of these problems, common risk factors, and their interrelationship. By the end of the first session, the therapist should collaboratively develop a safety plan with Cathy and her mother. The therapist will use motivational interviewing approaches to help establish rapport with the adolescent and her mother, to highlight ambivalence, to underscore self-efficacy, and to provide a foundation for steps taken toward change.

Over the course of therapy, the therapist will work with Cathy to help her become involved in activities that do not involve drugs and alcohol and, if possible, with new peer groups that are "safer" in terms of the behaviors they model and their avoidance of substances. Particularly given Cathy's low self-esteem and depression, as well as her hopelessness about the future, the therapist will help her to recognize and challenge overly negative thinking; consider her reasons for living, including aspirations for the future; and consider her good attributes. In tandem with reviewing the events that led to her current difficulties, the therapist can help Cathy to use better problem-solving skills so she can better consider the alternative behaviors and decisions she can make that might result in better outcomes. The therapist may use approaches described in Chapter 13, "Assessment and Treatment of Internalizing Disorders," to help with any posttraumatic stress symptoms related to Cathy's earlier abuse.

The therapist would work with Cathy's mother to monitor Cathy more closely and to more consistently administer consequences. If possible, the emphasis should be on reward-based consequences for positive steps taken toward change. Through work with the mother and Cathy together, the therapist can help the family improve the negative communication style and approach to resolving conflicts using problem-solving skills. The mother will be encouraged to "catch Cathy" making positive steps and to praise and reward these, and to try to limit negative expressed emotion, even when frustrated because Cathy is not making progress as quickly as hoped or has a setback.

As illustrated by Cathy, youths with both histories of suicidal behaviors and substance abuse often have multiple comorbidities. In addition to the psychotherapeutic approaches, Cathy's treatment may also involve pharmacotherapy aimed at reducing her level of depression and anxiety.

Conclusion

Youth with histories of suicidal thoughts and behaviors as well as substance abuse problems present challenges for the therapist, due to multiple psychiatric comorbidities and family difficulties, as well as risk of recurrent suicidal crises.

Clinicians must closely monitor each adolescent throughout the course of treatment for suicidal thoughts and behaviors, and maintain a flexible and individualized approach to intervention. Suicidal thoughts and behaviors are often interrelated, with common risk factors and triggers, and substance abuse may serve to increase the risk for suicidality. No large controlled study of psychosocial or pharmacological interventions for suicidal substance-abusing youths has yet been published, but it appears that motivational enhancement and cognitive-behavioral skills training approaches, particularly with a relapse-prevention focus, have potential utility with this population. Involvement of parents and caregivers is important in monitoring youths, reinforcing change, and collaborating in the intervention process.

Key Clinical Concepts

- There is heightened risk for suicidal thoughts and behavior in an adolescent substance-abusing population, and clinicians should routinely monitor for evidence and course of suicidality.
- Substance abuse and suicidality may have common triggers, risk factors, and even motives.
- Youth with suicidality and substance abuse problems often have multiple psychiatric comorbidities, family difficulties, and life problems, and a flexible approach to treatment is needed with this population.
- No large controlled studies have been published for alcohol- or substance-abusing and suicidal patients, although motivational enhancement and cognitive-behavioral skills training approaches, with the involvement of parents and caregivers and with an emphasis on relapse prevention, appear promising.

References

American Psychiatric Association: Diagnostic and Statistical Manual of Mental Disorders, 4th Edition, Text Revision. Washington, DC, American Psychiatric Association, 2000

Angle CR, O'Brien TP, McIntire MS: Adolescent self-poisoning: a nine year follow-up. J Dev Behav Pediatr 4:83–87, 1983

Arango V, Underwood MD, Boldrini M, et al: Serotonin 1A receptors, serotonin transporter binding and serotonin transporter mRNA expression in the brainstem of depressed suicide victims. Neuropsychology 25:892–903, 2001

Bailey JA, McCloskey LA: Pathways to adolescent substance abuse among sexually abused girls. J Abnorm Child Psychol 33:39–53, 2005

Beautrais AL, Joyce PR, Mulder RT: Risk factors for serious suicide attempts among youths aged 13 through 24 years. J Am Acad Child Adolesc Psychiatry 35:11–26, 1996

Beck A, Steer R: Beck Hopelessness Scale Manual. San Antonio, TX, Psychological Corporation, 1988

Beck A, Steer R: Manual for the Beck Scale for Suicide Ideation. San Antonio, TX, Psychological Corporation, 1991

Becker SJ, Curry JF: Interactive effect of substance abuse and depression on adolescent social competence. J Clin Child Adolesc Psychol 36:469–475, 2007

Berk MS, Henriques GR, Warman D, et al: A Cognitive Therapy Intervention for Suicide Attempters: An Overview of the Treatment and Case Examples. Cognitive and Behavioral Practice, Vol 11, No 3. New York, Association for Advancement of Behavior Therapy, 2004, pp 265–277

Berman AL, Schwartz RH: Suicide attempts among adolescent drug users. Am J Dis Child 144:310–314, 1990

Boergers J, Spirito A, Donaldson D: Reasons for adolescent suicide attempts: associations with psychological functioning. J Am Acad Child Adolesc Psychiatry 37:1287–1293, 1998

Boldrini M, Underwood MD, Mann JJ, et al: Serotonin-1A autoreceptor binding in the dorsal raphe nucleus of depressed suicides. J Psychiatr Res 42:433–442, 2008

Bovasso GB: Cannabis abuse as a risk factor for depression. Am J Psychiatry 158:2033–2037, 2001

Brent DA: Correlates of the medical lethality of suicide attempts in children and adolescents. J Am Acad Child Adolesc Psychiatry 26:87–89, 1987

Brent DA, Perper JA, Goldstein CE, et al: Risk factors for adolescent suicide: comparison of adolescent suicide victims with suicidal inpatients. Arch Gen Psychiatry 45:581–588, 1988

Brent DA, Kolko DJ, Allan MJ, et al: Suicidality in affectively disordered adolescent inpatients. J Am Acad Child Adolesc Psychiatry 29:586–593, 1990

Brent DA, Oquendo M, Birmacher B, et al: Familial pathways to early onset suicide attempts: risk factors for suicidal behavior in offspring of mood-disordered suicide attempters. Arch Gen Psychiatry 59:801–807, 2002

Breton JJ, Tousignant M, Bergeron L, et al: Informant-specific correlates of suicidal behavior in a community survey of 12- to 14-year-olds. J Am Acad Child Adolesc Psychiatry 41:723–730, 2002

Brown GK, Have TT, Henriques GR, et al: Cognitive therapy for the prevention of suicide attempts: a randomized controlled trial. JAMA 294:563–570, 2005

Burge V, Felts M, Chenier T, et al: Drug use, sexual activity and suicidal behavior in U.S. high school students. J Sch Health 65:222–227, 1995

Cantor C, McTaggart P, De Leo D: Misclassification of suicide: the contribution of opiates. Psychopathology 34:140–146, 2001

Carey MP, Kelley ML, Buss RR, et al: Relationship of activity to depression in adolescents: development of the Adolescent Activities Checklist. J Consult Clin Psychol 54:320–322, 1986

Cavaiola AA, Lavender N: Suicidal behavior in chemically dependent adolescents. Adolescence 34:735–744, 1999

Centers for Disease Control and Prevention: Suicide among black youths—United States, 1980–1995. MMWR Morb Mortal Wkly Rep 47:193–196, 1998

Centers for Disease Control and Prevention: Suicide attempts and physical fighting among high school students—United States, 2001. MMWR Morb Mortal Wkly Rep 53:473–476, 2004

Centers for Disease Control and Prevention: National Center for Injury Prevention and Control. Web-based Injury Statistics Query and Reporting System (WISQARS) Online. Available at: http://www.cdc.gov/ncipc/wisqars. Accessed January 3, 2010.

Clarke G, Hops H, Lewinsohn P, et al; Cognitive-behavioral group treatment of adolescent depression: prediction of outcome. Behav Ther 23:341–354, 1992

Conner KR, Goldston DB: Rates of suicide among males increase steadily from age 11 to 21: developmental framework and outline for prevention. Aggress Violent Behav 12:193–207, 2007

Costello EJ, Erkanli A, Federman E, et al: Development of psychiatric comorbidity with substance abuse in adolescents: effects of timing and sex. J Clin Child Psychol 28:298–311, 1999

Crockett LJ, Raffaeli M, Shen YL: Linking self regulation and risk proneness to risky sexual behavior: pathways through peer pressure and early substance abuse. J Res Adolesc 16:503–525, 2006

Deykin E, Buka S: Suicidal ideation and attempts among chemically dependent adolescents. Am J Public Health 84:634–639, 1993

Eaton DK, Kann L, Kinchen S, et al: Youth risk behavior surveillance—United States, 2007. MMWR Surveill Summ 57:1–131, 2008

Eggert LL, Herting JR: Drug involvement among potential dropouts and "typical" youth. J Drug Educ 23:31–55, 1993

Epstein J, Spirito A: Risk factors for suicidality among a nationally representative sample of high school students. Suicide Life Threat Behav 39:241–251, 2009

Esposito-Smythers C, Goldston DB: Challenges and opportunities in the treatment of adolescents with SUD and suicidal behavior. Subst Use 29:5–17, 2008

Esposito-Smythers C, Spirito A, Uth R, et al: Cognitive behavioral treatment for suicidal alcohol abusing adolescents: development and pilot testing. Am J Addict 15 (suppl 11):S126–S130, 2006

Esposito-Smythers C, Spirito A, et al: Treatment for adolescent alcohol other drug use disorders and suicidality: results of a randomized pilot trial. Poster presented at the Joint Scientific Meeting of the Research Society on Alcoholism and the International Society for Biomedical Research on Alcoholism, Washington, DC, June 2008

Foley DL, Goldston DB, Costello E, et al: Proximal psychiatric risk factors for suicidality in youth: the Great Smoky Mountains Study. Arch Gen Psychiatry 63:1017–1024, 2006

Garrison CZ, McKeown RE, Valois RF, et al: Aggression, substance use, and suicidal behaviors in high school students. Am J Public Health 83:179–184, 1993

Goldfried MR, Sprafkin JN: Behavioral Personality Assessment. Morristown, NJ, General Learning Press, 1974, pp 295–321

Goldston DB: Measuring Suicidal Behavior and Risk in Children and Adolescents. Washington, DC, American Psychological Association, 2003

Goldston DB: Conceptual issues in understanding the relationship between suicidal behavior and substance use during adolescence. Drug Alcohol Depend 76 (suppl 17):S79–S91, 2004

Goldston DB, Daniel SS, Reboussin DM, et al: Suicide attempts among formerly hospitalized adolescents: a prospective naturalistic study of risk during the first 5 years after discharge. J Am Acad Child Adolesc Psychiatry 38:660–671, 1999

Goldston D, Molock S, Whitbeck L, et al: Cultural considerations in adolescent suicide prevention and psychosocial treatment. Am Psychol 63:14–31, 2008

Goldston D, Daniel S, Erkanli A, et al: Psychiatric disorders as contemporaneous risk factors for suicide attempts among adolescents and young adults: developmental changes. J Consult Clin Psychol 77:281–290, 2009

Gould MS, Fisher P, Parides M, et al: Psychosocial risk factors of child and adolescent completed suicide. Arch Gen Psychiatry 53:1155–1162, 1996

Gould MS, King R, Greenwald S, et al: Psychopathology associated with suicidal ideation and attempts among children and adolescents. J Am Acad Child Adolesc Psychiatry 37:915–923, 1998

Hoberman HM, Garfinkel BD: Completed suicide in children and adolescents. J Am Acad Child Adolesc Psychiatry 27:689–695, 1988

Houston D, Hawton K, Shepperd R: Suicide in young people aged 15–24: a psychological autopsy study. J Affect Disord 63:159–170, 2001

Hufford MR: Alcohol and suicidal behavior. Clin Psychol Rev 21:797–811, 2001

Jacobs D; APA Work Group on Suicidal Behaviors: Practice guideline for the assessment and treatment of patients with suicidal behaviors. Am J Psychiatry 160 (suppl 11):S1–S60, 2003

Joe S, Kaplan MS: Firearm-related suicide among young African-American males. Psychiatr Serv 53:332–334, 2002

Joe S, Marcus SC: Datapoints: trends by race and gender in suicide attempts among U.S. adolescents, 1991–2001. Psychiatr Serv 54:454, 2003

Joiner TE Jr, Conwell Y, Fitzpatrick KK, et al: Four studies on how past and current suicidality relate even when "everything but the kitchen sink" is covaried. J Abnorm Psychol 114:291–303, 2005

Kaminer Y, Burleson JA, Goldston DB, et al: Suicidal ideation among adolescents with alcohol use disorders during treatment and aftercare. Am J Addict 15 (suppl 1): 43–49, 2006

Kaufman J, Birmaher B, Brent D, et al: Schedule for Affective Disorders and Schizophrenia for School-Aged Children—Present and Lifetime Version (K-SADS-PL): initial reliability and validity data. J Am Acad Child Adolesc Psychiatry 36:980–988, 1997

Kelly T, Lynch K, Donovan J, et al: Alcohol use disorders and risk factor interactions for adolescent suicidal ideation and attempts. Suicide Life Threat Behav 31:181–193, 2001

Khantzian EJ: The self-medication hypothesis of substance use disorders: a reconsideration and recent applications. Harv Rev Psychiatry 4:231–244, 1997

Kienhorst IC, De Wilde EJ, Diekstra RF, et al: Adolescents' image of their suicide attempt. J Am Acad Child Adolesc Psychiatry 34:623–628, 1995

King CA, Ghaziuddin N, McGovern L, et al: Predictors of comorbid alcohol and substance abuse in depressed adolescents. J Am Acad Child Adolesc Psychiatry 35:743–751, 1996

Klaus NM, Mobilio A, King CA: Parent-adolescent agreement concerning adolescents' suicidal thoughts and behaviors. J Clin Child Adolesc Psychol 38:245–255, 2009

Klimes-Dougan B: Screening for suicidal ideation in children and adolescents: methodological considerations. J Adolesc 21:435–444, 1998

Kovacs M, Goldston D, Gatsonis C: Suicidal behaviors and childhood-onset depressive disorders: a longitudinal investigation. J Am Acad Child Adolesc Psychiatry 32:8–20, 1993

Lane S, Cherek D, Pietras C, et al: Performance of heavy marijuana-smoking adolescents on a laboratory measure of motivation. Addict Behav 30:815–828, 2005

Latimer W, Winters K, D'Zurilla T, et al: Integrated family and cognitive-behavioral therapy for adolescent substance abusers: a stage I efficacy study. Drug Alcohol Depend 71:303–317, 2003

Lewinsohn PM, Rohde P, Seeley JR: Adolescent suicidal ideation and attempts: prevalence, risk factors and implications. Clinical Psychology: Science and Practice 3:25–36, 1996

Lewinsohn PM, Rohde P, Seeley JR, et al: Gender differences in suicide attempts from adolescence to young adulthood. J Am Acad Child Adolesc Psychiatry 40:427–434, 2001

Linehan MM, Comtois K: Lifetime Parasuicide Count. Seattle, WA, University of Washington, 1997

Linehan MM, Goodstein JL, Nielsen SL, et al: Reasons for staying alive when you are thinking of killing yourself: the Reasons for Living Inventory. J Consult Clin Psychol 51:276–286, 1983

Linehan M, Schmidt H, Dimeff L, et al: Dialectical behavior therapy for patients with borderline personality disorder and drug-dependence. Am J Addict 8:279–292, 1999

Linehan MM, Comtois KA, Murray AM, et al: Two-year randomized controlled trial and follow-up of dialectical behavior therapy vs therapy by experts for suicidal behaviors and borderline personality disorder. Arch Gen Psychiatry 63:757–766, 2006

Logan DE, King CA: Parental facilitation of adolescent mental health service utilization: a conceptual and empirical review. Clinical Psychology: Science and Practice 8:319–333, 2001

March JS, Silva S, Petrycki S, et al: The Treatment for Adolescents with Depression Study (TADS): long-term effectiveness and safety study. Arch Gen Psychiatry 64:1132–1144, 2007

Millsaps CL, Azrin RL, Mittenberg W: Neuropsychological effects of chronic cannabis use on the memory and intelligence of adolescents. J Child Adolesc Subst Abuse 3:47–55, 1994

Moeller FG, Barratt ES, Dougherty DM, et al: Psychiatric aspects of impulsivity. Am J Psychiatry 158:1783–1793, 2001

O'Carroll PW, Berman A, Maris RW, et al: Beyond the Tower of Babel: a nomenclature for suicidology. Suicide Life Threat Behav 26:237–252, 1996

Orvaschel H: Schedule for Affective Disorders and Schizophrenia for School-Aged Children—Epidemiologic Version 5 (K-SADS-E) (unpublished instrument). Ft Lauderdale, FL, Nova Southeastern University, 1994

Pinto E, Reggers J, Gorwood P, et al: The short allele of the serotonin transporter polymorphism influences relapse in alcohol dependence. Alcohol Alcohol 43:398–400, 2008

Posner K, Oquendo M, Gould M, et al: Columbia Classification Algorithm of Suicide Assessment (C-CASA): classification of suicidal events in the FDA's pediatric suicidal risk analysis of antidepressants. Am J Psychiatry 167:1035–1043, 2007

Prevette K, Mathias C, Marsh D, et al: Impulsivity in suicidal adolescent inpatients. Poster presented at the 2nd annual meeting of the International Society for Research on Impulsivity, Washington, DC, November 2005

Rathus JH, Miller AL: DBT for adolescents: dialectical dilemmas and secondary treatment targets. Cogn Behav Pract 7:425–434, 2000

Rathus JH, Miller AL: DBT adapted for suicidal adolescents. Suicide Life Threat Behav 32:146–157, 2002

Reynolds WM: Suicidal Ideation Questionnaire: Professional Manual. Odessa, FL, Psychological Assessment Resources, 1988

Reynolds WM: Development of a semistructured clinical interview for suicidal behavior in adolescents. Psychol Assess 2:382–390, 1990

Rudatsikara E, Muula AS, Siziya S: Variables associated with physical fighting among U.S. high-school students. Clin Pract Epidemiol Ment Health 4:16–24, 2008

Schuckit M, Schuckit J: Substance use and abuse: a risk factor in youth suicide, in Report of the Secretary's Task Force on Youth Suicide: Risk Factors for Youth Suicide, 2 (DHHS Publ No ADM-89-1622). Edited by Davidson L, Linnoila M. Rockville, MD, Alcohol, Drug Abuse, and Mental Health Administration, 1989

Shaffer D, Scott M, Wilcox H, et al: The Columbia Suicide Screen: validity and reliability of a screen for youth suicide and depression. J Am Acad Child Adolesc Psychiatry 43:71–79, 2004

Shneidman ES: The Suicidal Mind. New York, Oxford University Press, 1996

Speckens AE, Hawton K: Social problem–solving in adolescents with suicidal behavior: a systematic review. Suicide Life Threat Behav 35:365–387, 2005

Spirito A, Stark L, Fristad M, et al: Adolescent suicide attempters hospitalized on a pediatric unit. J Pediatr Psychol 12:171–189, 1987

Velez CN, Cohen P: Suicidal behavior and ideation in a community sample of children: maternal and youth reports. J Am Acad Child Adolesc Psychiatry 27:349–356, 1988

Waldron HB, Slesnick N, Brody JL, et al: Treatment outcomes for adolescent substance abuse at 4- and 7- month assessments. J Consult Clin Psychol 69:802–813, 2001

Walker M, Moreau D, Weissman MM: Parents' awareness of children's suicide attempts. Am J Psychiatry 147:1364–1366, 1990

Whitlow CT, Liguori A, Livengood L, et al: Long-term heavy marijuana users make costly decisions on a gambling task. Drug Alcohol Depend 76:107–111, 2004

Wilcox HC, Conner KR, Caine ED: Association of alcohol and drug use disorders and completed suicide: an empirical review of cohort studies. Drug Alcohol Depend 76(suppl):S11–S19, 2004

Wood A, Trainor G, Rothwell J, et al: Randomized trial of group therapy for repeated deliberate self-harm in adolescents. J Am Acad Child Adolesc Psychiatry 40:1246–1253, 2001

Wu NS, Lu Y, Sterling S, et al: Family environment factors and substance abuse severity in an HMO adolescent treatment population. Clin Pediatr (Phila) 43:323–333, 2004

Suggested Readings

Esposito-Smythers C, Goldston DB: Challenges and opportunities in the treatment of adolescents with SUD and suicidal behavior. Subst Use 29:5–17, 2008

Esposito-Smythers C, Spirito A, Uth R, et al: Cognitive behavioral treatment for suicidal alcohol abusing adolescents: development and pilot testing. Am J Addict 15 (suppl 11):S126–S130, 2006

Goldston DB: Conceptual issues in understanding the relationship between suicidal behavior and substance use during adolescence. Drug Alcohol Depend 76 (suppl 17):S79–S91, 2004

15

Assessment and Treatment of Comorbid Psychotic Disorders and Bipolar Disorder

Robert Milin, M.D., F.R.C.P.C.

Selena Walker, M.A.

Anne C. Duffy, M.D., F.R.C.P.C.

In this chapter, we address the relationship of psychotic disorders and bipolar disorder with substance use disorders (SUD). Case vignettes are used to illustrate key points raised in regard to assessment, differential diagnosis, and treatment.

Psychosis and SUD

In this section, we focus on 1) enhancing clinicians' understanding of the interrelationship between schizophrenia and SUD, and of the course of illness;

2) heightening the awareness of the value of assessment for substance-induced psychotic disorder and of outcome; and 3) increasing the knowledge in regard to treatment of schizophrenia and comorbid SUD. These objectives are addressed, as evidence permits, within the parameters of adolescents and young adults, for whom first-episode psychosis (FEP) is most representative. FEP refers, in principle, to first-episode psychotic disorders. Special attention is given to the impact of cannabis use as it relates to psychosis.

Association of Psychotic Disorders and SUD

The onset of schizophrenia is most common in young adulthood, with first psychotic symptoms often occurring before 20 years of age in 20%–40% of cases (Lehman et al. 2004). The period of onset of schizophrenia overlaps with the peak age at onset for SUD occurring in late adolescence/early adulthood (Brown et al. 2008; Compton 2007). Cannabis is the most common substance regularly used by adolescents, with 5.4% of 12th-grade students using daily (Monitoring the Future 2008). Cannabis would appear to be the most common and significant substance of dependence in adolescents, including being the most prevalent primary substance of abuse that leads to treatment admission (Dennis et al. 2002).

SUD is the most common comorbid disorder in schizophrenia and FEP. In clinical samples of patients with schizophrenia, current prevalence rates of SUD range from 20% to 40%, and lifetime prevalence rates range from 50% to 80% (Westermeyer 2006). Similar rates of lifetime and even higher rates of current comorbid SUD have been found in patients with adolescent-onset schizophrenia and FEP. In patients with FEP, current rates of SUD have been reported to be as high as 60% (Lambert et al. 2005; Milin 2008). In a highly representative large Canadian sample ($N=357$) of young adults with FEP, Van Mastrigt et al. (2004) reported that 44% had current comorbid SUD and 35% had a cannabis use disorder.

Cannabis is the most common substance of abuse in FEP, followed by alcohol, although polysubstance abuse is not uncommon. Younger age and male gender are the most consistent predictors of SUD, especially drug abuse (Milin 2008; Wade et al. 2005). Among other various correlates identified has been a history of criminal offenses (Cantor-Graae et al. 2001).

Patients with schizophrenia show remitting rates of comorbid SUD over the course of illness, as evidenced by the difference between lifetime and current prevalence rates. Remission rates are influenced by substance of abuse (alcohol having higher rates than cannabis and other drugs) and severity (abuse having higher rates than dependence) (Westermeyer 2006).

The incidence of psychotic disorders may not be reliably reported in the adolescent SUD population, and has been reported in only a few clinical studies. This lack of reporting may reflect the severity of the illness, as adolescents and young adults with psychotic symptoms and disorders would typically seek treatment with psychiatric services for care. It has been postulated that adolescence may be a unique period of vulnerability for the concurrent development of psychotic disorders and SUD. Van Nimwegen et al. (2005) suggested that specific psychosocial challenges and neurodevelopmental brain changes may increase the risk of onset of both psychosis and drug abuse in vulnerable adolescents.

Over the last decade, a growing body of evidence from international longitudinal and cohort studies, supported by a recent meta-analysis, indicates that cannabis use increases the risk of psychotic outcome. This outcome includes clinically relevant psychotic disorders, independent of confounding factors such as other substance abuse, preexisting psychotic symptoms and other psychopathology, and transient intoxication effects. The pooled analysis found an increased risk of psychosis of 40% for those who ever used cannabis, and a dose-dependent effect with a risk of psychosis of 50%–200% for those who used cannabis most frequently (Moore et al. 2007).

A similar significant relationship has been found for cannabis and schizophrenia, with accumulating evidence that cannabis use is an independent risk factor for the development of schizophrenia in adulthood and especially in vulnerable individuals. Findings across studies are consistent with an overall two- to threefold increase in the risk of developing schizophrenia with cannabis use in a dose-dependent manner, and a greater risk with onset of use in adolescence (Arseneault et al. 2004; Milin 2008; Semple et al. 2005). This increased risk is comparable to better-known associations, including the relationship of cigarette smoking and hypercholesterolemia in developing lung cancer and heart disease, respectively (D'Souza 2007).

Notwithstanding these findings, evidence to date does not support a causal link between cannabis use and schizophrenia (Degenhardt et al. 2003). Nevertheless, Moore et al. (2007) in their analysis concluded that sufficient evidence exists to warn young people that cannabis use may increase their risk for developing a psychotic illness later in adulthood. In essence, cannabis use in a dose-dependent manner is a significant independent risk factor in the complex interaction of genetic liability and environmental factors that leads to the expression of schizophrenia (Caspi et al. 2005; Henquet et al. 2005b).

Clinical studies show that for the most part, substance or cannabis abuse precedes the onset of psychosis or schizophrenia, but that abuse also may begin concurrently with or following the onset of schizophrenia. Drug abuse, particularly cannabis abuse, has been associated with an earlier age at onset of schizophrenia (Barnes et al. 2006; Van Mastrigt et al. 2004; Veen et al. 2004). Compton et al. (2009), in a cross-sectional study of FEP, examined the effect of pre-onset cannabis use on the age at onset of physicians and found that the progression to daily cannabis use, and not the frequency of cannabis use per se, was associated with an increased risk for onset of psychosis or prodromal symptoms. This association was found to show a gender bias and was stronger for females than for males with FEP.

A history of substance abuse has been identified as one of five factors that uniquely contribute to the prediction of psychosis in a high-risk population meeting criteria for prodromal syndrome (Cannon et al. 2008). Cannabis dependence has been identified as a common comorbid psychiatric disorder in a prodromal clinical population (Rosen et al. 2006).

Based on the balance of evidence, comorbid SUD imparts a negative effect on the course and outcome of schizophrenia and has been frequently associated with increased risk of psychotic relapse, hospitalization, criminality, violence, suicidality, homelessness, treatment nonadherence (including to pharmacotherapy), and poorer treatment response (including to pharmacotherapy) (Dixon 1999; Lambert et al. 2005; Milin 2008). In longitudinal studies of FEP, similar findings of poorer clinical outcomes have also been found for persisting comorbid SUD, including increased rates of relapse and hospitalization, decreased remission rates, and greater symptomatology, as well as poorer functional outcomes (Lambert et al. 2005; Sorbara et al. 2003; Wade et al. 2006). Wade et al. (2007) also demonstrated support for a relationship between substance severity and clinical outcomes in youth with FEP: heavy substance abuse showed a greater association with poorer symptomatic and functional outcomes, whereas mild substance abuse did not appear to have the same effect. Cannabis use disorders in FEP were highly prevalent in the high-severity SUD group and significantly more so than in the low-severity SUD group.

Cannabis abuse and severity have also been strongly implicated in poorer clinical outcomes in prospective studies of young adults with recent-onset psychosis or schizophrenia (Grech et al. 2005; Hides et al. 2006; Linszen et al. 1994).

Assessment and Differential Diagnosis

A wide variety of substances of abuse from different classes may induce a range of psychotic symptoms. These symptoms are typically associated with acute or chronic intoxication from the following classes of substances: alcohol, amphetamines, hallucinogens, cannabis, opioids, phencyclidine, cocaine, inhalants, sedative-hypnotics, and anxiolytics. Psychotic symptoms may also occur with substance withdrawal from heavy and prolonged use of alcohol and sedative-hypnotics and anxiolytics.

In individuals without serious mental health disorders, substances of abuse may produce psychotic symptoms that are similar to those of individuals with schizophrenia. In individuals with primary psychotic disorders, the use of substances of abuse may exacerbate, change, or temporarily decrease preexisting psychotic symptoms. Various substances of abuse, even from different classes, may produce similar psychotic symptoms and clinical features. Substance-induced psychotic symptoms are by far most commonly transient and resolve within several hours to days. However, some evidence suggests that chronic and heavy use of stimulants, cocaine, hallucinogens, phencyclidine, and cannabis may result in psychotic reactions that may last for weeks or longer (American Psychiatric Association 2000; Milin 2008). In a long-term follow-up study of young adult drug users, Perkins et al. (1986) concluded that those with psychotic symptoms suffered from a major psychotic disorder, whereas drug abusers with an acute course of psychotic symptoms were similar on all outcome measures to drug abusers without psychotic symptoms.

An important diagnostic distinction is between substance-induced psychotic disorder (SIPD) and substance intoxication or withdrawal with perceptual disturbance. The former diagnosis should be made when psychotic symptoms are assessed as being significantly more prominent than one would typically expect with intoxication or withdrawal and when the severity of symptoms warrants independent clinical attention. The latter diagnosis includes hallucinations (not delusions) that may occur in the course of intoxication or withdrawal, with intact reality testing (the individual is aware that the hallucinations are an effect of the substance) (American Psychiatric Association 2000).

The differential diagnosis between SIPD and a primary psychotic disorder with concurrent SUD is often challenging, and a history of significant substance abuse is typically common to both conditions. Mueser et al. (1992), in their review on the comorbidity of schizophrenia and substance abuse, reported that a diagnosis of schizophrenia and related disorders may be reliably made in the presence of symptoms of schizophrenia and the absence of substance abuse within the preceding month, even when the patient has a history of prior substance abuse. However, periods of abstinence of a month or longer are often difficult to achieve. Clinicians, therefore, may need to consider the onset, course, and other features of presentation. This differentiation is even more complex in the adolescent/young adult population as schizophrenia and SUD commonly have their onset in this age range. Other factors to be considered include the effect of substance use and cessation on psychotic symptoms, the severity of psychotic symptoms in relation to the degree of substance abuse, and the characteristic symptoms produced by the principal substance of abuse in relation to the full spectrum of positive and negative symptoms of schizophrenia. The clinical situation may be further confounded by a pattern of multiple substances of abuse. Where possible, urine drug analyses (both screening and quantitative levels) may be helpful in gauging the role of substance use.

Clinical support has been mounting for the construct that apparent substance-induced psychotic reactions that persist beyond a reasonable period of abstinence (from several days to a few weeks, depending on the known characteristics of the substance) without significant improvement of psychotic symptoms should be treated as a functional psychotic disorder (Milin 2008). A diagnosis of psychotic disorder not otherwise specified (NOS) may be given when the clinician is uncertain whether the psychotic condition is a primary or a substance-induced disorder. Addington and Addington (1998) recommended that treatment for schizophrenia be initiated even though a diagnosis of drug-induced psychosis cannot be ruled out.

In assessing concurrent psychotic and substance-related disorders, the clinician should explore both the cross-sectional and longitudinal course of illness. A collateral and family history, where possible, are often helpful in assessing the course of illness and differentiating etiology, especially in adolescents and young adults.

In the most substantive study to date, Caton et al. (2005) examined the differences between early-phase primary psychotic disorders with concurrent substance use and substance-induced psychosis. The most common SIPD was found to be due to cannabis, followed by alcohol and cocaine. Several significant predictive factors were found to distinguish between SIPD and primary psychotic disorders with concurrent substance use. The SIPD group had greater prevalence of diagnosis of drug dependence, parental history of substance abuse, and visual hallucinations, whereas the primary psychotic disorder group had a greater degree of total psychopathology, including both positive and negative symptoms. In the 1-year follow-up study of this sample, Caton et al. (2007) assessed diagnostic change and stability. The SIPD group showed a greater instability of diagnosis, with 25% having received a change in diagnosis to a primary psychotic disorder. The primary psychotic disorder group remained diagnostically stable. A family history of parental mental illness was found to be an additional key predictor differentiating primary psychotic disorders from SIPD, with greater prevalence in the primary psychosis group. Parental substance abuse was no longer found to be significant, although the odds ratio remained elevated, and the other three characteristics remained key predictors.

In a Danish longitudinal cohort study (Arendt et al. 2005), the incidence rate for cannabis-induced psychotic disorder was estimated at 2.7 per 100,000 person-years, indicating that it is a relatively uncommon event. However, of the patients who received a diagnosis of and treatment for cannabis-induced psychotic disorder with no prior history of psychosis, nearly 50% subsequently received a diagnosis of a schizophrenia spectrum disorder on follow-up of at least 3 years. Male gender and younger age were associated with an increased risk for the development of schizophrenia spectrum disorders.

In a broader Danish cohort study, Arendt et al. (2008) examined history of treatment of psychiatric and psychotic disorders in first-degree relatives as an indicator of predisposition to psychiatric disorder. This association was compared in those who developed first-presentation cannabis-induced psychosis and those who developed a schizophrenia spectrum disorder. Similar rate ratios for family history of general psychiatric and psychotic disorders were found for both groups. This data, coupled with results from the previous study (Arendt et al. 2005), led the authors to suggest that cannabis-induced psychosis is neither a random occurrence nor a benign condition. They concluded that cannabis-induced psychotic disorder (defined as requiring treatment and as involving psychotic symptoms lasting more than 48 hours) may be an early sign of schizophrenia. Caton et al. (2006) also found evidence to strongly endorse the likelihood that drug-induced psychotic disorder requiring treatment represents a cogent vulnerability marker for development of schizophrenia.

In summary, there is no certain way to differentiate SIPD from a primary psychotic disorder with concurrent SUD. For the most part, a clinical judgment is necessary, based on knowledge about current and longitudinal history of the individual's psychotic symptoms and substance use, about the course of illness of schizophrenia, and about the pharmacological properties of the principal substance in question. Differentiation is made even more complex in adolescents and young adults by the severity of SUD and the early age at onset, as well as the often unclear course of premorbid symptoms, with both abrupt and insidious onset of psychosis. The following predictive factors have been identified as being helpful in the differential diagnosis: diagnosis of drug dependence, parental mental illness (as well as parental substance abuse), visual hallucinations, and severity of psychotic or psychiatric symptoms. However, one must keep in mind that the vast majority of those presenting with FEP do not have a positive family history for a psychotic disorder (D'Souza 2007). Despite best efforts to differentiate the diagnosis of SIPD versus FEP, diagnostic ambiguity may remain. Irrespective of differential diagnosis, a growing body of evidence suggests that SIPD, especially cannabis-induced psychosis, among individuals presenting for treatment is a strong marker for the development of schizophrenia, with the highest risk in young males. The serious clinical implications warrant longitudinal follow-up of SIPD and specifically cannabis-induced psychosis in adolescents and young adults, given diagnostic instability and as a cogent marker for schizophrenia. However, clinicians should keep in mind that in epidemiological surveys, it is not uncommon for cannabis users to report transient psychotic symptoms (B. Green et al. 2003), whereas substance- or cannabis-induced psychosis is a relatively uncommon diagnosis made in individuals requiring clinical attention and treatment.

Treatment

In this subsection, we focus mainly on treatment findings of FEP as they relate to comorbid SUD. First, however, we have a few comments on the treatment of SIPD.

In essence, no established guidelines are available regarding the treatment or follow-up of SIPD apart from behavioral and supportive management. Patients with SIPD have shown a greater rate of remission than those with primary psychotic disorders at 1-year follow-up (Caton et al. 2006). In "Treatment of Patients With Substance Use Disorders," Kleber et al. (2007) described that individuals with certain substance-induced psychotic symptoms may benefit from the short-term use of antipsychotic medication.

In cases of diagnostic uncertainty, proceeding with treatment for a functional psychotic disorder is recommended even though drug-induced psychosis cannot be excluded. Overlooking a primary psychotic disorder may lead to a longer duration of untreated psychosis associated with poorer prognosis and poorer treatment outcome in FEP (Marshall et al. 2005). Comorbid SUD has been linked to a longer duration of psychosis in FEP (Marshall et al. 2005). On the other hand, inaccurate diagnosis of SIPD as a primary psychotic disorder may lead to unnecessary stress of diagnosis and treatment for a psychotic disorder and to the omission of SUD treatment. Clinicians in psychiatric emergency services may have a tendency to overdiagnose primary psychotic disorder in lieu of SIPD, affecting treatment and referral patterns (Schanzer et al. 2006).

The current emerging gold standard of care for FEP involves specialized early intervention (SEI) treatment services. SEI services were developed to enhance course of illness outcomes as defined by such parameters as symptom remission, relapse rates, and quality of life/functioning. A variety of factors may influence outcome, including such potentially malleable factors as duration of untreated psychosis, duration of untreated illness, substance abuse, and adherence to medication and/or treatment, and nonmalleable factors such as premorbid adjustment, age at onset of psychosis, and positive family history of psychotic disorders (Malla et al. 2008).

Models of SEI services vary across countries and programs. However, certain common elements have been identified, which include a form of assertive case management, use of low-dose second-generation antipsychotic (SGA) medication regimens, close monitoring of treatment progress, family intervention, and individual and group psychotherapeutic and cognitive-behavioral intervention. These intensive treatment programs typically range from 18 months to 2 years. Preliminary evidence from a small number of randomized controlled studies and open studies supports the effectiveness of SEI for FEP.

The relative benefit of SEI over routine care has been identified through higher rates of remission, lower relapse rates, better control of symptoms, and greater adherence to and retention in treatment, as well as through some improvement on broadly defined outcomes of functioning and quality of life over the course of intensive treatment (1–2 years) (Malla et al. 2005). In a Cochrane review, Marshall and Rathbone (2006) supported the ethical use of SEI for FEP but considered the evidence insufficient for support of its effectiveness. A randomized controlled study in the United Kingdom found policy support for the provision of SEI for early psychosis over standard care, with SEI achieving better outcomes (Garety et al. 2006). The optimal duration and long-term effectiveness of SEI services remain to be determined. Two 5-year follow-up studies of SEI services for patients with FEP, one being the largest randomized controlled study to date (Bertelsen et al. 2008) and the other an uncontrolled study of an older adolescent sample (Linszen et al. 2001), found that positive clinical outcomes were not sustained with transition to routine care following programs of 2 years and 15 months, respectively.

In a study comparing adolescents and young adults with FEP entering an SEI program, findings suggested that patients with adolescent-onset FEP were more likely to present with characteristics associated with poorer outcome, including greater duration of untreated psychosis and degree of primary negative symptoms. Apart from these differences, these two patient groups shared many similar clinical features, including level of substance abuse (Ballageer et al. 2005). More important, in a follow-up study of patients receiving SEI, adolescents with FEP showed both clinical and functional improvement equivalent to adult patients with FEP, except that the adolescents used more cannabis and had more relapses (Pencer et al. 2005). The adolescent group did demonstrate a significant reduction in cannabis use over time, and by the end of the 2-year follow-up period, their level of cannabis use did not differ from that of the adults. Pencer et al. (2005) noted that attention to substance abuse is a major focus of this SEI program. The most robust predictors of outcome were persisting residual symptoms, including both positive and negative symptoms in adolescents.

Wade et al. (2006) followed the course of comorbid SUD in a sample of FEP patients with a high rate of SUD (about 70%) over the initial 15-month treatment period, during which time the patients received either standard mental health care or SEI with at least basic counseling on the negative impact of SUD on psychosis, and found substance abuse to persist in a large majority of patients. However, by the end of the follow-up period, a significant minority of patients had experienced a remission of SUD. Furthermore, for those patients in whom SUD persisted, there was a likelihood of a significant reduction in level of substance use in terms of severity and/or frequency. Very few patients developed SUD after entering treatment. Persistent SUD was associated with younger age and with greater severity of cannabis use upon entry into treatment for FEP.

Studies have shown that patients with FEP receiving SEI have had a significant and meaningful reduction in SUD over the course of treatment. Reduction in SUD has been associated with improved clinical outcome, and SEI has been shown to be significantly more likely than routine care to reduce SUD (Lambert et al. 2005; Petersen et al. 2005). Despite these promising findings, patients with FEP and comorbid SUD have shown increased relapse rates in the context of high medication adherence and controlling for other predictive factors over a 2-year follow-up in an SEI program (Malla et al. 2008).

There appears to be a window of opportunity in the early course of treatment of FEP to address the significant negative impact of SUD on outcome. Two Australian pilot studies have examined the benefit of adding a specific brief intervention for SUD to treatment as usual for young adults in the early course of a psychotic disorder with comorbid SUD. These studies showed evidence of preliminary support for treatment effectiveness of brief intervention for SUD, with greater reduction of substance use at 6 months and up to 12 months posttreatment compared with treatment as usual (Kavanagh et al. 2004; R. Kemp et al. 2007). A similar approach with favorable results has been found for adult patients with schizophrenia and comorbid SUD in a randomized controlled study. This pilot study found that adding integrated treatment for SUD was more effective than treatment as usual, with improvement of functioning and reduction of positive symptoms, relapse rate, and substance use (Barrowclough et al. 2001).

In another randomized controlled study of young people with FEP receiving SEI services from Australia, Edwards et al. (2006) compared a cannabis-focused intervention (cannabis and psychosis therapy, a cognitive-behavioral approach) and a clinical control condition defined as psychoeducation on psychotic disorder for FEP patients who continued to use cannabis. No differences in cannabis use were found between treatment groups 6 months posttreatment. Both interventions resulted in a significant reduction in cannabis use. However, the study had several methodological limitations that may have affected the findings and the ability to have discriminated responses between integrated treatments. A significant factor that may have confounded findings was the low level of cannabis use required for inclusion in the study, with a reported median level prior to entering the study of 4 days of use in 4 weeks (Edwards et al. 2006). Addington and Addington (2001), based on FEP preliminary outcome evidence, suggested the benefit of an integrated approach of addressing the impact of substance abuse through the various components of SEI services and reserving SUD-specific treatment for those with persisting substance abuse in later stages of the program. Numerous studies have noted the reluctance of FEP patients, or for that matter any patient with a psychotic disorder and comorbid SUD, to engage in concurrent SUD-specific treatment.

Pharmacotherapy remains the mainstay of treatment for schizophrenia and other related psychotic disorders with or without comorbid SUD. Clinically, SGAs remain the first choice of treatment for adolescents and young adults with FEP. As of this writing, four SGAs—risperidone, aripiprazole, quetiapine, and olanzapine—have received U.S. Food and Drug Administration approval for the treatment of schizophrenia in adolescents. In treating FEP, SGAs are typically initiated at low dosage and gradually titrated to response within standard therapeutic dosage range. Careful monitoring for adverse effects is required, especially in adolescents and those with comorbid SUD, because adverse effects may be potentiated by active substance abuse.

In general, SGAs may hold some advantage over first-generation antipsychotics in treating patients with schizophrenia-related disorders (including those with recent onset) and comorbid SUD in terms of reduced substance use. However, these findings in favor of SGAs should be considered tentative, given the inability to differentiate an effect between SGAs and specific substances as well as the absence of long-term outcome studies (Swanson et al. 2007; Van Nimwegen et al. 2005).

In patients with schizophrenia-related disorders, studies have associated comorbid SUD with higher antipsychotic dosage and poorer response to antipsychotic treatment, even when patients were adherent to medication. Comorbid SUD is also associated with nonadherence with pharmacotherapy, which further exacerbates its negative influence on outcome (Hunt et al. 2002). Similar poorer treatment response and adherence, irrespective of first- or second-generation antipsychotic medication use, have been found for patients with FEP and a lifetime history of comorbid SUD (A.I. Green et al. 2004). Interestingly, in one study, medication adherence was linked to a modest reduction in cannabis relapse in patients with recent-onset psychosis who were predominantly receiving SGAs (Hides et al. 2006). One should not overlook the potential benefit of long-acting injectable antipsychotic medication in FEP patients with comorbid SUD, who are at increased risk of medication nonadherence (A.I. Green et al. 2007). Risperidone is the only SGA that is available to date as a long-acting injectable medication.

In summary, in treating adolescents with FEP and comorbid SUD, clinicians are challenged with a variety of confounding and competing factors over time, including problematic treatment adherence. The advent of SEI and the addition of integrated SUD treatment hold considerable promise in improving outcomes for this complex population. A model to be considered in addressing comorbid SUD, especially cannabis use disorders, is working with the adolescent in treatment for FEP with SEI services, integrating an enhanced focus on the negative impact of SUD in the various facets of the treatment program, including emphasis on harm reduction and treatment adherence. Those patients who show persisting substance abuse/dependence or SUD relapse would be encouraged to further engage in SUD-specific treatment, preferably a combination of individual motivational enhancement therapy and cognitive-behavioral therapy that is integrated into overall treatment. This model could also be applied to adolescents with FEP and comorbid SUD who are not readily receiving SEI services.

Case Vignette

Eric, a 16-year-old male living with his mother, has not been attending school due to safety concerns. He presented to a youth psychiatric program accompanied by his mother and youth criminal justice caseworker for outpatient assessment of possible psychotic disorder. He had been released on probation about 2 months earlier from a youth detention center, where he was in custody for 3 months charged with two counts of indecent exposure and one count of resisting a police officer. Documentation included multiple reports, including a comprehensive court-ordered youth offender assessment completed during his stay in detention. Eric's behavior at the time of his offenses and arrest was reported as erratic, bizarre, and agitated. He was assessed in the emergency room of a teaching hospital and described as delusional, having used marijuana. He was discharged to police custody. No formal diagnosis was provided; however, he was described as seriously disturbed, suffering from severe thought disorder consistent with a psychotic disorder. Eric had an extensive prior history of assessment and involvement in psychiatric and mental health services dating back to childhood. In the year prior to incarceration, he had on several occasions been briefly admitted to hospital-based child and adolescent psychiatric services, including once for a suicide attempt. His discharge diagnoses included conduct disorder (with aggressivity) and substance abuse, with possible underlying attention-deficit/hyperactivity disorder (ADHD) and posttraumatic stress disorder. Eric had received treatment with stimulant medication for ADHD, combined with a low-dose SGA for management of aggressive behavior. The court-ordered assessment recommended that Eric, being at high risk, receive psychiatric care, intense supervision, and pharmacotherapy in a secure treatment facility for his serious mental health disorder.

When seen, Eric was not currently receiving any formal treatment, including pharmacotherapy. He presented as a physically well-developed and well-groomed youth who was restrained but articulate. He showed no evidence of thought process disorder or overt psychosis. Eric was guarded and evasive. Identified at-risk behaviors included reinforcing the locked apartment door with a chair, sleeping with a large knife at his bedside, and burning a picture of himself. Eric reported a history of daily marijuana use for 1 year prior to entering youth detention. He had also experimented with ecstasy and acid, and used alcohol excessively on weekends. During this period of heavy marijuana and other substance use, Eric demonstrated aggressive, out-of-control behavior and experienced significant negative consequences in multiple life areas secondary to his marijuana use. Eric had been abstinent from all substances for the past 5 months since his placement in detention and release.

Prompted by a collateral history of psychotic symptoms from his mother and caseworker, Eric disclosed a system of predominantly paranoid and persecutory delusions, sexual delusions, and delusions of reference. Eric identified male pedophiles living in his building who would break into their apartment to rape and castrate him. He also reported that people believed he was a homosexual or "fag." Eric endorsed hearing voices making a running commentary on his behavior and events. His mother reported that he first disclosed the onset of intermittent voices at age 12. Eric showed poor insight into his illness, relating that he just wanted to get on with things and go to school. Eric had no history of manic or hypomanic episodes, and he did not endorse current symptoms of major depressive disorder.

The family's psychiatric history was negative for schizophrenia or substance dependence. Eric's mother and maternal grandmother each had a history of recurrent depression. Other background information was noncontributory to presentation.

Case Discussion

Eric presented as a youth offender with a significant history of serious behavioral problems and extensive prior involvement with specialized psychiatric and mental health services for children and adolescents. Eric's course of substance abuse clearly exacerbated his behavioral problems and confounded his presentation. It was subsequently discovered that he had in the past reported often becoming intensely paranoid and hearing voices when using marijuana; nevertheless, he continued to use heavily. Cross-sectional and longitudinal history pointed to a prolonged duration of untreated psychosis. Eric's clinical picture was consistent with FEP and comorbid SUD supported by an extended period of substance abstinence.

Eric declined admission and need for treatment. He was certified and admitted as an involuntary patient. Once admitted, Eric agreed to pharmacotherapy with an SGA, in context of the court order to comply with treatment. The urine drug screen on admission was negative for substances of abuse. Eric showed good response to SGA treatment, with resolution of psychotic symptoms. However, evidence of negative symptoms persisted. He was discharged to attend a specialized school-based adolescent psychiatric day treatment program with the capacity for integrated concurrent disorder treatment (Milin et al. 2000). His discharge diagnoses included 1) schizophrenia, paranoid type (first episode), 2) cannabis dependence in early remission, and 3) conduct disorder by history.

Bipolar Disorder and SUD

In this section, we review the association between bipolar disorder and SUDs, with an emphasis on the effect of the clinical course, differential diagnosis, and intervention implications.

Substance abuse and dependence have long been recognized as associated with mood disorders. Compared with major depression, bipolar disorder has a particularly strong association with SUD, and substance (both alcohol and drug) dependence is more strongly associated with mood disorders than are problems of heavy use or abuse. This specificity of risk for SUD extends to individuals with broader diagnoses of bipolar disorder, including subthreshold hypomania (Angst et al. 2006; Glantz et al. 2008; Merikangas et al. 2008).

Epidemiological studies have consistently reported that bipolar disorder is the second most highly associated disorder with SUD, after antisocial personality disorder (for review, see Salloum and Thase 2000). Specifically, both the Epidemiologic Catchment Area study and the National Comorbidity Survey reported six- to tenfold elevated rates of SUD in patients with bipolar disorder compared with the general population, and a lifetime history of SUD in approximately 50% of patients with bipolar disorder (Kessler et al. 1997; Regier et al. 1990).

In a prospective epidemiological study, Henquet et al. (2006) found that cannabis use increased the risk of later manic symptoms, even after adjusting for the use of other substances and the presence of depressive, manic, and psychotic symptoms. The findings were suggestive of a dose-response relationship between frequency of cannabis use and mania outcome. However, considerably more research is called for to elucidate any role that cannabis use may have in the subsequent risk of bipolar disorder.

Clinical studies have also reported similarly high rates of SUD among patients with bipolar disorder (for reviews, see Cassidy et al. 2001; Merikangas et al. 2008). Alcohol and cannabis are the first and second most frequent substances of abuse or dependence, respectively, and a substantial proportion of alcoholic patients with bipolar disorder are thought to abuse at least one other substance. In reports of younger clinical populations, cannabis appears to be overtaking alcohol as the most prevalent substance of abuse or dependence (Goldstein et al. 2008b; Wilens et al. 2008). Also, patients with bipolar disorder are estimated to have a fourfold increased risk of sedative-hypnotic and opiate addictions compared with those in the general population (Salloum and Thase 2000).

Most epidemiological and clinical studies have relied on cross-sectional and retrospective data to investigate the association between mood disorders and SUD. In a recent analysis by Merikangas et al. (2008) of the Zurich cohort study, the association between bipolar disorder and subsequent onset of alcohol abuse (odds ratio = 9.1) and dependence (odds ratio = 21.1) was replicated. Furthermore, manic symptoms (subthreshold hypomania) were found to be a risk factor for the future development of all categories of SUD studied (alcohol, cannabis, benzodiazepines). A lack of association was found between major depression and later cannabis abuse or dependence. This and previous studies underscore the specificity of risk of bipolar disorder for the subsequent development of SUD.

SUD are well known to negatively impact the course of illness and all manner of measured outcomes in patients with bipolar disorder. (For a comprehensive review, see Salloum and Thase 2000.) Briefly, comorbid SUD has been associated with an earlier age at onset; shortened cycle length; delayed time to recovery; shortened time to relapse; higher number of recurrences; more mixed and rapid-cycling presentations; more chronicity, disability, cognitive impairment, and mortality attributed to increased suicide risk; and more medical complications. Furthermore, SUD is strongly associated with treatment nonadherence, a factor correlated with the poor outcomes cited above.

Course of Bipolar Disorder

SUD may precede or start early in the course of bipolar disorder. Bipolar disorder typically has an onset during adolescence and early adulthood (Leboyer et al. 2005) and has a strong genetic basis (Alda and Grof 2000). The most robust characteristic of bipolar disorder is the nature of the clinical course, characterized by recurrent episodes of major depression and hypomania or mania. Patients vary greatly in the frequency of episodes and in the quality of remission; some patients experience a spontaneous completely remitting episodic course, whereas others have residual symptoms between episodes. In approximately 15% of cases, the illness is chronic and nonremitting (Grof et al. 1995). Although there is a high individual difference in the ratio of depressed to activated episodes, most patients over their life course experience more depressive episodes, which are longer in duration than the manic episodes. In fact, depression is typically the first major mood episode, and some patients even experience many years of recurrent major depression before their first identified hypomanic, manic, or mixed episode (Angst 1998). Evidence from epidemiological and clinical studies suggests that subthreshold mood episodes (depression NOS, bipolar NOS, mood NOS) and mood symptoms are common antecedents to the full-blown mood episodes (Angst and Preisig 1995; Lewinsohn et al. 2000).

First-Episode Mania and SUD

Early-onset bipolar disorder, particularly during adolescence, has a reportedly strong association with SUD (Joshi and Wilens 2009). In a 24-month prospective study of patients admitted for a first-episode mania/mixed bipolar I episode, Baethge et al. (2005) reported a 33% prevalence rate of SUD (mostly substance dependence) at baseline, with 40% of these patients having polysubstance use and 60% having monosubstance use disorders. Compared with first-episode patients without an SUD, polysubstance users were younger, less well educated, more likely to present in a mixed state, and more likely to have a positive family history of psychiatric illness. Furthermore, substance use in this patient population was associated with a lifetime history of an anxiety disorder. On follow-up, cannabis-dependent patients spent more time in mania, whereas alcohol-dependent patients spent more time depressed. Overall, morbidity was much greater among polysubstance users.

The Cincinnati First-Episode Mania Study reported a lifetime prevalence of 42% and 46% for alcohol and cannabis use disorders, respectively (Strakowski et al. 2007). Substance use disorders in this cohort were associated with treatment noncompliance and a longer time to recovery. In a study reported by DelBello et al. (2007), the rate of either an alcohol or a cannabis use disorder at baseline was only 15%; however, the age of the cohort was much younger (mean age of 15 years at enrollment) than in the previous study.

In a large cohort of adolescents diagnosed with bipolar disorder who were selected from the Course and Outcome of Bipolar Youth study, Goldstein et al. (2008b) described a lifetime rate of SUD of 16%. Cannabis use disorders were most prevalent, with lifetime rates of 12% in the entire adolescent bipolar disorder cohort and 73% in those with an SUD. Alcohol use disorders had prevalence rates of 8% in the entire cohort and 50% in those with an SUD. Finally, 5% of all adolescents with bipolar disorder and 30% of those with an SUD met lifetime criteria for both cannabis and alcohol use disorders. In this study, bipolar disorder anteceded SUD in 60% of subjects, whereas both conditions had concurrent onset in an additional 10%. Conduct disorder, suicide attempt, and age were significant positive predictors of SUD in these adolescents with bipolar disorder. Furthermore, adolescents with bipolar disorder and comorbid SUD were more likely to report trouble with police, teenage pregnancy, and abortion.

A recent case control study of subjects ranging in age from 10 to 18 years examined the relationship between bipolar disorder and SUD, including nicotine dependence, and other psychiatric comorbidity. Wilens et al. (2008) reported a higher age-adjusted rate of any SUD among subjects with bipolar disorder compared with controls (hazard ratio [HR] = 8.68)—in particular, higher rates of alcohol abuse (HR = 7.66), drug abuse (HR = 18.5), drug dependence (HR = 12.1), and cigarette smoking (HR = 12.3). The association between bipolar disorder and SUD remained significant when controlling for other comorbidities, including conduct disorder, ADHD, and anxiety disorders. Furthermore, adolescent-onset bipolar disorder (compared to pediatric-onset bipolar disorder) was strongly associated with an elevated risk of SUD (Joshi and Wilens 2009). In 67% of subjects, the onset of bipolar disorder preceded the onset of SUD, and an additional 24% experienced the onset of bipolar disorder and SUD within the same year.

Daily cigarette smoking occurs at a very high rate among adult patients with bipolar disorder, and has been associated with elevated cardiovascular morbidity, as well as with psychosis, suicidal behavior, and other SUD. Goldstein et al. (2008a) investigated cigarette smoking in over 400 subjects ages 7–17 participating in the Course and Outcome of Bipolar Youth study. The authors reported that 11% of these youth with bipolar disorder smoked at least one cigarette daily at study entry (daily group), and an additional 14% of subjects reported a lifetime history of smoking. The mean age at regular smoking onset among the daily group was estimated at 12.9 years. Bipolar disorder onset occurred prior to or in the same year as regular cigarette smoking in 69% of the subjects. A regression analysis comparing ever-smoked to never-smoked subgroups of youth with bipolar disorder found that age, lifetime SUD, lifetime suicide attempt, and a positive family history of SUD were most strongly associated with having ever smoked. The authors concluded that compared with epidemiological studies, the lifetime prevalence of having ever smoked may be similar for youths with a bipolar disorder as for youths in the general population, although those with bipolar disorder have an increased rate of daily smoking.

Cigarette smoking has been reported as highly prevalent in samples of inpatients with first-episode mania. Heffner et al. (2008) recently reported that over 45% of first-episode patients diagnosed with bipolar disorder smoked cigarettes within 30 days of admission. The mean age at smoking onset was estimated to be 14 years. Current smokers were more likely to report recent alcohol and marijuana use and to meet criteria for alcohol and cannabis use disorders. Almost 40% of the subjects indicated a lifetime history of both cannabis and cigarette use, the majority (over 65%) initiating use of both within the same year. For subjects with a lifetime history of regular use of both alcohol and cigarettes (over 35%), most initiated use of cigarettes first.

Temporal Association Between Bipolar Disorder and SUD

Most studies have found that psychiatric illnesses typically have earlier onset than do SUD, although this temporal relationship is less clear for mood disorders. A recent analysis of the National Comorbidity Survey Replication data assessed retrospectively the reported age at onset of substance use and psychiatric disorders (Glantz et al. 2008). The age at onset distributions showed that SUD typically occurred in young adults and that externalizing and anxiety disorders were more likely to precede nicotine, alcohol, and other drug dependence. Mood disorders were only slightly more likely to precede nicotine dependence and somewhat less likely to precede dependence on alcohol (46%) and other drugs (45.9%). However, most studies, particularly those with a longitudinal prospective design, have found that the onset of bipolar disorder precedes or is concurrent with the onset of SUD, especially if the onset of the mood disorder is defined as the first manifestation of the syndrome (Angst et al. 2006; Biederman et al. 1999; Merikangas et al. 2008). In a report by Angst et al. (2006) investigating the temporal sequence of bipolar II disorder and alcohol use disorders, the affective episodes preceded SUD in the majority of cases. The onset of bipolar disorder was typically prior to age 20, whereas the use of alcohol was "a minor problem" at this age. However, very rapidly over the next decade, alcohol use disorders became a substantial comorbid diagnosis.

At the time of writing, there was an estimated 18% lifetime prevalence of SUD in a cohort of longitudinally studied offspring (age 12 and older) of parents with a confirmed diagnosis of bipolar disorder (Table 15–1). In this cohort, the most frequently used drug was cannabis. Comparing high-risk offspring with and without a lifetime SUD (Table 15–2), there was a significant association of SUD with comorbid mood disorder and with lifetime history of psychosis and hospitalization.

We recently reported that bipolar disorder among these offspring of well-characterized bipolar parents evolves in a series of recognizable and predictable clinical stages (Duffy et al. 2010). Not all offspring manifest all stages, but when they start to develop psychopathology, it unfolds in accordance with the predicted staging sequence (i.e., individuals can enter the sequence at any stage). Specifically, we noted that the first stage includes nonspecific (non-mood) anxiety and sleep disorders in childhood, followed by minor mood disorders (depression NOS, mood NOS) and adjustment disorders (sensitivity to stress) in early adolescence. Later, in mid-adolescence, major depressive episodes manifest, followed by activated episodes (hypomania, mania).

In a preliminary analysis, we found that SUDs began either concurrently with or following the first major mood episode in the majority (67%) of high-

Table 15–1. Substance use disorders in adolescent/young adult high-risk offspring (N=202)

Characteristic	n	%
Lifetime SUD (abuse or dependence)	36	17.8
SUD distribution		
Alcohol abuse/dependence	7	3.5
Cannabis abuse/dependence	19	9.4
Alcohol and cannabis abuse	9	4.5
Other substance abuse (cocaine, ecstasy)	1	0.5
	Mean	SD
SUD onset age (years)	17.20	2.87
Age at last interview (years)	23.88	4.98

Note. SUD=substance use disorder.

risk offspring. Furthermore, offspring without a history of mood disorder had an 18% age-adjusted morbid risk of SUD, whereas offspring with a history of a major mood disorder had a 35% age-adjusted morbid risk of SUD (HR= 2.4; 95% confidence interval=1.20–4.76) (Duffy et al. 2010).

Explaining Association Between Bipolar Disorder and SUD

The association between bipolar disorder and SUD has not as yet been worked out, although a number of possibilities have been discussed. There is generally good agreement, from a number of different researchers, that the association cannot be explained by a shared genetic diathesis (Duffy et al. 1998; Merikangas et al. 2008; Winokur et al. 1995); that is, there is no difference in familial loading for SUD among the relatives of patients with bipolar disorder and SUD versus those of patients with bipolar disorder but not SUD. Put another way, no evidence supports the independent transmission of SUD in patients with bipolar disorder and their family members, and SUD in these families typically occur as a secondary complication to the bipolar disorder. Therefore, most discussion has focused on causal models and pathways.

Some evidence supports the view that patients use substances to self-medicate specific symptoms. In a study presented, but not yet published, at a

Table 15–2. Clinical characteristics of high-risk offspring with and without lifetime history of substance use disorders (N=202)

Characteristic	With SUD (n=36)	Without SUD (n=166)	χ^2	df	P
	%	%			
Internalizing disorders					
Major mood disorder	72.2	28.9	23.9	1	0.0001
Minor mood disorder	19.4	9.6	2.8	1	0.142
Anxiety disorder	25.0	15.1	2.1	1	0.149
Comorbid externalizing disorders					
ADHD	5.6	4.8			
Oppositional/conduct	8.3	0.6	3.3	1	0.138
	Years	Years	t	df	P
Major mood onset age	17.8±3.8	17.5±3.8	0.32	72	0.749
Minor mood onset age	16.2±6.9	16.5±5.1	1.14	41	0.260
	%	%	χ^2	df	P
Hospitalized ever	11	2	7.7	1	0.020
Psychotic features ever	22	4	14.0	1	0.001

Note. ADHD=attention-deficit/hyperactivity disorder; SUD=substance use disorder.

national conference by Lorberg et al. (2008; cited in Joshi and Wilens 2009), youth with bipolar disorder reported initiating substances to treat mood symptoms, whereas controls without mood disorders used substances to get high. This model would require a match between specific symptoms and the properties of the substance used. In a prospective study of 166 first-episode patients, Baethge et al. (2008) reported that cannabis use selectively and strongly preceded or coincided with activated episodes, whereas alcohol use preceded or coincided with depression. As discussed by Salloum and Thase (2000), anergic depressive symptoms may be indicative of hypofunction of dopaminergic circuits, and dopamine has a central role in the highly reinforcing effects of alcohol and other drugs of abuse, including opiates and cocaine. Therefore, several examples implicate neurotransmitter systems as being involved in both the pathophysiology of bipolar disorder and the neurobiology of SUD.

Another possibility is that certain temperamental, personality, and behavioral factors are associated with the risk of SUD, as well as bipolar disorder. Specifically, arousal, novelty seeking, impulsivity, happiness, and nervousness have been reported as highly predictive of alcohol consumption (Merikangas et al. 2008) and as characteristics of those at risk for and diagnosed with bipolar disorder (Cassano et al. 1992). Moreover, anxiety symptoms and disorders occur frequently in patients with bipolar disorder and also have a well-recognized association with SUD. The possibility that unstable personality characteristics and anxiety might mediate the relationship between bipolar disorder and subsequent SUD would also explain the comprehensive risk for a number of different substances in bipolar disorder.

The variable pattern of substance use between individuals with the same diagnosis (bipolar disorder) and over time (cannabis increasing in popularity relative to alcohol in younger age groups) suggests that several mechanisms likely underlie the association between bipolar disorder and SUD. In addition to large-scale studies describing general trends, smaller detailed longitudinal studies of individual patients can clarify certain associations. In one such qualitative study of SUD in patients with bipolar disorder, Healey et al. (2009) reported that patients' reasons for SUD derived from their own personal experiences and that personal experience of alcohol and drugs was idiosyncratic; that is, some found that specific substances enhanced activated episodes, whereas others found a dampening effect. Furthermore, subjects' experiences and beliefs regarding the effects of substances on their mood symptoms were formulated early in the course of illness and provided evidence of early self-medication and self-titration. In addition, some subjects stopped taking prescribed medication and used substances to feel a part of the normal peer group (social conformity). The latter point may be of particular relevance early in the course of illness, when experimentation with substances is a common adolescent experience and at the same time a developmental and clinical course stage at which acceptance of an illness is most challenging, yet effective treatment may have its largest impact on preventing the substantial burden of illness associated with established illness.

Treatment

The primary treatment for bipolar disorder, both acute episodes and prophylaxis, is pharmacotherapy, and a number of efficacious agents for these indications have been outlined in various published guidelines (Yatham et al. 2009). However, growing evidence suggests that outcome is significantly improved if the mood stabilizer chosen for prophylactic indications is selected based on the individual patient profile (Garnham et al. 2007; Grof 2003; Grof and Müller-Oerlinghausen 2009; Passmore et al. 2003). Selective response reflects the heterogeneity of bipolar disorder; for example, responders to lithium are characterized by an episodic remitting course, with good quality of remission both clinically and on psychological testing, and have a family history of recurrent mood disorders and not chronic psychotic illnesses (Alda 2004; Grof et al. 1993). Despite a paucity of studies examining the treatment of bipolar disorder in adolescents, authors have based treatment guidelines on the available research (Garland and Duffy, in press; Kowatch et al. 2005). Preliminary evidence suggests that at least a subgroup of youth with bipolar disorder may respond very well early in the course of illness to selected monotherapy based on the nature of the clinical course (episodic vs. nonepisodic), family history (recurrent mood disorders vs. chronic psychosis), and the response to mood stabilizers in affected family members (lithium responsive vs. lithium nonresponsive) (Duffy et al. 2007, 2009; Grof et al. 2002).

Few randomized controlled studies have examined the effectiveness of pharmacotherapies in patients with comorbid bipolar disorder and SUD. Valproate was studied using a 24-week, randomized, double-blind, placebo-controlled, parallel-group design in adults with bipolar disorder and alcoholism receiving treatment as usual with lithium and psychosocial intervention

(Salloum et al. 2005). The authors reported that adjunctive valproate improved alcohol use outcomes but not symptoms of depression or mania. Recently, D. E. Kemp et al. (2009) compared lithium to lithium and divalproate in adults with rapid-cycling bipolar disorder and comorbid SUD using a 6-month double-blind randomized controlled study of maintenance therapy for bipolar disorder. Attrition rates were high, and no benefit was found for combined pharmacotherapy over monotherapy.

Only one randomized controlled study of adolescents with bipolar disorder and SUD has been conducted. Geller et al. (1998) investigated 6 weeks of lithium treatment in a small group of adolescents presenting with bipolar spectrum disorders and comorbid substance dependence and receiving interpersonal therapy. Compared with placebo, lithium resulted in a reduced number of positive drug urine screens and increased scores on the Children's Global Assessment Scale. To our knowledge, there are no studies of SGA or valproate in adolescents with bipolar disorder and comorbid SUD with which to compare.

A frequently reported issue in treating patients with bipolar disorder is nonadherence to medication regimens. Treatment nonadherence has been associated with poorer treatment outcome, including relapse (Manwani et al. 2007). Nonadherence is exacerbated if the patient has comorbid SUD, and may result in delayed recovery (Cerullo and Strakowski 2007). Preliminary findings have suggested that alcohol abuse may be associated with the duration of bipolar depression and that cannabis may be associated with the duration of mania (Strakowski et al. 2000).

Adult studies of the effects of psychosocial therapies on patients with bipolar disorder and comorbid SUD are few. Weiss et al. (2007) developed integrated group therapy, a manualized approach based on cognitive-behavioral therapy, designed specifically for patients with bipolar disorder and comorbid substance dependence. They conducted a randomized controlled study of 20 weeks of integrated group therapy compared with group drug counseling for adults with bipolar disorder and current substance dependence who were receiving mood stabilizers. Compared with group drug counseling, integrated group therapy reduced substance use but increased symptoms of depression and mania (Weiss et al. 2007). No studies of psychosocial therapies have been conducted in adolescent populations with bipolar disorder and comorbid SUD.

A significant gap remains in the evidence-based knowledge and treatment of bipolar disorder in adolescents with and even without SUD. Also, few conclusions can be drawn from the limited treatment studies of adults with bipolar disorder and comorbid SUD. It remains important to address stabilization of the underlying primary disorder, in this case bipolar disorder, to understand the nature of the relationship with SUD, and if necessary to include specific treatment for SUD, with the promise of benefit of integrated treatment for both disorders.

Summary Remarks

SUD is a major complicating factor for patients with bipolar disorder. SUD has been associated with a higher burden of illness, increased treatment refractoriness, and increased morbidity and mortality. The onset of SUD appears in close temporal contiguity with the onset of the first major mood episodes, early in the course of bipolar illness. Antecedent SUD in adolescent and early adult patients may be temporally associated with subthreshold mood symptoms and prodromal presentations. Clearly, adolescents at familial risk for bipolar disorder are a target group for further studies of the relationship between the evolving mood disorder and SUD and the development of effective early intervention and prevention strategies.

Case Vignette

Helene, age 24 years, was referred for psychiatric consultation after discharge from the emergency department of a local hospital. She had been taken to the emergency department by a family member for assessment of bizarre behavior and impaired judgment.

Specifically, Helene gave a several-week history of insomnia, agitation, a subjective feeling of her mind racing with many new ideas and thoughts, elevated mood with an increasingly irritable edge, mild paranoid ideation with no fixed delusions, and poor insight. There was no evidence of thought insertion/ withdrawal, ideas of reference, bizarre delusions, or hallucinations. She had not been attending university and was unable to focus on her schoolwork. Helene felt it necessary to write notes to herself because her ideas were coming to her so quickly that she was afraid of forgetting them, but the ideas were more plans and were not necessarily bizarre in nature. The patient was admitted to the hospital, and her activated state settled with benzodiazepines and lithium.

When a complete history from the patient and family members was ascertained, it was clear that this illness began in adolescence. At age 16, Helene abruptly developed a major depressive episode. Uncharacteristically, she felt profoundly sad and forlorn, was often tearful, ruminated about the pointlessness of life, and blamed herself for the strife between her parents. This episode, which lasted for several weeks, was clearly a different and unpleasant experience for this individual but completely remitted without treatment. The next episode came abruptly at age 18; the patient was a first-year university student away from home. Her parents had since separated. Helene again became clinically depressed with suicidal ideation, and sought help through student health services at the university she was attending and was referred to psychiatry. The psychiatrist diagnosed adjustment disorder with depressed mood related to the stress of attending university and the parental separation; psychotherapy was recommended and instituted. The major depressive episode resolved after several months. The next episode occurred 18 months later, with similar abruptness of onset of major depressive symptoms associated with incapacity. The patient began to self-medicate with alcohol and marijuana. Eventually, she reengaged with the previous psychiatrist, who diagnosed major depression and instituted an antidepressant (selective serotonin reuptake inhibitor). There was a relatively abrupt change in the clinical picture, with worsened substance abuse, mild paranoid ideation, poor insight and judgment, insomnia, and mixed mood symptoms. The patient left the university and started to travel the world. This episode finally subsided after approximately 1 year, but not as completely as in the past. The patient continued to self-medicate with marijuana on a daily basis.

In terms of family history, Helene had a first-degree relative diagnosed with bipolar I disorder, responsive to lithium prophylaxis, and a history of secondary alcoholism. There was an extended family history of recurrent mood disorder, and some affected individuals had developed comorbid SUD. There was no family history of schizophrenia or primary SUD.

Helene went on to experience several years of non-completely remitting illness characterized by fluctuating mood symptoms and impaired concentration and motivation. She continued to use substances and started to feel that her major problem was actually SUD, and consequently was ambivalent about taking lithium. This view (primary diagnosis of SUD with secondary mood problems) was actually reinforced in an assessment for admission to a substance use program, in which Helene elected not to participate. She was unsuccessful in securing regular employment and was involved with a partner who also abused marijuana. After Helene successfully stopped substance use and began taking lithium regularly, the underlying bipolar disorder stabilized. The patient reinvented her life, took on a new job, and moved to a new city, and when last seen was adjusting very well.

Case Discussion

Helene's case illustrates a number of key points: 1) the onset of major mood episodes in the context of a confirmed first-degree family member with lithium-responsive bipolar I disorder was completely missed by the initial clinicians, who appeared to be focusing on the presenting symptoms and circumstances in the diagnostic formulation, rather than on the clinical course or familial risk; 2) the patient began to self-medicate with cannabis and alcohol, and in this context the prior episodic course was converted to a rapid-cycling nonepisodic course; and 3) the classical mood episodes converted into mixed symptoms with psychotic features in association with substance use. The substance use contributed to confusion around diagnosis, an increase in the duration of active bipolar disorder, a decrease in compliance with and engagement in effective treatment, and perhaps a reduction in efficacy of the lithium treatment while the patient was actively using substances.

Key Clinical Concepts

- SUD is the most common comorbid disorder with first-episode psychosis, first-episode mania, and other psychotic disorders, and it has a significant negative impact on outcome.

- Cannabis use has been linked to an increased risk for psychosis- and schizophrenia-related disorders in young people, with cannabis-induced psychosis being a cogent marker of vulnerability.

- Cross-sectional, longitudinal, and family history, with knowledge of the inherent pharmacological properties of substances of abuse, will assist in differentiating substance-induced psychotic disorder from a primary psychotic disorder with comorbid SUD.

- Optimal treatment for patients with first-episode psychosis and comorbid SUD includes specialized early intervention services with integrated SUD-focused treatment. Treatment for first-episode psychosis should be initiated even though drug-induced psychosis cannot be excluded.

- Clinical course and family history are essential to accurately diagnosing bipolar disorder early in its course and to differentiating a primary from a secondary SUD.

- Substance use complicates the acute presentation, clinical course, and treatment responsivity of bipolar disorder.

References

Addington J, Addington D: Effect of substance misuse in early psychosis. Br J Psychiatry Suppl 172:134–136, 1998

Addington J, Addington D: Impact of an early psychosis program on substance use. Psychiatr Rehabil J 25:60–67, 2001

Alda M: The phenotypic spectra of bipolar disorder. Eur Neuropsychopharmacol 14 (suppl 2):94–99, 2004

Alda M, Grof P: Genetics and lithium response in bipolar disorders, in Basic Mechanisms and Therapeutic Implications of Bipolar Disorder. Edited by Soares JC, Gershon S. New York, Marcel Dekker, 2000, pp 529–543

American Psychiatric Association: Diagnostic and Statistical Manual of Mental Disorders, 4th Edition, Text Revision. Washington, DC, American Psychiatric Association, 2000

Angst J: The emerging epidemiology of hypomania and bipolar II disorder. J Affect Disord 50:143–151, 1998

Angst J, Preisig M: Course of a clinical cohort of unipolar, bipolar and schizoaffective patients. Results of a prospective study from 1959 to 1985. Schweiz Arch Neurol Psychiatr 146:5–16, 1995

Angst J, Gamma A, Endrass J, et al: Is the association of alcohol use disorders with major depressive disorder a consequence of undiagnosed bipolar-II disorder? Eur Arch Psychiatry Clin Neurosci 256:452–457, 2006

Arendt M, Rosenberg R, Foldager L, et al: Cannabis-induced psychosis and subsequent schizophrenia-spectrum disorders: follow-up study of 535 incident cases. Br J Psychiatry 187:510–515, 2005

Arendt M, Mortensen PB, Rosenberg R, et al: Familial predisposition for psychiatric disorder: comparison of subjects treated for cannabis-induced psychosis and schizophrenia. Arch Gen Psychiatry 65:1269–1274, 2008

Arseneault L, Cannon M, Witton J, et al: Causal association between cannabis and psychosis: examination of the evidence. Br J Psychiatry 184:110–117, 2004

Baethge C, Baldessarini RJ, Khalsa HM, et al: Substance abuse in first-episode bipolar I disorder: indications for early intervention. Am J Psychiatry 162:1008–1010, 2005

Baethge C, Hennen J, Khalsa HM, et al: Sequencing of substance use and affective morbidity in 166 first-episode bipolar I disorder patients. Bipolar Disord 10:738–741, 2008

Ballageer T, Malla A, Manchanda R, et al: Is adolescent-onset first-episode psychosis different from adult onset? J Am Acad Child Adolesc Psychiatry 44:782–789, 2005

Barnes TR, Mutsatsa SH, Hutton SB, et al: Comorbid substance use and age at onset of schizophrenia. Br J Psychiatry 188:237–242, 2006

Barrowclough C, Haddock G, Tarrier N, et al: Randomized controlled trial of motivational interviewing, cognitive behavior therapy, and family intervention for patients with comorbid schizophrenia and substance use disorders. Am J Psychiatry 158:1706–1713, 2001

Bertelsen M, Jeppesen P, Petersen L, et al: Five-year follow-up of a randomized multicenter trial of intensive early intervention vs standard treatment for patients with a first episode of psychotic illness. Arch Gen Psychiatry 65:762–771, 2008

Biederman J, Mick E, Prince J, et al: Systematic chart review of the pharmacologic treatment of comorbid attention deficit hyperactivity disorder in youth with bipolar disorder. J Child Adolesc Psychopharmacol 9:247–256, 1999

Cannon TD, Cadenhead K, Cornblatt B, et al: Prediction of psychosis in youth at high clinical risk: a multisite longitudinal study in North America. Arch Gen Psychiatry 65:28–37, 2008

Cantor-Graae E, Nordstrom LG, McNeil TF: Substance abuse in schizophrenia: a review of the literature and a study of correlates in Sweden. Schizophr Res 48:69–82, 2001

Caspi A, Moffitt TE, Cannon M, et al: Moderation of the effect of adolescent-onset cannabis use on adult psychosis by a functional polymorphism in the catechol-O-methyltransferase gene: longitudinal evidence of a gene x environment interaction. Biol Psychiatry 57:1117–1127, 2005

Cassano GB, Akiskal HS, Savino M, et al: Proposed subtypes of bipolar II and related disorders: with hypomanic episodes (or cyclothymia) and with hyperthymic temperament. J Affect Disord 26:127–140, 1992

Cassidy F, Ahearn EP, Carroll BJ: Substance abuse in bipolar disorder. Bipolar Disord 3:181–188, 2001

Caton CL, Drake RE, Hasin DS, et al: Differences between early phase primary psychotic disorders with concurrent substance use and substance-induced psychosis. Arch Gen Psychiatry 62:137–145, 2005

Caton CL, Hasin DS, Shrout PE, et al: Predictors of psychosis remission in psychotic disorders that co-occur with substance use. Schizophr Bull 32:618–625, 2006

Caton CL, Hasin DS, Shrout PE, et al: Stability of early phase primary psychotic disorders with concurrent substance use and substance-induced psychosis. Br J Psychiatry 190:105–111, 2007

Cerullo MA, Strakowski SM: The prevalence and significance of substance use disorders in bipolar type I and II disorder. Subst Abuse Treat Prev Policy 2:29, 2007

Compton MT, Kelley ME, Ramsay CE, et al: Association of pre-onset cannabis, alcohol, and tobacco use with age at onset of prodrome and age at onset of psychosis in first-episode patients. Am J Psychiatry 166:1251–1257, 2009

Degenhardt L, Hall W, Lynskey M: Testing hypotheses about the relationship between cannabis use and psychosis. Drug Alcohol Depend 71:37–48, 2003

DelBello MP, Hanseman D, Adler CM, et al: Twelve-month outcome of adolescents with bipolar disorder following first hospitalization for a manic or mixed episode. Am J Psychiatry 164:582–590, 2007

Dennis M, Babor TF, Roebuck MC, et al: Changing the focus: the case for recognizing and treating cannabis use disorders. Addiction 97 (suppl 1):4–15, 2002

Dixon L: Dual diagnosis of substance abuse in schizophrenia: prevalence and impact on outcomes. Schizophr Res 35:S93–S100, 1999

D'Souza DC: Cannabinoids and psychosis. Int Rev Neurobiol 78:289–325, 2007

Duffy A, Grof P, Grof E, et al: Evidence supporting the independent inheritance of primary affective disorders and primary alcoholism in the families of bipolar patients. J Affect Disord 50:91–96, 1998

Duffy A, Alda M, Milin R, et al: A consecutive series of treated affected offspring of parents with bipolar disorder: is response associated with the clinical profile? Can J Psychiatry 52:369–376, 2007

Duffy A, Milin R, Grof P: Maintenance treatment of adolescent bipolar disorder: open study of the effectiveness and tolerability of quetiapine. BMC Psychiatry 9:4, 2009

Duffy A, Alda M, Hajek T, et al: Early stages in the development of bipolar disorder. J Affect Disord 121:127–135, 2010

Edwards J, Elkins K, Hinton M, et al: Randomized controlled trial of a cannabis-focused intervention for young people with first-episode psychosis. Acta Psychiatr Scand 114:109–117, 2006

Garety PA, Craig TKJ, Dunn G, et al: Specialised care for early psychosis: symptoms, social functioning and patient satisfaction: randomised controlled trial. Br J Psychiatry 188:37–45, 2006

Garland JE, Duffy A: Treating bipolar disorder in the early stages of the illness, in Practical Management of Bipolar Disorder: A Guide for Clinicians. Edited by Young A, Ferrier N, Michalak E. Cambridge University Press (in press)

Garnham J, Munro A, Slaney C, et al: Prophylactic treatment response in bipolar disorder: results of a naturalistic observation study. J Affect Disord 104:185–190, 2007

Geller B, Cooper TB, Sun K, et al: Double-blind and placebo-controlled study of lithium for adolescent bipolar disorders with secondary substance dependency. J Am Acad Child Adolesc Psychiatry 37:171–178, 1998

Glantz MD, Anthony JC, Berglund PA, et al: Mental disorders as risk factors for later substance dependence: estimates of optimal prevention and treatment benefits. Psychol Med 2:1–13, 2008

Goldstein BI, Birmaher B, Axelson DA, et al: Significance of cigarette smoking among youths with bipolar disorder. Am J Addict 17:364–371, 2008a

Goldstein BI, Strober MA, Birmaher B, et al: Substance use disorders among adolescents with bipolar spectrum disorders. Bipolar Disord 10:469–478, 2008b

Grech A, van Os J, Jones PB, et al: Cannabis use and outcome of recent psychosis. Eur Psychiatry 20:349–353, 2005

Green AI, Tohen MF, Hamer RM, et al: First episode schizophrenia-related psychosis and substance use disorders: acute response to olanzapine and haloperidol. Schizophr Res 66:125–135, 2004

Green AI, Drake RE, Brunette MF, et al: Schizophrenia and co-occurring substance use disorder. Am J Psychiatry 164:402–408, 2007

Green B, Kavanagh D, Young R: Being stoned: a review of self-reported cannabis effects. Drug Alcohol Rev 22:453–460, 2003

Grof P: Selecting effective long-term treatment for bipolar patients: monotherapy and combinations. J Clin Psychiatry 64 (suppl 5):53–61, 2003

Grof P, Müller-Oerlinghausen B: A critical appraisal of lithium's efficacy and effectiveness: the last 60 years. Bipolar Disord 11 (suppl 2):10–19, 2009

Grof P, Alda M, Grof E, et al: The challenge of predicting response to stabilising lithium treatment: the importance of patient selection. Br J Psychiatry 163:16–19, 1993

Grof P, Alda M, Ahrens B: Clinical course of affective disorders: were Emil Kraepelin and Jules Angst wrong? Psychopathology 28 (suppl 1):73–80, 1995

Grof P, Duffy A, Cavazzoni P, et al: Is response to prophylactic lithium a familial trait? J Clin Psychiatry 63:942–947, 2002

Healey C, Peters S, Kinderman P, et al: Reasons for substance use in dual diagnosis bipolar disorder and substance use disorders: a qualitative study. J Affect Disord 113:118–126, 2009

Heffner JL, DelBello MP, Fleck DE, et al: Cigarette smoking in the early course of bipolar disorder: association with ages-at-onset of alcohol and marijuana use. Bipolar Disord 10:838–845, 2008

Henquet C, Krabbendam L, Spauwen J, et al: Prospective cohort study of cannabis use, predisposition for psychosis, and psychotic symptoms in young people. BMJ 330:11, 2005a

Henquet C, Murray R, Linszen D, et al: The environment and schizophrenia: the role of cannabis use. Schizophr Bull 31:608–612, 2005b

Henquet C, Krabbendam L, de Graaf R, et al: Cannabis use and expression of mania in the general population. J Affect Disord 95:103–110, 2006

Hides L, Dawe S, Kavanagh DJ, et al: Psychotic symptom and cannabis relapse in recent-onset psychosis. Br J Psychiatry 189:137–143, 2006

Hunt GE, Bergen J, Bashir M: Medication compliance and comorbid substance abuse in schizophrenia: impact on community survival 4 years after a relapse. Schizophr Res 54:253–264, 2002

Joshi G, Wilens T: Comorbidity in pediatric bipolar disorder. Child Adolesc Psychiatr Clin N Am 18:291–319, 2009

Kavanagh DJ, Young R, White A, et al: A brief motivational intervention for substance misuse in recent-onset psychosis. Drug Alcohol Rev 23:151–155, 2004

Kemp DE, Gao K, Ganocy SJ, et al: A 6-month, double-blind, maintenance trial of lithium monotherapy versus the combination of lithium and divalproex for rapid-cycling bipolar disorder and co-occurring substance abuse or dependence. J Clin Psychiatry 70:113–121, 2009

Kemp R, Harris A, Vurel E, et al: Stop using stuff: trial of a drug and alcohol intervention for young people with comorbid mental illness and drug and alcohol problems. Australas Psychiatry 15:490–493, 2007

Kessler RC, Crum RM, Warner LA, et al: Lifetime co-occurrence of DSM-III-R alcohol abuse and dependence with other psychiatric disorders in the National Comorbidity Survey. Arch Gen Psychiatry 54:313–321, 1997

Kleber HD, Weiss RD, Anton RF Jr, et al; Work Group on Substance Use Disorders; American Psychiatric Association: Treatment of patients with substance use disorder, second edition. Am J Psychiatry 164(suppl):5–123, 2007

Kowatch RA, Fristad MA, Birmaher B, et al: Treatment guidelines for children and adolescents with bipolar disorder. J Am Acad Child Adolesc Psychiatry 44:213–235, 2005

Lambert M, Conus P, Lubman DI, et al: The impact of substance use disorders on clinical outcome in 643 patients with first-episode psychosis. Acta Psychiatr Scand 112:141–148, 2005

Leboyer M, Henry C, Paillere-Martinot ML, et al: Age at onset in bipolar affective disorders: a review. Bipolar Disord 7:111–118, 2005

Lehman AF, Lieberman JA, Dixon LB, et al; American Psychiatric Association; Steering Committee on Practice Guidelines: Practice guideline for the treatment of patients with schizophrenia, second edition. Am J Psychiatry 161(suppl):1–56, 2004

Lewinsohn PM, Klein DN, Seeley JR: Bipolar disorder during adolescence and young adulthood in a community sample. Bipolar Disord 2:281–293, 2000

Linszen DH, Dingemans PM, Lenior ME: Cannabis abuse and the course of recent-onset schizophrenic disorders. Arch Gen Psychiatry 51:273–279, 1994

Linszen D, Dingemans P, Lenior M: Early intervention and a five year follow up in young adults with a short duration of untreated psychosis: ethical implications. Schizophr Res 51:55–61, 2001

Malla AK, Norman RM, Joober R: First-episode psychosis, early intervention, and outcome: what have we learned? Can J Psychiatry 50:881–891, 2005

Malla A, Norman R, Bechard-Evans I, et al: Factors influencing relapse during a 2-year follow-up of first-episode psychosis in a specialized early intervention service. Psychol Med 38:1585–1593, 2008

Manwani SG, Szilagyi KA, Zablotsky B, et al: Adherence to pharmacotherapy in bipolar disorder patients with and without co-occurring substance use disorders. J Clin Psychiatry 68:1172–1176, 2007

Marshall M, Rathbone J: Early intervention for psychosis. Cochrane Database Syst Rev CD004718, 2006

Marshall M, Lewis S, Lockwood A, et al: Association between duration of untreated psychosis and outcome in cohorts of first-episode patients. Arch Gen Psychiatry 62:975–983, 2005

Merikangas K, Herrell R, Swendsen J, et al: Specificity of bipolar spectrum conditions in the comorbidity of mood and substance use disorders: results from the Zurich cohort study. Arch Gen Psychiatry 65:47–52, 2008

Milin R: Comorbidity of schizophrenia and substance use disorders in adolescents and young adults, in Adolescent Substance Abuse: Psychiatric Comorbidity and High Risk Behaviors. Edited by Kaminer Y, Bukstein O. New York, Routledge/Taylor & Francis, 2008, pp 355–378

Milin R, Coupland K, Walker S, et al: Outcome and follow-up study of an adolescent psychiatric day treatment school program. J Am Acad Child Adolesc Psychiatry 39:320–328, 2000

Monitoring the Future: Various stimulant drugs show continuing gradual declines among teens in 2008, most illicit drugs hold steady. December 2008. Available at: http://monitoringthefuture.org/pressreleases/08drugpr.pdf. Accessed January 2, 2010.

Moore TH, Zammit S, Lingford-Hughes A, et al: Cannabis use and risk of psychotic or affective mental health outcomes: a systematic review. Lancet 370:319–328, 2007

Mueser KT, Bellack AS, Blanchard JJ: Comorbidity of schizophrenia and substance abuse: implications for treatment. J Consult Clin Psychol 60:845–856, 1992

Passmore MJ, Garnham J, Duffy A, et al: Phenotypic spectra of bipolar disorder in responders to lithium versus lamotrigine. Bipolar Disord 5:110–114, 2003

Pencer A, Addington J, Addington D: Outcome of a first episode of psychosis in adolescence: a 2-year follow-up. Psychiatry Res 133:35–43, 2005

Perkins KA, Simpson JC, Tsuang MT: Ten-year follow-up of drug abusers with acute or chronic psychosis. Hosp Community Psychiatry 37:481–484, 1986

Petersen L, Jeppesen P, Thorup A, et al: A randomised multicentre trial of integrated versus standard treatment for patients with a first episode of psychotic illness. BMJ 331:602, 2005

Regier DA, Farmer ME, Rae DS, et al: Comorbidity of mental disorders with alcohol and other drug abuse. Results from the Epidemiologic Catchment Area (ECA) study. JAMA 264:2511–2518, 1990

Rosen JL, Miller TJ, D'Andrea JT, et al: Comorbid diagnoses in patients meeting criteria for the schizophrenia prodrome. Schizophr Res 85:124–131, 2006

Rybakowski JK, Chlopocka-Wozniak M, Suwalska A: The prophylactic effect of long-term lithium administration in bipolar patients entering treatment in the 1970s and 1980s. Bipolar Disord 3:563–67, 2001

Salloum IM, Thase ME: Impact of substance abuse on the course and treatment of bipolar disorder. Bipolar Disord 2:269–280, 2000

Salloum IM, Cornelius JR, Daley DC, et al: Efficacy of valproate maintenance in patients with bipolar disorder and alcoholism. Arch Gen Psychiatry 62:37–45, 2005

Schanzer BM, First MB, Dominquez B, et al: Diagnosing psychotic disorders in the emergency department in the context of substance use. Psychiatr Serv 57:1468–1473, 2006

Semple DM, McIntosh AM, Lawrie SM: Cannabis as a risk factor for psychosis: systematic review. J Psychopharmacol 19:187–194, 2005

Sorbara F, Liraud F, Assens F, et al: Substance use and the course of early psychosis: a 2-year follow-up of first-admitted subjects. Eur Psychiatry 18:133–136, 2003

Strakowski SM, DelBello MP, Fleck DE, et al: The impact of substance abuse on the course of bipolar disorder. Biol Psychiatry 48:477–485, 2000

Strakowski SM, DelBello MP, Fleck DE, et al: Effects of co-occurring cannabis use disorders on the course of bipolar disorder after a first hospitalization for mania. Arch Gen Psychiatry 64:57–64, 2007

Swanson J, Van Dorn A, Swartz MS: Effectiveness of atypical antipsychotics for substance use in schizophrenia patients. Schizophr Res 94:114–118, 2007

Van Mastrigt S, Addington J, Addington D: Substance misuse at presentation to an early psychosis program. Soc Psychiatry Psychiatr Epidemiol 39:69–72, 2004

Van Nimwegen L, de Haan L, van Beveren N, et al: Adolescence, schizophrenia and drug abuse: a window of vulnerability. Acta Psychiatr Scand Suppl 427:S35–S42, 2005

Veen ND, Selten J-P, van der Tweel I, et al: Cannabis use and age at onset of schizophrenia. Am J Psychiatry 161:501–506, 2004

Wade D, Harrigan S, Edwards J, et al: Patterns and predictors of substance use disorders and daily tobacco use in first-episode psychosis. Aust N Z J Psychiatry 39:892–898, 2005

Wade D, Harrigan S, Edwards J, et al: Substance misuse in first-episode psychosis: 15-month prospective follow-up study. Br J Psychiatry 189:229–234, 2006

Wade D, Harrigan S, McGorry PD, et al: Impact of severity of substance use disorder on symptomatic and functional outcome in young individuals with first-episode psychosis. J Clin Psychiatry 68:767–774, 2007

Weiss RD, Griffin ML, Kolodziej ME, et al: A randomized trial of integrated group therapy versus group drug counseling for patients with bipolar disorder and substance dependence. Am J Psychiatry 164:100–107, 2007

Westermeyer J: Comorbid schizophrenia and substance abuse: a review of epidemiology and course. Am J Addict 15:345–355, 2006

Wilens TE, Biederman J, Adamson JJ, et al: Further evidence of an association between adolescent bipolar disorder with smoking and substance use disorders: a controlled study. Drug Alcohol Depend 95:188–198, 2008

Winokur G, Coryell W, Akiskal HS, et al: Alcoholism in manic-depressive (bipolar) illness: familial illness, course of illness, and the primary-secondary distinction. Am J Psychiatry 152:365–372, 1995

Yatham LN, Kennedy SH, Schaffer A, et al: Canadian Network for Mood and Anxiety Treatments (CANMAT) and International Society for Bipolar Disorders (ISBD) collaborative update of CANMAT guidelines for the management of patients with bipolar disorder: update 2009. Bipolar Disord 11:225–255, 2009

Young SE, Corley RP, Stallings MC, et al: Substance use, abuse and dependence in adolescence: prevalence, symptom profiles and correlates. Drug Alcohol Depend 68:309–322, 2002

Suggested Readings

D'Souza DC: Cannabinoids and psychosis. Int Rev Neurobiol 78:289–325, 2007

Duffy A, Alda M, Hajek T, et al: Early stages in the development of bipolar disorder. J Affect Disord 121:127–135, 2010

Goldstein BI, Bukstein OG: Bipolar disorder and adolescent substance use disorders, in Adolescent Substance Abuse: Psychiatric Comorbidity and High-Risk Behaviors. Edited by Kaminer Y, Bukstein O. New York, Routledge/Taylor & Francis, 2008

Milin R: Comorbidity of schizophrenia and substance use disorders in adolescents and young adults, in Adolescent Substance Abuse: Psychiatric Comorbidity and High-Risk Behaviors. Edited by Kaminer Y, Bukstein O. New York, Routledge/Taylor & Francis, 2008

16

Management of Youth With Substance Use Disorders in the Juvenile Justice System

Peter B. Rockholz, M.S.S.W., L.C.S.W.

This chapter addresses a distinct subgroup of adolescents with substance use disorders (SUDs) who come into contact with the juvenile justice system[1] and whose substance use histories and patterns, co-occurring mental disorders, and related needs are similar to those of adolescents not involved in the juvenile justice system. Therefore, much of what has been presented in earlier chapters

---

[1]Although the term *juvenile justice system* can be inferred to represent an organized, coordinated infrastructure and processes, the norm is quite the opposite. Most states and jurisdictions lack a clearly defined, systemic approach to handling juveniles, and certainly to providing comprehensive services to meet the complex needs of these youth.

415

applies to juveniles.[2] However, there are clearly identifiable characteristics, clinical presentations, and psychosocial needs that distinguish juveniles from other adolescents.

Compared with other adolescents with SUDs, many juveniles present with measurably greater acuity and earlier onset of SUDs, have a higher prevalence and different combinations of co-occurring mental disorders, and require greater attention and sensitivity to cultural, gender-specific, trauma-related, environmental, and circumstantial factors. The very fact of their involvement with law enforcement, judicial, and custody processes and personnel can be stigmatizing—often exacerbating their existing mental disorders. The additional dynamics created by the authority of the court and, for those who become incarcerated, correctional staff affect the nature of therapeutic relationships (for both client and clinician), especially during engagement and the formation of a trusting, therapeutic alliance. Settings in which services are provided range from open "free-world" residential and nonresidential placements to high-security environments that can place significant restrictions on what would be considered ideal clinical circumstances, including active family participation. Although research supports the relatively equal effectiveness of voluntary and mandated treatment, the latter requires accommodation, compromise, and acceptance by practitioners of the constraints inherent in the public safety imperative of the justice system in order for treatment to be successful.

Although most correctional (e.g., security) personnel genuinely want juveniles to get their lives in order and neither to return to the correctional system nor to graduate into the adult criminal justice system (both of which, they know, occur all too often), their primary mandate remains to ensure public safety above all else. High caseloads, understaffed institutional settings, and a lack of available services for juveniles both within institutions and in the community (National Center on Addiction and Substance Abuse 2004b) tend, in many cases, to force these staff to expend much of their energy on the basics of enforcement, supervision, and sanctioning of juveniles. This unfortunate reality, combined with historically punitive and at times dehumanizing environ-

---

[2]The term *juveniles* is used here to refer to minors who have been subject to arrest and therefore come into contact with the juvenile justice system. In this chapter, juveniles include those who are more deeply involved in the system, including juvenile detainees, juvenile delinquents, juvenile offenders, and serious juvenile offenders.

ments and practices, contributes to an institutional culture that unless actively addressed perpetuates values that are at odds with those of treatment practitioners. For treatment to be effective, particularly in containment settings, security and program (e.g., clinical, educational, vocational) personnel should ideally participate together in experiential, cross-disciplinary, team-building exercises to examine their values, assumptions, beliefs, and attitudes—toward finding common ground, understanding each other's roles and responsibilities, and achieving mutual respect leading to cooperation. Despite the limitations posed by the juvenile justice system, treatment is effective and generally results in reductions in both recidivism and substance abuse, when programs are implemented properly.

The objectives of this chapter are to 1) introduce practitioners to some of the typical life experiences, unique environmental realities, and psychosocial needs of the modal youth who becomes involved with the juvenile justice system; 2) provide information that identifies the distinctive clinical needs of juveniles with SUDs (and co-occurring mental disorders), compared with other adolescents, along with practical responses; 3) increase awareness of approaches to assessment and treatment of juveniles within a range of settings; and 4) provide insight into the challenges and solutions inherent in working with adolescents involved with the juvenile justice system.

In this chapter, I avoid, to the extent possible, repeating otherwise applicable information presented in previous chapters. I also limit description of the intricacies and vagaries of what is loosely referred to as the juvenile justice system, because this concept varies from state to state, county to county, and even within localities. I also avoid entertaining important policy recommendations that might reduce the increased overreliance on the juvenile justice system to address societal, developmental, behavioral health, and public health needs. I hope that the reader with particular interest in treatment of juveniles with SUDs will return to previous chapters to incorporate the information presented here with that describing the basic needs of and approaches to adolescents in need of treatment for SUDs. Also, the end-of-chapter list of recommended readings should be useful for readers seeking more detailed information.

Socioeconomic, Cultural, and Environmental Factors Associated With SUDs and Unlawful Behavior Among Juveniles

It is valuable, when working with juveniles, to first understand the environments from which they come and their perceptions of them. I recall vividly a 14-year-old black male appearing for the first time outside his urban environment at a primarily white, suburban community substance abuse treatment center for a court evaluation. He arrived wearing a bulletproof vest. His explanation for this protection was that not only did he believe he would be lucky to live to the end of any given week in his drug- and crime-infested neighborhood, but he had no idea what to expect "far" away from it. This single action spoke volumes about the internal experience of this child. One needs to imagine what his daily life and interpersonal interactions were like to fully appreciate what his values, beliefs, and assumptions were, and what place his use of substances held in that context, from his viewpoint. The standard treatment industry approach would be to first address his addictive disorder. Such a step would likely end any possibility of connecting with this juvenile, because it would be not only clinically inappropriate but also culturally offensive.

Although some adolescents with SUDs may have genetic predisposition or biological vulnerability to addiction, there is no evidence to suggest that the higher SUD rates among those youth who become involved in the juvenile justice system are reflective of a higher prevalence of such factors. Rather, the disproportionate substance use prevalence may more likely be associated with socioeconomic, cultural, environmental, and circumstantial factors. Compared with adolescents with SUDs who are not involved with the juvenile justice system, juveniles are more likely disenfranchised, disengaged from academic achievement, living in single-parent and abusive homes, embedded in environments that lack nurturing and are emotionally and psychologically toxic, limited in their views of the world and its available opportunities, and experiencing lives of hopelessness, lawlessness, constant fear, poverty, violence, distrust, and anomie. Despite these realities, posttraumatic stress disorder among juveniles is significantly underdiagnosed (Guchereau et al. 2009).

There are many relevant views of the etiology of juvenile delinquency, with one sociological theory continuing to capture the core factors. Independent of the sociocultural factors described above, the impact of limited opportunity for traditional success in mainstream society, described in the classic work *Delinquency and Opportunity* (Cloward and Ohlin 1960)—as expanded by Cloward to include limited opportunity also for the expression of deviant behavior, and still later to include the concept of the social structuring of deviance (R. Cloward, personal communication, 1976)—is enduring. This view has been validated empirically through such examples as the economic impact of the crack epidemic beginning in 1985—which provided instant growth in fast, cash-making opportunities for urban, poor youth—and the disproportionate, national increase in violent, gang-related, and other criminal behavior among girls—which paralleled the increase in legitimate opportunities for women to achieve empowerment within mainstream U.S. society. Changes in the social structure of mainstream society do appear to have correlates in the social structuring of deviance. The underlying message for practitioners is the importance of understanding, and remaining current in knowledge about, both the mainstream culture and deviant subcultures of groups of youth from the full socioeconomic range in order to effectively engage them.

Many juveniles are surrounded by multigenerational family and community influences that transmit values and attitudes that view substance use—especially use of alcohol and marijuana—and antisocial behavior in general as acceptable. American society is entering the second generation of parents whose parents themselves have high prevalence of lifetime and current illicit substance use. It is not uncommon, particularly among families of juveniles, for parents to get high with their children or to involve them in low-level drug dealing and similar unlawful behavior (e.g., shoplifting). I recall a 15-year-old, mainland-born, Puerto Rican male who sought treatment for SUD at a long-term, residential therapeutic community program while facing several charges, including sale of marijuana, possession of a deadly weapon, and attempted manslaughter. His explanation for shooting at a police officer was simply (and matter-of-factly) that the "cop" was trying to interfere with his drug deal, so he did the only thing he knew to do in that situation. This child lived in an impoverished, urban neighborhood as a third-generation gang member. He was raised and immersed in a multigenerational family and community culture that imparted a sense of morality that accepts actions such as his—and their potential consequences—as merely how life is lived. He could not imagine any other way to behave. The intent here of course is to explain, not excuse, his behavior.

For many youth, becoming subjects of the juvenile justice system is highly associated with their low socioeconomic status. According to the National Survey on Drug Use and Health (National Center on Addiction and Substance Abuse 2004a), juvenile arrestees are significantly more likely than other youth to come from poverty. Youth who come from families with sufficient economic resources are generally better able to afford private legal representation and to subsequently avoid involvement in the judicial system for all but the most serious criminal acts. They are better able to access the (albeit limited) range of private and public adolescent substance abuse treatments in lieu of retributive consequences. Those living in poverty, however, typically perceive—if not experience in reality—that they will be able to obtain (or certainly afford) such treatment only after becoming involved in the judicial system, and often only when ultimately incarcerated. This reality speaks to the importance of actively providing early intervention services to urban communities through culturally appropriate service delivery involving clinicians indigenous to local subpopulations (Rockholz et al. 1996).

The disproportionate representation of youth from lower socioeconomic groups overlaps with a disproportionate representation of black youth in the justice system. For example, the total case rate for blacks ages 12–17 in juvenile courts was more than twice the rate for whites; the further their involvement in the system, the greater this disparity became and the more it broadened to other minority groups (Puzzanchera et al. 2003). The juvenile residential placement rate for black youth was nearly 5 times higher, for American Indians 3 times higher, and for Latino youth 2 times higher than for white juveniles (Sickmund 2004). The salient point here is that racial and ethnic minority juveniles and their families continue to experience institutional racism and discrimination within the juvenile justice system. Practitioners must acknowledge and respond to these societal factors in a culturally competent manner if they are to effectively engage juveniles. It is also important to recognize that constructs of culture should extend beyond those of racial and ethnic minority groups to the distinct cultures of poverty, drug lifestyles, and "street" and urban society, among others.

Circumstantial factors add to the environmental stressors influencing juveniles' use of substances, co-occurrence of mental disorders, and involvement in illegal behaviors. These factors include street and gang violence, witnessing (including at early ages) murders and other violent crimes against persons, other forms of trauma, and hypervigilance associated with familial and community violence. Additionally, as with many adolescents with SUDs, juveniles experience high prevalence of sexual, physical, and emotional abuse—mostly within extended families (Hoffmann et al. 2004). For many victims, substance use is viewed by experienced practitioners as both adaptive and symptomatic, often as self-medication for emotional pain—providing a helpful, though maladaptive, solution to their emotional and psychological distress, and developmental struggles. For others, substance abuse and drug-trade involvement often only increase their exposure to dangerous situations and participation in high-risk behaviors, placing them at greater risk for negative health, social, legal, and academic consequences.

Consideration of these sociocultural and environmental influences should not disregard the consequences of substance use and abuse alone. Young persons are taking very powerful drugs, with high physical and psychological dependence potential—often leading rapidly to addiction. This has become increasingly evident since 1985 with the introduction of crack cocaine, and through recent national epidemics of methamphetamine abuse and the opioid analgesic–to–heroin dependence phenomenon that is currently ravaging middle-class suburbia. The latter underscores that in the end, drug abuse is not limited to the poor and victimized, and that the brain is nondiscriminating in its susceptibility to addictive disease. Also, mental distress should not be underrecognized as a more significant correlate of criminal behavior than is substance abuse alone (Hubbard et al. 1985).

My primary intent in this section was to establish a lens through which the remainder of this chapter can be viewed. I did not intend to provide a comprehensive review of the literature on either the causes of juvenile delinquency or the sociocultural correlates of SUDs among juveniles. Rather, my goal was to provide a sampling of such factors that collectively make the point that the cultural context within which SUD emerges, and is associated with unlawful behavior among juveniles, should inform practitioners regarding important prerequisites to client engagement and effective service delivery.

Unique Clinical Needs of Juveniles With Substance Use Disorders

Comparing Prevalence Rates: Juvenile Justice System–Involved Youth and Other Youth

The association between substance abuse among adolescents and behavior that brings them into contact with the juvenile (and in some cases adult) justice system is strong and has been well established in the professional literature (Dembo et al. 1993; Deschenes and Greenwood 1994; Elliot et al. 1989; Winters 1998). Juvenile delinquents and offenders represent a subgroup with among the highest prevalence rates of substance use of all youth. Data from the National Survey on Drug Use and Health (National Center on Addiction and Substance Abuse 2004a) indicate that compared with youth ages 12–17 who were never arrested, juvenile arrestees were about 3 times more likely to have used alcohol, 6 times more likely to have used marijuana, 16 times more likely to have used heroin, and 18 times more likely to have used cocaine in the past month. Among arrestees ages 12–17, compared with those never arrested, 61% versus 32% used alcohol, 43% versus 13% used marijuana, 24% versus 8% misused prescription medications, and 12% versus 1% used crack/cocaine in the past year. Data from the 1997 National Longitudinal Survey of Youth (Barnes et al. 2002) indicate that of those juveniles reporting three or more delinquent acts, only 6% reported no history of drug or alcohol use.

Regional differences should be monitored over time to determine which substances are being used by any youth cohort. The federal government has recently reinstituted the Arrestee Drug and Alcohol Monitoring program after a hiatus. This study identifies regional trends in drugs of abuse at the first point of contact with the juvenile justice system; data from arrestees are predictive of emerging trends. As of the time of this writing, the survey had documented the continuation of a decade-long trend of significantly greater methamphetamine abuse in the western United States, and a continued dominance of opiate abuse in the eastern United States, particularly in the Northeast (Office of National Drug Control Policy 2009). Knowing current primary drugs of choice among juveniles is important in shaping effective treatment responses at the local level.

The National Survey on Drug Use and Health data (National Center on Addiction and Substance Abuse 2004a) also indicate that juveniles initiate alcohol, tobacco, and other drug use at younger ages than youth who do not come to the attention of the judicial system. This earlier use greatly increases the likelihood of being arrested, developing SUD (including later in adulthood), recidivating (e.g., rearrest and reincarceration) following incarceration, and committing increasingly serious crimes, any of which may lead to adult, criminal lifestyles. Dembo et al. (1998) found that substance-abusing juveniles were more likely to recidivate than non-using juveniles. Whereas substance abuse and criminal activity are closely associated, so too are the likelihood of both relapse to SUD and recidivism to justice system involvement. Continuing clinical and recovery-supportive care, combined with community supervision, are necessary in tandem for successful outcomes to be realized for juveniles with SUDs.

Substance abuse and criminal activity are associated, both independently and in combination, with progression to more serious SUDs and crime, and increasingly so with earlier ages of initiation. This connection highlights the importance of intervening at the earliest possible point in the initiation of substance use and/or juvenile justice system involvement. Prevention and early intervention, especially prior to juvenile justice system involvement, are addressed earlier in this volume (see Chapter 2, "Prevention of Substance Use and Substance Use Disorders: Role of Risk and Protective Factors") and in Suggested Readings appearing at the end of this chapter.

One subgroup of juvenile offenders with SUD that deserves mention consists of those involved in the drug trade—through selling (mostly low-level, street retail) or occasionally serving as transports (i.e., "mules") for illegal drugs (primarily marijuana and crack cocaine). There has been a belief, held widely by many formally trained chemical dependency and correctional counselors, that most youth involved in the drug trade do not use drugs or alcohol, and therefore require treatment in specialized programs separate from those primarily designed for SUDs. Data from the 1997 National Longitudinal Survey of Youth support the view held by other, relatively more experienced (including "streetwise") counselors that this is merely a myth (Farlie 1999).

Of all youth ages 12–17 years, 8% reported they "ever sold drugs." Compared with youth who never sold drugs, those who ever sold drugs were much more likely, within the past month, to have used alcohol (68% vs. 19%), marijuana (54% vs. 6%), or both alcohol and marijuana (46% vs. 4%). Of the 9% of all youth in this age group who used marijuana, 45% sold drugs. In contrast, of the 91% who did not use marijuana, only 4% sold drugs, although half of those reported they drank alcohol (National Center on Addiction and Substance Abuse 2004a). The average reported number of drug sales in the previous year was 10.5 times for youth ages 12–14 and 16.7 times for youth ages 15–17; therefore, the incidence of any significant drug-selling behavior requiring specialized treatment appears minimal (McCurley and Snyder 2008). This point is emphasized to raise awareness of the underreporting and identification of SUDs among juveniles involved in the drug trade, and the need to treat them for SUDs. For those relatively few juveniles with no reported substance use but immersion in the drug subculture, treatment programs that address drug lifestyles, healthy socialization, and habilitation needs may be the most suitable options (e.g., therapeutic communities).

Co-occurring Mental Disorders in Juveniles

The range of mental disorders that coexist with adolescent SUDs has been thoroughly described in this volume. National attention to the need to address co-occurring mental disorders within the juvenile justice system peaked in the 1990s through local grassroots and national coalitions, academic institutions, and both state and federal governmental agencies. These included, among others, the Coalition for Juvenile Justice (Hubner and Wolfson 2000), the National Coalition for the Mentally Ill in the Criminal Justice System (Cocozza 1992), the National GAINS Center (Peters et al. 1997), and the U.S. Department of Justice's Office of Juvenile Justice and Delinquency Prevention (Bilchik 1998; Cocozza and Skowyra 2000; Sickmund 2004; Snyder and Sickmund 1999; Teplin 2001). Overall rates of serious emotional disturbance and mental illness and rates for specific disorders among adolescent substance abusers involved with the juvenile justice system have not been measured systematically on a national basis, and results of local studies vary according to study populations. However, some recent estimates have emerged through two multisite studies, the Cannabis Youth Treatment (CYT) study (Dennis et al. 2004) and the Adolescent Treatment Model (ATM; Dennis 2005) study, and a meta-analysis that included 25 studies of juvenile detainees (Fazel et al. 2008). Estimates of co-occurring mental disorders among juveniles in local studies range from 20% to 80%. Much of this variation is due to differing definitions of mental disorders and differences in instrumentation.

The Adolescent Treatment Model study provides multisite data that are beginning to more clearly define national prevalence rates. For example, Dennis (2005) reported that juveniles present with higher rates of co-occurring externalizing versus internalizing disorders. Although external disorders only are, on average, reported at more than twice the rate of internal disorders only (approximately 25% and 10%, respectively), most internal distress is reportedly multimorbid with external (and substance use) disorders. The prevalence of any external disorder among juveniles is approximately 70%, and any internal disorder about 50%. Combined, an estimated 80% had some diagnosable mental disorder. Clearly, multiple co-occurring mental disorders and SUDs are the norm among juveniles, requiring treatment approaches that address co-occurring disorders concurrently.

In a meta-analysis, Fazel et al. (2008) reported on 25 studies involving 13,778 boys and 2,972 girls in detainment. About 3% of juvenile boys and girls met criteria for psychotic disorder (reportedly about 10 times the prevalence of the general adolescent population); juvenile girls were diagnosed with major depression at nearly 3 times the rate in boys (29.2% vs. 10.6%) and were about 50% more likely to have attention-deficit/hyperactivity disorder (ADHD) (18.5% vs. 11.7%); and juvenile boys and girls presented with conduct disorder at identical rates of 52.8%.

Dennis (2005) reported that conduct disorder is the most frequent diagnosis among juveniles (approximately 65%), followed by ADHD (approximately 50%), with these two coexisting at an overlapping rate of approximately 90%. Specific internalizing disorders (e.g., major depression, generalized anxiety disorder, traumatic stress disorder) were reported individually at rates of approximately 30%.

In one study of detainees in Cook County (Chicago area), Illinois, Teplin et al. (2002) found that when conduct disorder was excluded, nearly 60% of juvenile males and more than two-thirds of females met diagnostic criteria for one or more mental disorders, using the Diagnostic Interview Schedule for Children (DISC). In a similar study, using the Voice DISC Version IV, the National Center for Mental Health and Juvenile Justice, in collaboration with the Council of Juvenile Correctional Administrators, found the rate for all juveniles to be 66.3% (Skowyra and Cocozza 2007). Some of the lower incidence rates reported in these studies, compared with others, may be related to instrumentation. As Fazel et al. (2008) specifically indicated, surveys using the

DISC reported lower prevalence estimates for depression, ADHD, and conduct disorder compared with those using other assessment instruments.

Despite inconsistent findings and the lack of a reliable, regularly administered, national survey of SUDs and co-occurring mental disorders among juvenile populations, it is clear that this subgroup has significantly higher rates of both SUDs and mental disorders. Additionally, as Hoffmann et al. (2004) pointed out, given the high prevalence of co-occurring mental disorders among juveniles, juvenile centers should conduct routine screening and assessment for both SUDs and co-occurring mental disorders. Finally, the existing evidence strongly suggests the need for substance abuse treatment programs, in both institution- and community-based settings, to be competent in treating co-occurring disorders in juveniles.

Screening and Assessment Approaches With Juveniles

Historically, juveniles who entered the justice system were assessed solely for the level of security needed to address their risk of violence and other behavioral disorders during and following their period of detainment and postrelease supervision. Juvenile courts across the country, although generally more sensitive to treatment needs than adult courts, have been inconsistent in their methods of screening, assessing, and referring juveniles to treatment for SUDs. This has been, in large part, attributable to the dearth of treatment options for adolescents, especially for juveniles. With the increasing recognition by state, federal, and county governments of the need for and value afforded by treatment of SUDs and co-occurring mental disorders, there has been an increase in both screening and assessment—but not necessarily a corresponding increase in the availability of treatment services. As a result, most juvenile justice systems have tended to provide screening only, and then to refer juveniles (often regardless of assessment result) to what is typically available—most often self-help groups, alcohol and drug education, and counseling.

With a growing movement supporting judicial diversion options and the development of in-home, family-based services that are effective with SUDs, the use of assessment instruments in juvenile justice systems has become more widespread, as well as more appropriate for and sensitive to the comprehensive needs of juveniles. In addition, national consensus groups have identified best practice components of screening and assessment processes in juvenile justice systems. For example, the Center for Substance Abuse Treatment (1999) of the Substance Abuse and Mental Health Services Administration (SAMHSA) recommended making screening available not only at intake but at all points in the system, by comprehensively assessing every juvenile who screens positive for potential substance abuse problems and making assessment an ongoing process throughout the juvenile's involvement with the system. SAMHSA also urged that all screening and assessment instruments used show evidence of being normed with a juvenile population.

Substance Use Screening With Juveniles

Substance use screening of juveniles can be realistically considered a matter of screening out those who do *not* require a more complete substance abuse assessment, given the fact that over 90% of juveniles will likely screen positive. The selection of a particular screening instrument is less a matter of attempting to achieve higher levels of accuracy than an effort to be able to compare aggregate results over time and across sites using a standardized instrument. As Hoffmann et al. (2004) pointed out, the use of any of the several commonly used screening instruments (highlighted in Chapter 3, "Screening and Brief Interventions for Adolescent Substance Use in the General Office Setting") produced results that varied without measurable differences from the others. Hoffmann et al. also indicated that most such instruments were developed using samples in academic models rather than juveniles in naturalistic settings, perhaps affecting their validity to some extent.

Rockholz et al. (1996) reported a cultural effect when using academic research assistants to administer a screening instrument with at-risk youth in an urban setting. The wording of basic questions can result in inaccurate results if the local, "street" terminology is not incorporated into the instrument and application process. For example, when asked, "Do you drink alcohol?" one youth answered, "No"; however, when asked a follow-up question not on the instrument (i.e., "Do you drink Colt 45"s?"), he answered, "Yes, of course." His association to the word *alcohol* was limited to distilled spirits. The same youth, when asked "Do you smoke marijuana?" again answered negatively, but when asked "Do you smoke 'illy'?" (a preparation of small, hollowed-out cigars filled with marijuana laced with formaldehyde), he answered affirmatively. In addition to the cultural competence issue demonstrated in this study, an important point is that underreporting of substance use is not always an indication of denial, deception, or minimization.

The federal Office of Juvenile Justice and Delinquency Prevention (1997) recommends the combination of three methods for assessing SUDs with adolescents, including juveniles. These methods include the use of an assessment instrument, drug recognition techniques (e.g., identifying physical signs such as needle marks, changes in the eyes, performance on motor tests including movements that indicate muscle rigidity), and drug testing (e.g., breath, urine, saliva, hair, sweat).

Substance Use Assessment With Juveniles

Some of the same issues raised above regarding screening instruments and their application also apply to the selection of substance abuse assessments. However, more useful information clearly results from assessment, depending on when it is conducted. Thought should be given to the practicality of identifying the severity and patterns of a juvenile's SUD at intake, during confinement, in community-based settings, and at release. For the results to have utility for juveniles, a range of services that align with the findings should ideally be available. There should also be flexibility in placements based on clinical/case management judgment and environmental realities. For example, a juvenile who scores in the low to moderate range on an SUD assessment instrument but who lacks a viable (e.g., safe, substance-free) housing alternative at release might require residential placement despite scoring in a range suggesting the need for outpatient counseling.

Juvenile justice systems typically use the same instruments used for all adolescents to assess for potential substance use problems (see Appendix A). These include the Personal Experience Inventory (Winters and Henly 1989), Teen Addiction Severity Index (Kaminer et al. 1993), and Global Appraisal of Individual Needs (Dennis 1999), among others.

Adding mental health assessments for juveniles changes the consideration of timing and utility of the substance use assessment. It is generally more important to have information about mental disorders at the earliest possible time, to begin appropriate treatment, whereas it is preferable to provide SUD treatment in institutional settings so it ends just prior to release (assuming abstinence is actually occurring). Many states have simply added mental health–specific assessment instruments to existing SUD instruments. For example, the Massachusetts Youth Screening Instrument Version 2 has been validated using a national sample, and is widely used in over 42 states as a stand-alone mental health assessment instrument (Vincent et al. 2008). With growing understanding of the prevalence of co-occurring mental disorders, especially among juveniles, the use of those instruments that incorporate assessment of SUDs and co-occurring mental disorders is becoming more popular. In community settings, however, it is important for the combined assessment to occur at the point of diversion or placement, to ensure a proper match and comprehensive treatment and case planning.

Evolution of Risk Assessment

The combination of SUD and risk assessment instrumentation is becoming the norm in juvenile justice systems because of improved predictive validity regarding both relapse to substance abuse and recidivism to criminal behavior. Bonta and Wormith (2008) defined four generations of risk assessment processes that have helped to join together the treatment and public safety worlds to foster effective placement and case planning decisions. They described the first generation as based solely on professional judgment, lacking even the most basic of actuarial assessment. The second generation focused on static risk factors—those that are historical and otherwise unchangeable (e.g., age, criminal history). Although these factors have demonstrated reasonable predictive accuracy for future criminal behavior, they are limited in their ability to provide guidance to practitioners toward targeting interventions to effect behavioral and psychological change with juveniles.

The third generation of risk assessment introduced the addition of dynamic risk factors (also referred to as criminogenic needs) to the assessment of static risk factors. These dynamic risk factors include variables that are changeable and amenable to intervention, such as unemployment, substance abuse, and the lack of high school completion. The introduction of dynamic risk factors, while being questioned in terms of predictive validity, offers the practitioner some practical direction to work with malleable conditions that may have an impact on future behavior.

Gendreau and Goggins (1997) emphasized the importance of addressing dynamic risk factors (e.g., attitudes, values, behaviors) in determining treatment placement. The combination of SUD screening/assessment and level of risk assessment instruments has become recognized as a best practice that enables juvenile justice personnel to consider treatment needs and public safety requirements concurrently. Most recently, this practice has been evaluated by Lipsey (1992, 2005), using the combination of the Substance Problem Scale and the Crime and Violence Scale, as reported by Dennis (2005). Findings indicated that the Substance Problem Scale, but not the Crime and Violence Scale, predicted the probability of residential placement and the probability of relapse at 12 months. Each scale predicted recidivism, but the best predictor of both relapse and recidivism was the combination of the two instruments. Although popular, practical, and laden with face validity, this combination (referred to as risk-needs assessment) has been challenged for its scientific validity, leading to an active debate regarding the comparative value of static versus dynamic risk factors (Rice et al. 2002).

In the fourth generation of risk assessment, and perhaps ahead of the evidence, assessment instruments that not only combine static and dynamic risk factors but go further to include protective factors and case management planning represent the most promising of assessment instruments. One example of this is the Youth Assessment and Screening Instrument, which combines assessment of risks, needs, and protective factors in youth populations with a case planning component that has been designed to help caseworkers identify and monitor priority targets for behavioral change (Orbis Partners 2007). More study on this instrument will be informative.

Another example that has been found effective is a combination of the Simple Screening Instrument and the Youth Level of Service/Case Management Inventory (Hoge and Andrews 2002). This particular combination is being used widely and has additional utility for assisting in case planning, juvenile offender classification, and avoiding unnecessary residential placements (Hoge et al. 2002). The evidence that supports the use of both substance abuse instruments that are normed for juveniles and level-of-risk instruments that include dynamic risk factors is only beginning to emerge. Nevertheless, this approach is beginning to be widely implemented.

The use of instruments that assess SUDs, co-occurring mental disorders, and both risk and protective factors, and that do so in a manner that provides practical guidance to placement and case management planning, holds much promise to connect with the emerging view of addiction as a chronic health condition requiring sustained abstinence and long-term recovery supports following release. Linking this process to postrelease supervision (i.e., parole, probation) and peer recovery supports holds promise for reducing the historically high rates of relapse to substance use and recidivism to the juvenile justice system. For example, the Crime/Violence Scale of the Global Appraisal of Individual Needs has shown early efficacy (Dennis 2005) and will be looked to for its ability to inform case management.

Educational achievement is one critical area that has received only minimal attention as one of many protective factors. Only occasional obscure studies, including an unpublished revisit to data from the national Drug Abuse Treatment Outcome Study (funded by the National Institute on Drug Abuse in 1990), have identified positive academic experience and, in young adults, high school completion as highly associated with positive outcomes. These findings, combined with extensive empirical evidence, suggest the potential value in ensuring that juveniles are engaged in effective, individualized, success-based learning opportunities and, if necessary, providing motivational incentives for their attaining high school completion.

Treatment Approaches and Program Settings for Juveniles

Prior to the past two decades, the only treatment options widely available for the publicly supported juvenile population were long-term residential programs (e.g., therapeutic communities) and outpatient counseling. Those individuals and families with financial means typically sought help through private hospitalization or individual practitioners in the community. Treatment services within juvenile institution settings were all but nonexistent. In the late 1960s, when a young adult heroin and methamphetamine epidemic began and lower-level drug use (e.g., marijuana) became widespread among youth, many adolescents were referred to community-based treatment under coercion of the juvenile courts as a result of their having been charged and detained for status offenses (e.g., runaway, truancy, incorrigibility). This practice fell out of favor, leading to the deinstitutionalization of status offenders movement of the mid-1970s; what had been in all practicality an early intervention/court diversion option for youth with SUD was essentially lost. Although placing status offenders in confinement was not a desirable practice, its loss as an option did result afterward in many young persons with emerging SUD developing higher severity of SUD and criminal behavior before receiving treatment. Not until the 1990s did juvenile justice systems develop widespread diversion programs, such as juvenile drug courts.

Traditional Approaches

Both scientific and empirical evidence have consistently shown that merely adopting or, in many cases, slightly modifying adult treatment philosophies and approaches for juveniles usually produces poor results. For example, the medical "disease" approach, which has shown some effectiveness with segments of the general adolescent population, has not had measurable success with juveniles; this may be attributable in part to the cultural, environmental, and circumstantial factors noted at the beginning of this chapter. Similarly, 12-step facilitation—an otherwise evidence-supported practice in "free-world" settings—has not demonstrated effectiveness in juvenile justice populations, yet has been used as a mandated "program" in some states for all juveniles who screen positive for SUDs. A more practical solution might be for juvenile programs to avoid blanket requirements of participation in Alcoholics Anonymous (AA), Narcotics Anonymous (NA), and other self-help meetings and instead to encourage those with the highest levels of severity and risk, as measured near release, to be exposed to the 12 steps as a framework to help them to manage their sobriety after discharge.

Another common approach that has not been at all successful with juveniles, despite its popularity with those providing it, is drug and alcohol education. This dissonance is an example of how leaving juveniles (i.e., the so-called consumers) out of the program design process often results in a waste of precious resources. Policy-makers and practitioners are well advised to include individuals in recovery in the shaping of effective programs for juveniles. This might help bring balance to the reliance on the use of some "evidence-based" practices that may have demonstrated effectiveness in research studies but not necessarily with juveniles in naturalistic settings.

In a presentation to a state legislative body, a chief state's attorney commented on the then-spreading national methamphetamine epidemic. Following a motivational presentation by a recovering "meth addict," who had shot himself in the face, the attorney declared, "If only young people had the information about what 'meth' does to them, I am sure they wouldn't use it." Such remarkable naïveté is often, and unfortunately, effective in shaping public policy and the selection of ineffective programs in both juvenile and adult justice systems. Input from juveniles, families, and former juveniles has an important place.

Other examples of programs and services deemed by some policy-makers to be worthy of funding have been found by research to be minimally effective, ineffective, or negatively effective (obviously, with scattered stories of "success" in some isolated cases). These include Scared Straight and similar "shock" incarceration programs, drug and alcohol counseling, juvenile boot camps, routine practice, and wilderness programs (Lipsey 2005).

Institution-Based Programs

Substance abuse treatment for juveniles is generally delivered in three settings: institutional, community-based residential/inpatient, and nonresidential (e.g., outpatient, in-home). Institutional settings mostly provide physically secure (locked) confinement for the short term (e.g., pretrial detention centers) or long term (e.g., training schools or secure treatment centers) for juveniles who are dangerous to others or themselves. Since the mid-1900s, many youth have been transferred to adult court and sentenced to prison for serious juvenile offenses, felonies against persons, and even non-person offenses. This segment of juveniles has the highest level of need for treatment, yet only 37% of juvenile correctional facilities provide on-site SUD treatment (SAMHSA 2002).

Some states allocated federal resources that were made available beginning in the 1990s through the Residential Substance Abuse Treatment (RSAT) program (administered by the Corrections Program Office, Office of Justice Programs, U.S. Department of Justice) to establish juvenile residential programs in institutional settings—modified from adult programs—most of which adopted the therapeutic community model that had demonstrated effectiveness in studies of prisons across the country (Field 1989; Inciardi et al. 1997; Knight et al. 1997; Wexler 1996; Wexler et al. 1988). Although these studies were conducted with adult populations, a review of the RSAT programs in Ohio revealed that the Mohican Youth Center, a youthful offender therapeutic community, performed better than the adult therapeutic community programs. Pealer et al. (2002) concluded that "participation in Mohican's therapeutic community RSAT program significantly reduced the probability of being incarcerated after termination" (p. 64). A national review of institution-based therapeutic community programs found that there were 252 such programs in state prisons and jails, but only six were reported in facilities for juveniles (Rockholz 2004).

Most other juvenile institutions offer only basic drug and alcohol education programs (77%), although 42% offer voluntary self-help programs (e.g.,
AA, NA) and 5% offer detoxification (SAMHSA 2002). Cognitive-behavioral therapies, although not inventoried nationally, are also increasingly used
in juvenile correctional facilities in most states. These include manual-driven
variations of cognitive-behavioral therapy, such as aggression replacement
training (Glick and Goldstein 1987), moral reconation therapy (Burnette et
al. 2004), and Thinking for a Change (Bush et al. 1996), among others. Such
programs not only have been well received by both staff and juveniles, but
have demonstrated effectiveness equal to that of therapeutic communities.

Although parent involvement in institutional treatment of juveniles is necessarily very limited, organized support programs for parents while their children
are confined can contribute to improved postrelease adjustment. One evidence-
based example is the Denver Juvenile Justice Integrated Treatment Network
(CSAT 1998). Among many points of intervention, the Denver network mobi-
lized the collective resources of more than 40 public and private agencies to
adopt 116 points of intervention. One such intervention involved parent support during incarceration. It also addressed the critical point of postrelease, or
reentry, when most jurisdictions leave juveniles to their own means and resources—generally falling short of addressing needs. One example of an innovative approach to targeting juvenile postrelease is the Vera Institute's "Portable
Substance Abuse Treatment Model" (Callahan 2001), which provides a therapist
to span across the detention, incarceration, and, most important, postrelease
periods.

Differing cultural characteristics within the judicial and treatment systems can pose challenges that are surmountable, if managed properly. Both es-
poused and enacted values, beliefs, attitudes, and resultant behaviors, which
can appear conflictual on the surface, need not impede the opportunity for
therapeutic and behavioral gains by juveniles. However, when ineffectively addressed (or simply ignored), these can result in polarization, conflict, and
splitting that only bring stress to both staff and juveniles. The most basic di-
chotomy is inherent in the opposing views of the need for punishment versus
the need for rehabilitation. Some staff are viewed as "punitive," whereas others
are viewed as "bleeding hearts." When, for example, effective cross-disciplinary team-building training is provided, these views can be synthesized into a
philosophy of "discipline without punishment; love without enabling." The

value placed in offender accountability is the most commonly shared among even the most polarized of staffs.

For some clinicians, mandated treatment, including accountability (e.g., through urine drug screening and required reporting to juvenile authorities), can create conflict with their professional values. Clinicians working with juvenile justice clients must resolve their issues with being placed in somewhat of an authority role, with the boundary issues inherent in such activities as collecting urine samples (especially observed collection), and with the exceptions to confidentiality regulations allowing disclosures to judicial authorities without written consent.

For correctional practitioners, security and safety are paramount. However, both rigid and flexible interpretations occur in practice. "Hard-liners" can be inflexible, enacting the belief that juveniles are contained in order to *be* punished, whereas others (primarily treatment staff) take the view that juveniles' simply being there *is* punishment. This can lead to tension, because correctional practitioners are trained to hold a firm boundary between themselves and offenders—where being "friendly" or sharing personal information can be construed as a breach of security, referred to as "fraternization." For clinicians, forming a therapeutic alliance in an otherwise dehumanizing environment is best accomplished by occasionally "crossing the line" while reinforcing the need for juveniles to accept responsibility and learn healthy discipline.

Community-Based Programs

For moderate to serious juvenile offenders with low risk of violence, substance abuse treatment is increasingly being provided in community-based residential settings that range from state-operated, secure facilities to staff-secure or open residential treatment centers—the latter primarily operated under contract by private provider organizations. These settings range in capacity from 6 to over 100 residents. They are primarily treatment focused, as compared to institutional programs that focus on security and behavioral compliance (the "public safety imperative"). In addition to therapeutic communities, therapeutic boarding schools are considered evidence-based residential options. (A directory of many of these programs is published annually by the National Association of Therapeutic Schools and Programs; see http://www.natsap.org.) Although a shift has occurred toward shorter durations of residential treatment (driven primarily by cost containment), this may be counterproductive, because time in treatment remains the most significant predictor of positive outcomes. Also, although the National Institute on Drug Abuse (1999) has identified 90 days as a benchmark for minimal effective duration, empirical wisdom consistently supports stays of 9–18 months for adolescents (and juveniles in particular).

Community-based, nonresidential treatment programs (e.g., in-home, family-focused, and outpatient treatment; therapeutic foster homes) are growing rapidly across the country, because evidence increasingly supports the effectiveness (and cost benefit) of these strengths-based programs over the deficits-based programs of the past, most of which were originally developed for adult offenders and adapted for adolescents. These programs can be utilized at several points in the judicial process to divert juveniles from court, sentencing, and potential confinement. Comprehensive diversion programs provide a range of interventions, services, and treatments that are designed to address both clinical and criminogenic needs, aligned with findings of the combined assessment instruments mentioned earlier in this chapter.

In addition to approaches used with juveniles in institutional and residential settings, as well as with non-justice-involved adolescents (e.g., Aggression Replacement Training, Moral Reconation Therapy, and Thinking for a Change, as mentioned earlier), other cognitive-behavioral group therapies have demonstrated effectiveness with juveniles in community settings, reducing recidivism by an average of 25%, with some versions exceeding 50%, according to a meta-analysis conducted by Landenberger and Lipsey (2005). These include, but are not limited to, Dialectical Behavior Therapy (Linehan et al. 1999), Interpersonal Social Problem Solving, Motivational Enhancement Therapy/Cognitive-Behavioral Therapy (Sampl and Kadden 2001), and Reasoning and Rehabilitation (Ross 1988).

With heightened recognition of the need for and benefits of working with families, community-based programs for juveniles increasingly include evidence-based treatments such as Functional Family Therapy (Barton et al. 1985), Multidimensional Family Therapy (Liddle 1998), and Multisystemic Therapy (Henggeler et al. 2002), along with others described in Chapter 9, "Brief Motivational Interventions, Cognitive-Behavioral Therapy, and Contingency Management for Youth Substance Use Disorders."

States and other jurisdictions that are shifting toward community- and family-based treatments as alternatives to incarceration are seeing barriers reduced, and more effective outcomes are resulting in increased return-on-investment of taxpayer dollars (Fass and Pi 2002). For example, the Washington State Institute for Public Policy (2007) presents a comprehensive cost-benefit review for various juvenile programs.

Collaborative Community Partnership Approaches
The importance and value of involving both families and communities in all aspects of the juvenile justice system, ideally throughout the treatment and supervision process—and especially during the transition of juveniles back home—have spawned an increase in community initiatives involving case management and coordinated efforts that surround juveniles with needed supports. Early efforts, such as the Juvenile Assessment Centers developed in Florida (Dembo et al. 1998) and juvenile versions of the federal Treatment Alternatives for Safe Communities (TASC) program, demonstrated the effectiveness of this approach (Anglin et al. 1996).

These early efforts were followed by the development of juvenile drug courts, juvenile reentry courts, and comprehensive managed service delivery networks, such as the Adolescent Community Reinforcement Approach (Godley et al. 2001), Iowa Case Management Program (Hall et al. 2002), PEPNet: Connecting Juvenile Offenders to Education and Employment (Office of Juvenile Justice and Delinquency Prevention 2001), The 8% Solution: Reducing Chronic Repeat Offenders (Schumacher and Kurz 1999), and Wrap-Around Milwaukee (Kamradt 2001), a unique health maintenance organization model of behavioral health care.

Juvenile drug courts have been the focus of much attention and anticipation. However, results of several local evaluations range widely, from suggesting that participants have significantly lower rates of recidivism within 1 year, to increased drug use compared with matched juveniles who did not participate in drug court programs (Belenko 2003). Clearly, this is an area that requires further research. The federal Office of Juvenile Justice and Delinquency Prevention has provided training and technical assistance to jurisdictions to develop and enhance juvenile drug courts. The challenge with juvenile drug courts may be the dearth of an available range of services. Several juvenile drug courts have, out of necessity, focused on a single approach rather than on a continuum of services, as has been a factor in the success of such programs for adults, mostly in highly populated areas.

Issues Related to Community-Based Programs

One of the most basic challenges to community-based programs is simply where to put them, in light of understandable community safety concerns that become generalized into the "not in my backyard" syndrome. Working proactively with parent-driven, grassroots advocacy groups can help mitigate this challenge. A related concern is that physical security and surveillance are often necessary, not only to protect (or appease) the surrounding community, but also to protect the integrity of programs from intrusion and confidentiality breaches. Private providers must cooperatively adapt to the needs of those public agencies ultimately responsible for such security and supervision.

Service providers in the community must be prepared to coordinate actively, often with multiple agencies and other interested parties. Cross-system collaboration, especially between clinical, judicial/correctional, educational, and social welfare agencies, is essential for effective engagement of youth and their families, treatment retention, and sustained community-based recovery. Some of the tension experienced between treatment and judicial supervision staff does extend into community juvenile programs, but to a much lesser extent. One approach that serves to mitigate this is the on-site location of dedicated probation officers whose caseloads are rearranged to include all residents of these facilities and who help join both juveniles and staff in a more cooperative and productive manner. This also fosters improved coordination with community-based practitioners.

Perhaps a more important requirement when working with juveniles is the need to competently respond to culture-linked, gender-specific, and trauma-related issues, as well as educational and vocational needs, all of which are often more pronounced among the juvenile population (these essential and primary issues are too extensive for the space allotted for this chapter). This challenge becomes incrementally more difficult as area population (and therefore service) densities decrease. Rural localities understandably provide limited options for juveniles. One emerging solution is the use of telemedicine, an option that has been successful in long-distance health and behavioral health service delivery in correctional institutions, and with remote populations.

Despite being excellent models, the TASC and juvenile drug court programs are effective largely to the extent that a range of community resources is available. They function best in high-density population areas (e.g., cities) and must be creative in less populous areas.

The increased participation by families afforded in community-based programs creates an important opportunity to work with the entire family and to have greater impact on the success of juveniles. At the same time, given the high prevalence of SUDs, co-occurring mental disorders, and other problems within families, the community providers must be prepared to also ensure that parents and significant others receive their own treatment, when needed. For example, parental substance abuse alone is a significant factor associated with adolescent SUDs and juvenile offending. At times, it may be necessary to address the active addiction of a parent before attempting to address SUD with the juvenile.

Case Vignette

Katie (a pseudonym for an actual patient) is a 16-year-old girl from an intact white, middle-class, Irish Catholic family. She was referred through the juvenile court, due to charges associated with an alcohol-related automobile crash. As an alternative to sentencing, she was conditionally diverted to treatment for chronic alcohol dependence at a short term (45-day) inpatient program for adolescents with co-occurring SUDs and mental disorders; the program was located in her suburban, home community. Conditions of her diversion included that she complete all treatment recommended by the program, and that she continue on community supervision by the court (i.e., probation) until her 18th birthday.

The father was described as chronically alcoholic, having recently relapsed, yet able to keep his two jobs. The mother was reportedly involved in Al-Anon. Katie had received prior inpatient treatment three times, once in a chemical dependency rehabilitation center and twice in a psychiatric hospital. She was not diagnosed with a co-occurring mental disorder. Her father had reportedly been in alcohol detoxification five times in the past 20 years and was attending AA sporadically; he explained that his need to work two jobs interfered with regular attendance. This case was viewed with great interest by the clinical staff, who had not previously had the opportunity to work with a "classic" multigenerational, alcoholic family.

Upon arrival, on time, at the program, the family displayed striking behavior that gave clues into the significant disease processes that were longstanding and deeply embedded in the family functioning. Mother, father, and Katie entered the unit smiling, joking, and hugging one another. Katie was proudly holding a bouquet of flowers given by her parents to celebrate her entering treatment. Her mother was somewhat subdued and deferential to her husband. Katie's father, born in Ireland and speaking with a heavy brogue, made mention of his recent "terrible relapse" that "happened" to him—with an attitude that it was something that might have simply fallen out of the sky.

He was wearing a green sweater with an embroidered Guinness (famous Irish brewery) logo on his chest. Katie's 17-year-old sister was unable to attend.

In the initial interview, Katie's father indicated that he had a long history of alcohol abuse; that despite his recent unfortunate relapse, he felt he was able to manage things without needing to enter treatment; and that he tried his hardest to get to AA meetings when he could. He was obviously still drinking regularly (the sweater logo was an interesting, clear signal). Katie's mother surprisingly indicated she had been attending Al-Anon religiously for 16 years. Her lack of action regarding her husband's obvious, active alcoholism was indicative of deeply ingrained (and, perhaps, culturally reinforced) codependency in need of intensive treatment. Katie, who was an above-average student, had only recently been making lower grades. She minimized her alcohol abuse severity, pointing to her active functioning as a high school cheerleader and participation on the field hockey team. She was not resistant to entering treatment in the slightest.

Katie's course of inpatient treatment was mostly unremarkable. She participated fully, achieved increasing behavioral status, and was essentially a "model" patient, until she reported to staff that she "messed up" and drank one drink (by her reporting) during her sole overnight home visit at week 5. After consultation between program staff and Katie's probation officer, her treatment stay was extended by 2 weeks. [Note: At the time, it was more common for court staff to "pull the trigger," insisting that—even upon the first positive urine screen or other evidence of a single "slip"—the client be brought back to court for sentencing. Or, in the case of postsentencing diversion from incarceration, the juvenile would likely have been locked up without a graduated sanction. The field has since moved toward the use of graduated sanctions, supporting treatment interventions—especially in the case of juvenile drug courts.]

Katie's mother participated in weekly family psychoeducational groups (as required for family visitation to be allowed) and family therapy sessions. Her father and sister attended family therapy sessions on occasion (again, her father often pointed to his need to hold down two jobs). Consistent with the family dynamics, despite being told about Katie's slip, neither parent mentioned Katie's slip to the program staff.

Only when Katie approached the final week of her treatment was significant clinical progress able to be made. Her expression of the normal predischarge anxiety and regression was to become quiet and somewhat sad. The clinical staff seized this opportunity to actively explore her feelings and concerns about returning to her family. She was able to divulge more of the true picture of her alcoholic family and its disease process. The staff offered to keep her in treatment even longer (at the nonprofit agency's expense) to facilitate an effective intervention. The next day, Katie's mother called to ask whether Katie could have an extra home visit to attend her sister's high school graduation party at the family's house. When asked if there would be alcohol at the party, the mother initially and unconvincingly answered, "No." However, when questioned further, she admitted, somewhat ashamedly, "Well, there will be some in the punch." The family was subsequently scheduled for an administrative case meeting following the weekend. They attended and were informed that Katie would not be discharged until the entire family completed a 1-week residential family treatment program out of state. The probation officer, again, supported the program's intervention. With only half-hearted objection by Katie's father regarding his job, the family agreed. Katie was visibly relieved and made impressive progress during the wait for admission, identifying her codependent role as the heroic identified family patient, the systemic family dysfunction driven by her father's untreated alcoholism, and her mother's inability to effectively place demands on her husband.

The family completed residential family treatment and participated in 2 more weeks of family therapy, while Katie remained in the program until she felt confident enough to begin effectuating both her personal individuation and her continuing treatment and recovery plans.

Case Discussion

This case clearly illustrates the importance not only of including family members in the juvenile's treatment planning, but also of fully assessing the entire family. Parental substance abuse should be addressed in order for the juvenile identified patient to be expected to maintain sobriety and achieve sustained personal recovery.

Emerging Approaches: The New Recovery Movement

Similar to earlier efforts to provide opportunities for persons in recovery to anonymously "give back" by, for example, serving as sponsors for others in recovery (a hallmark of the 12-step approach used in AA and NA) and volunteering at treatment facilities and hospitals, the past decade has seen a major expansion of the roles and services conducted by peers in the recovery community. Known as the "new recovery movement" (White 2000), this has included the development of recovery support centers, recovery (e.g., sober) housing, telephone recovery supports, transportation, recovery management checkups, recovery mentoring, recovery social networking, and similar peer-to-peer recovery supports. Although mostly available for adults, these supports are becoming increasingly available for youth.

Three models of providing recovery supports for adolescents, including juveniles, are emerging:

1. *Model recovery community partnerships.* For example, the Free Mind program in Tucson, Arizona (funded through the federal Recovery Community Supports Program; CSAT 2008), targets adjudicated youth, ages 14–18, from multiethnic communities, providing a range of peer-led recovery support services in collaboration with the University of Arizona and the Pima County Juvenile Court.

2. *Grassroots youth and family recovery support and advocacy groups.* For example, Connecticut Turning to Youth and Families, a peer-owned and -operated nonprofit organization (www.ctyouthandfamilies.org), provides a range of recovery supports for young persons and parents, including organizing local recovery communities and student assistance groups, providing recovery coaching/mentoring, and community organizing for advocacy on behalf of the need for adolescent substance abuse treatment and recovery services.

3. *Internet-based recovery supports and resource linkages.* Several organizations are currently developing web-based supports, including searchable, nationally geomapped inventories of adolescent treatment and recovery supports, "virtual recovery communities" via online social networking for youth in recovery and parents, and both online and telephone guidance to assist youth and families to locate local treatment and recovery services (White 2010).

These resources are especially valuable for juveniles who are recovering from SUDs and co-occurring mental disorders and are returning to the community from juvenile institutions and residential placements. For those practitioners who will be involved with juveniles, in institution- or community-based settings, knowledge about the types of locally available recovery supports is essential to enhancing long-term recovery for youth.

Key Clinical Concepts

- A prerequisite for treatment engagement and retention with juveniles is to understand the unique cultural, environmental, familial, and circumstantial variables they present.

- Compared with adolescents not involved in the juvenile justice system, adolescents involved with the juvenile justice system (juveniles) have significantly higher prevalence and severity as well as earlier onset of SUDs and co-occurring mental disorders (including multiply comorbid conditions).

- Assessment of the severity of SUDs and co-occurring mental disorders, combined with risk and case management, results in identification of more appropriate treatment levels of care and better-coordinated transitional placements.

- Strengths-based and family-focused community interventions (including diversion programs) demonstrate superior outcomes and save limited resources.

- Systems coordination is essential; treatment and security must be complementary, with treatments integrating accountability and graduated sanctions.

- Gender-specific (both females and males), trauma-informed, and culturally competent services are essential, and require greater attention.

- Fostering educational success that is responsive to individual learning styles, and to learning and attentional disorders, is critical to recovery but is not being adequately recognized or addressed.

References

Anglin MD, Longshore S, Turner S, et al: Studies of the Functioning and Effectiveness of Treatment Alternatives to Street Crime (TASC) Programs: Final Report. Los Angeles, UCLA Drug Abuse Research Center, 1996

Barnes GM, Welte JW, Hoffman JH: Relationship of alcohol use to delinquency and illicit drug use in adolescents: gender, age, and racial/ethnic differences. J Drug Issues, Winter 2002, pp 153–178

Barton C, Alexander JF, Waldron H, et al: Generalizing treatment effects of Functional Family Therapy: three replications. American Journal of Family Therapy 13(3):16–26, 1985

Belenko S: Delivering more effective treatment to adolescents: improving the juvenile drug court model. J Subst Abuse Treat 25:189–211, 2003

Bilchik S: Office of Juvenile Justice and Delinquency Prevention Fact Sheet. Rockville, MD, U.S. Government Printing Office, July 1998

Bonta J, Wormith SJ: Risk and need assessment, in Developments in Social Work With Offenders. Edited by McIvor G, Raynor P. London, Jessica Kingsley Publishers, 2008, pp 131–152

Burnette KD, Swan ES, Robinson KD, et al: Treating youthful offenders with moral reconation therapy: a recidivism and pre- posttest analysis. Cognitive Behavioral Treatment Review 3:14-15, 2004

Bush J, Glick B, Taymans J: Thinking for a Change: An Integrated Cognitive Behavior Change Program. Longmont, CO, National Institute of Corrections, 1996

Callahan J: Adolescent Portable Therapy for the Juvenile Justice System. New York, Vera Institute of Justice, 2001

Center for Substance Abuse Treatment: Continuity of offender treatment for substance use disorders from institution to community. Treatment Improvement Protocol (TIP) Series 30 (DHHS Publ No SMA-98-3245). Rockville, MD, Substance Abuse and Mental Health Services Administration, 1998

Center for Substance Abuse Treatment: Screening and assessing adolescents for substance use disorders. Treatment Improvement Protocol (TIP) Series 31 (DHHS Publ No SMA-99-3282). Rockville, MD, Substance Abuse and Mental Health Services Administration, 1999

Center for Substance Abuse Treatment: Recovery Community Services: Project Profiles. Rockville, MD, Substance Abuse and Mental Health Services Administration, 2008

Cloward R, Ohlin LE: Delinquency and Opportunity: A Theory of Delinquent Gangs. Glencoe, IL, Free Press, 1960

Cocozza JJ (ed): Responding to the Mental Health Needs of Youth in the Juvenile Justice System. Seattle, WA, The National Coalition for the Mentally Ill in the Criminal Justice System, 1992

Cocozza J, Skowyra K: Office of Juvenile Justice and Delinquency Prevention. Juvenile Justice Journal 7, April 2000

Dembo R, Williams L, Schmeidler J: Addressing the problems of substance abuse in juvenile corrections, in Drug Treatment and Criminal Justice. Edited by Inciardi J. Newbury Park, CA, Sage, 1993, pp 97–126

Dembo R, Schmeidler J, Nini-Gough, et al: Predictors of recidivism to a juvenile assessment center: a three-year study. J Child Adolesc Subst Abuse 7(3):57–77, 1998

Dennis ML: Global Appraisal of Individual Needs (GAIN): Administration Guide for the GAIN and Related Measures. Bloomington, IL, Lighthouse, 1999

Dennis ML: Juvenile justice, substance abuse and mental disorders. Presentation at the Southeast Conference on Co-occurring Mental and Substance Related Disorders, Orlando, FL, June 2005

Dennis ML, Godley SH, Diamond G, et al: The Cannabis Youth Treatment (CYT) study: main findings from two randomized trials. J Subst Abuse Treat 27:197–213, 2004

Deschenes E, Greenwood P: Treating the juvenile drug offender, in Drugs and Crime: Evaluating Public Policy Initiatives. Edited by MacKenzie D, Uchida C. Thousand Oaks, CA, Sage, 1994, pp 253–280

Elliot D, Huizinga D, Menard S: Multiple Problem Youth: Delinquency, Substance Use and Mental Health Problems. New York, Springer-Verlag, 1989

Farlie RW: Drug dealing and legitimate self-employment. JCPR Working Paper 88. Chicago, IL, Joint Center for Parenting Research, Northwestern University/University of Chicago, April 1999

Fass SM, Pi C-R: Getting tough on juvenile crime: an analysis of costs and benefits. J Res Crime Delinq 39:363–399, 2002

Fazel S, Doll H, Långström N: Mental disorders among adolescents in juvenile detention and correctional facilities: a systematic review and metaregression analysis of 25 surveys. J Am Acad Child Adolesc Psychiatry 47:1010–1019, 2008

Field G: The effects of intensive treatment on reducing the criminal recidivism of addicted offenders. Fed Probat 53:51–56, 1989

Gendreau P, Goggin C: Correctional treatment: accomplishments and realities, in Correctional Counseling and Rehabilitation. Edited by VanVourhis P, Broswell M, Lester D. Cincinnati, OH, Anderson, 1997, pp 271–279

Glick B, Goldstein A: Aggression replacement training. J Couns Dev 65:356–362, 1987

Godley SH, Meyers RJ, Smith JE, et al: The Adolescent Community Reinforcement Approach for Adolescent Cannabis Users (Cannabis Youth Treatment Series, Vol 4; DHHS Publ No 01-3489). Rockville, MD, Center for Substance Abuse Treatment, Substance Abuse and Mental Health Services Administration, 2001

Guchereau M, Jourkiv O, Zametkin A: Mental disorders among adolescents in juvenile detention and correctional facilities: posttraumatic stress disorder is overlooked (letter). J Am Acad Child Adolesc Psychiatry 48:340, 2009

Hall J, Carswell C, Walsh E, et al: Iowa Case Management: innovative social casework. Social Work 47:132–141, 2002

Henggeler SW, Clingempeel WG, Brondino MJ, et al: Four-year follow-up of Multisystemic Therapy with substance-abusing and substance-dependent juvenile offenders. J Am Acad Child Adolesc Psychiatry 41:868–874, 2002

Hoffmann NG, Abrantes AM, Anton R: Problems identified by the Practical Adolescent Dual Diagnostic Interview (PADDI) in a juvenile detention center population, in Treating Addicted Offenders: A Continuum of Effective Practices. Edited by Knight K, Farabee D. Kingston, NJ, Civic Research Institute, 2004

Hoge RD, Andrews DA: Youth Level of Service/Case Management Inventory: User's Manual. Toronto, Ontario, Canada, Multi-Health Systems, 2002

Hoge RD, Andrews DA, Leschied AW: Youth Level of Service/Case Management Inventory. North Tonawanda, NY, Multi-Health Systems, 2002

Hubbard R, Cavanaugh E, Craddock S, et al: Characteristics, behaviors and outcomes for youth in the TOPS, in Treatment Services for Adolescent Substance Abusers. Edited by Friedman AS, Beschner GM. Washington, DC, U.S. Department of Health and Human Services, National Institute on Drug Abuse, 1985, pp 49–65

Hubner J, Wolfson J: Handle With Care: Serving the Mental Health Needs of Young Offenders: Annual Report of the Coalition for Juvenile Justice. Washington, DC, Coalition for Juvenile Justice, 2000

Inciardi JA, Martin SS, Butzin CA, et al: An effective model of prison-based treatment for drug-involved offenders. J Drug Issues 27:261–278, 1997

Kaminer Y, Wagner E, Plummer B, et al: Validation of the Teen Addiction Severity Index (T-ASI): preliminary findings. Am J Addict 2:221–224, 1993

Kamradt B: Wraparound Milwaukee: aiding youth with mental health needs. Juvenile Justice 7:14–23, 2001

Knight K, Simpson DD, Chatham LR, et al: An assessment of prison-based drug treatment: Texas' in-prison therapeutic community program. J Offender Rehabil 24:75–100, 1997

Landenberger N, Lipsey M: The positive effects of cognitive behavioral programs for offenders: a meta-analysis of factors associated with effective treatment. Journal of Experimental Criminology 1:451–476, 2005

Liddle HA: Multidimensional Family Therapy Treatment Manual. Miami, FL, Center for Treatment Research on Adolescent Drug Abuse, University of Miami School of Medicine, 1998

Linehan MM, Schmidt H, Dimeff LA, et al: Dialectical behavior therapy for patients with borderline personality disorder and drug dependence. Am J Addict 8:279–292, 1999

Lipsey M: Juvenile delinquency treatment: a meta-analytic inquiry into the variability of effects, in Meta-Analysis for Explanation: A Casebook. Edited by Cook TD, Cooper H, Cordray DS, et al. New York, Russell Sage Foundation, 1992, pp 83–127

Lipsey M: What works with juvenile offenders: translating research into practice. Paper presented at the Adolescent Treatment Issues Conference, Tampa, FL, 2005

McCurley C, Snyder HN: Co-occurrence of substance use behaviors in youth. November 2008. Available at: http://www.ncjrs.gov/pdffiles1/ojjdp/219239.pdf. Accessed January 4, 2010.

National Center on Addiction and Substance Abuse (CASA) at Columbia University: CASA analysis of the National Survey on Drug Use and Health (NSDUH). Rockville, MD, U.S. Department of Health and Human Services, Substance Abuse and Mental Health Services Administration, Office of Applied Studies, 2004a

National Center on Addiction and Substance Abuse (CASA): Criminal Neglect: Substance Abuse, Juvenile Justice and the Children Left Behind. New York, Columbia University, October 2004b

National Institute on Drug Abuse: Principles of Drug Addiction Treatment: A Research-Based Guide (NIH Publ No 09-4180). Rockville, MD, National Institutes of Health, 1999

Office of Juvenile Justice and Delinquency Prevention: Capacity building for juvenile substance abuse treatment. OJJDP Juvenile Justice Bulletin, December 1997

Office of Juvenile Justice and Delinquency Prevention: PEPNet: Connecting Juvenile Offenders to Education and Employment. OJJDP Fact Sheet #29. Washington, DC, Office of Justice Programs, U.S. Department of Justice, July 2001

Office of National Drug Control Policy: ADAM II 2008 Annual Report. 2009. Available at: http://www.whitehousedrugpolicy.gov/publications/pdf/adam2008.pdf. Accessed January 4, 2010.

Orbis Partners: Long-term validation of the Youth Assessment and Screening Instrument (YASI) in New York State juvenile probation. 2007. Available at: http://dpca.state.ny.us/pdfs/nyltyasifullreport20feb08.pdf. Accessed January 4, 2010.

Pealer JA, Latessa EJ, Winesburg M: Final report, Mohican Youth Center RSAT Outcome Evaluation. Submitted to the National Institute of Justice, September 2002

Peters RH, Bartoi MG, Sherman PB: Screening and Assessment of Co-occurring Disorders in the Justice System. Delmar, NY, CMHS National Gains Center, 1997

Puzzanchera C, Stahl AL, Finnegan TA, et al: Juvenile Court Statistics 1999: Celebrating 100 years of the juvenile court, 1899–1999 (NCJ Publ No 201241). Pittsburgh, PA, National Center for Juvenile Justice, 2003

Rice ME, Harris GT, Quinsey VL: The appraisal of violence risk. Curr Opin Psychiatry 15:589–593, 2002

Rockholz PB: National update on therapeutic community programs for substance abusing offenders in state prisons, in Treating Addicted Offenders: A Continuum of Effective Practices. Edited by Knight K, Farabee D. Kingston, NJ, Civic Research Institute, 2004, pp 1–10

Rockholz PB, McMahon TJ, Luthar SS: Improving residential substance abuse treatment for inner-city teens: New Haven ACTS, in Adolescents and Substance Abuse. Edited by Crowley TJ, Beal JM. San Juan, PR, College on Problems of Drug Dependence, 1996, p 135

Ross RR: Reasoning and rehabilitation. International Journal of Offender Therapy and Comparative Criminology 32:29–35, 1988

Sampl S, Kadden R: MET and CBT for adolescent cannabis users: 5 sessions. CYT Series, Vol 1 (BKD384). Rockville, MD, Center for Substance Abuse Treatment, Substance Abuse and Mental Health Services Administration, 2001

Schumacher M, Kurz GA: The 8% Solution: Preventing Serious, Repeat Juvenile Crime. Thousand Oaks, CA, Sage, 1999

Sickmund M: Juveniles in corrections (NCJ Publ No 202885). Washington, DC, U.S. Department of Justice, Office of Justice Programs, Office of Juvenile Justice and Delinquency Prevention, 2004

Skowyra KR, Cocozza JJ: Blueprint for Change: A Comprehensive Model for the Identification and Treatment of Youth With Mental Health Needs in Contact With the Juvenile Justice System. Delmar, NY, National Center for Mental Health and Juvenile Justice, 2007

Snyder H, Sickmund M: Juvenile Offenders and Victims: 1999 National Report. Washington, DC, Office of Juvenile Justice and Delinquency Prevention, 1999

Substance Abuse and Mental Health Services Administration (SAMHSA), Office of Applied Studies: Drug and alcohol treatment in juvenile correctional facilities: the DASIS report. Rockville, MD, U.S. Department of Health and Human Services, 2002

Teplin L: Assessing Alcohol, Drug and Mental Disorders in Juvenile Detainees. Washington, DC, Office of Juvenile Justice and Delinquency Prevention, 2001

Teplin L, Abram KM, McClelland GM, et al: Psychiatric disorders in youth in juvenile detention. Arch Gen Psychiatry 59:1133–1143, 2002

Vincent GM, Grisso T, Terry A, et al: Sex and race differences in mental health symptoms in juvenile justice: the MAYSI-2 national meta-analysis. J Am Acad Child Adolesc Psychiatry 47:282–290, 2008

Washington State Institute for Public Policy: Evidence-based juvenile offender programs: program description, quality assurance, and cost. June 2007. Available at: http://www.wsipp.wa.gov/rptfiles/07-06-1201.pdf. Accessed February 11, 2010.

Wexler HK: The Amity Prison TC evaluation: inmate profiles and reincarceration outcomes. Presentation for the California Department of Corrections, Sacramento, CA, 1996

Wexler HK, Falkin GP, Lipton DS: A model prison rehabilitation program: an evaluation of the Stay'n Out therapeutic community. A final report to the National Institute on Drug Abuse by Narcotic and Drug Research, August 31, 1988. New York, Narcotic and Drug Research, 1988

White WL: Toward a new recovery movement: historical reflections on recovery, treatment and advocacy. Paper prepared for the Center for Substance Abuse Treatment, Recovery Community Support Program Conference, Arlington, VA, April 3–5, 2000. Available at: http://www.bhrm.org/advocacy/newrecmove.pdf. Accessed January 6, 2010.

White WL: The future of AA, NA and other recovery mutual aid organizations. www.counselormagazine.com, March 29, 2010.

Winters K: Kids and drugs: treatment recognizes link between delinquency and substance abuse. Corrections Today 60:118–121, 1998

Winters KC, Henly GA: Personal Experience Inventory and Manual. Los Angeles, CA, Western Psychological Services, 1989

Suggested Readings

Center for Substance Abuse Treatment, Denver Juvenile Justice Integrated Treatment Network: Strategies for integrating substance abuse treatment and the juvenile justice system: a practice guide (DHHS Publ No SMA-00-3369). Rockville, MD, Substance Abuse and Mental Health Services Administration, U.S. Department of Health and Human Services, 1999

Elliot D, Huizinga D, Ageton S: Explaining Delinquency and Drug Use. Beverly Hills, CA, Sage, 1985

Knight K, Farabee D (eds): Treating Addicted Offenders: A Continuum of Effective Practices. Kingston, NJ, Civic Research Institute, 2004

Lipsey MW, Wilson DB, Cothern L: Effective intervention for serious juvenile offenders. OJJDP Juvenile Justice Bulletin, April 2000

McPhail MW, Wiest BM (co-chairs): Combining alcohol and other drug abuse treatment with diversion for juveniles in the justice system. Treatment Improvement Protocol (TIP) Series 21 (DHHS Publ No SMA-95-305). Rockville, MD, U.S. Department of Health and Human Services, Substance Abuse and Mental Health Services Administration, Center for Substance Abuse Treatment, 1995

Robert Wood Johnson Foundation: Reclaiming Futures: Building Solutions to Substance Abuse and Delinquency. Princeton, NJ, Robert Wood Johnson Foundation, 2001

Substance Abuse and Mental Health Services Administration (SAMHSA), Office of Applied Studies: Drug and alcohol treatment in juvenile correctional facilities: the DASIS report. Rockville, MD, U.S. Department of Health and Human Services, 2002

Select Drug Abuse Screening and Comprehensive Instruments

Assessment	Purpose	Clinical utility	Example group used	Norms?
Screens				
Assessment of Substance Misuse in Adolescence (Willner 2000)	Screen for drug use problem severity	Quick screen	Adolescents referred for emotional or behavioral disorders	Yes
CRAFFT (Knight et al. 2003)	Screen for drug use problem severity	Quick screen	Adolescents referred for emotional or behavioral disorders	Yes
Drug Abuse Screening Test for Adolescents (Martino et al. 2000)	Screen for drug use problem severity	Quick screen	Adolescents referred for emotional or behavioral disorders	Yes
Global Appraisal of Individual Needs— Short Screener (Dennis et al. 2006)	Screen for substance use problem severity and related problems	Screen	Adolescents referred for emotional or behavioral disorders	NA
Massachusetts Youth Screening Instrument–2 (Grisso and Barnum 2000)	Screen for substance use problem severity and related problems	Screen	Adolescents referred for emotional or behavioral disorders	Yes
Personal Experience Screening Questionnaire (Winters 1992)	Screen for substance use problem severity	Quick screen	Adolescents referred for emotional or behavioral disorders	Yes
Substance Abuse Subtle Screening Inventory— Adolescent Version (Miller 1985)	Screen for substance use problem severity and related problems	Screen	Adolescents referred for emotional or behavioral disorders	Yes

Normed groups	Format	Time (min)	Training needed?	Scoring time (min)	Computer scoring?	Fee for use?
Normals	8 items, questions	5	No	2	No	No
Normals; substance abusers	6 items, questions	5	No	2	No	No
Substance abusers	27 items, questions	5	No	5	No	No
NA	20 items, interview	5	No	5	Yes	No
Juvenile offenders	52 items, questions	15	No	10–15	In progress	No
Normals; substance abusers	40 items, questions	10	No	5	No	Yes
Normals; substance abusers	81 items, questions	10–15	No	5	Yes	Yes

Assessment	Purpose	Clinical utility	Example group used	Norms
Comprehensive questionnaires				
Adolescent Self-Assessment Profile (Wanberg 1992)	Multiscale measure of substance involvement and related psychosocial factors	Aids in identification, referral, and treatment	Adolescents suspected of substance use problems	Yes
Hilson Adolescent Profile (Inwald et al. 1986)	Multiscale measure of substance involvement and related psychosocial factors	Aids in identification, referral, and treatment	Adolescents suspected of substance use and related problems	Yes
Juvenile Automated Substance Abuse Evaluation (Ellis 1987)	Multiscale measure of substance involvement and related psychosocial factors	Aids in identification, referral, and treatment	Adolescents suspected of substance use problems	Yes
Personal Experience Inventory (Winters and Henly 1989)	Multiscale measure of substance involvement and related psychosocial factors	Aids in identification, referral, and treatment	Adolescents suspected of substance use problems	Yes

Normed groups	Format	Time (min)	Training needed?	Scoring time (min)	Computer scoring?	Fee for use?
Normals; substance abusers	225 items, question-naire	45–60	No	5	Yes	Yes
Normals; substance abusers	310 items, question-naire	45	No	5	Yes	Yes
Normals; substance abusers	108 itcms, question-naire	20	No	5	Yes	Yes
Normals; substance abusers	276 items, question-naire	45–60	No	5	Yes	Yes

Assessment	Purpose	Clinical utility	Example group used	Norms
Comprehensive interviews				
Adolescent Diagnostic Interview (Winters and Henly 1993)	Assess DSM-IV substance use disorders and other life areas	Aids in case identification, referral, treatment	Adolescents suspected of substance use problems	NA
Comprehensive Addiction Severity Index for Adolescents (Meyers et al. 1995)	Assess substance use and other life problems	Aids in case identification, referral, and treatment	Adolescents suspected of substance use problems	NA
Global Appraisal of Individual Needs (Dennis 1999)	Assess substance use and other life problems	Aids in case identification, referral, treatment	Adolescents suspected of substance use problems	NA
Practical Adolescent Dual Diagnostic Interview (Hoffman et al. 2004)	Assess DSM-IV-TR substance use disorders and other disorders	Aids in case identification, referral, treatment	Adolescents suspected of substance use problems	NA
Teen Addiction Severity Index (Kaminer et al. 1993)	Assess substance use and other life problems	Aids in case identification, referral, treatment	Adolescents at risk for substance use problems	NA
Teen Treatment Services Review (Kaminer et al. 1998)	Assess type and number of program services	Aids in describing services received	Adolescents receiving treatment for substance use problems	NA

Note. The requirements for inclusion in the table are that 1) the instrument was specifically developed for youth, 2) its psychometric data were published in a detailed manual or a peer-reviewed publication, and 3) the instrument's author(s) or publisher was available to address questions by users. Information about the instruments is based on published literature and correspondence with instrument authors.

NA = not available; normals = nonclinical comparison group.

Normed groups	Format	Time (min)	Training needed?	Scoring time (min)	Computer scoring?	Fee for use?
NA	Structured interview	45	Yes	15–20	No	Yes
NA	Semistructured interview	45–55	Yes	15	Yes	Yes (computer)
NA	Semistructured interview	90–120	Yes	15	Yes	Yes
NA	Structured interview	60–90	Yes	15–20	No	Yes
NA	Semistructured interview	20–45	Yes	10	No	No
NA	Semistructured interview	10–15	Yes	5	No	No

References

Dennis ML: Global Appraisal of Individual Needs (GAIN): Administration Guide for the GAIN and Related Measures. Bloomington, IL, Lighthouse, 1999

Dennis ML, Chan Y-F, Funk RR: Development and validation of the GAIN Short Screener (GAIN-SS) for psychopathology and crime/violence among adolescents and adults. Am J Addict 15 (suppl 1):S80–S91, 2006

Ellis BR: Juvenile Automated Substance Abuse Evaluation. Clarkston, MI, ADE, 1987

Grisso T, Barnum R: Massachusetts Youth Screening Instrument–2: User's Manual and Technical Report. Worcester, MA, University of Massachusetts Medical School, 2000

Hoffmann NG, Bride BF, MacMasters SA, et al: Identifying co-occurring conditions in adolescent clinical populations. J Addict Dis 23:41–53, 2004

Inwald RE, Brobst MA, Morissey RF: Identifying and predicting adolescent behavioral problems by using a new profile. Juvenile Justice Digest 14:1, 1986

Kaminer Y, Wagner E, Plummer B, et al: Validation of the Teen Addiction Severity Index (T-ASI): preliminary findings. Am J Addict 2:221–224, 1993

Kaminer Y, Blitz C, Burleson JA, et al: The Teen Treatment Services Review (T-TSR). J Subst Abuse Treat 15:291–300, 1998

Knight J, Sherritt L, Harris SK, et al: Validity of brief alcohol screening tests among adolescents: a comparison of the AUDIT, POSIT, CAGE and CRAFFT. Alcohol Clin Exp Res 27:67–73, 2003

Martino S, Grilo CM, Fehon DC: Development of the Drug Abuse Screening Test for Adolescents (DAST-A). Addict Behav 25:57–70, 2000

Meyers K, McLellan AT, Jaeger JL, et al: The development of the Comprehensive Addiction Severity Index for Adolescents (CASI-A): an interview for assessing multiple problems of adolescents. J Subst Abuse Treat 12:181–193, 1995

Miller G: The Substance Abuse Subtle Screening Inventory—Adolescent Version. Bloomington, IN, SASSI Institute, 1985

Wanberg K: Adolescent Self-Assessment Profile (ASAP). Arvada, CO, Center for Addictions Research and Evaluation, 1992

Willner R: Further validation and development of a screening instrument for the assessment of substance misuse in adolescents. Addiction 95:1691–1698, 2000

Winters KC: Development of an adolescent alcohol and other drug abuse screening scale: Personal Experience Screening Questionnaire. Addict Behav 17:479–490, 1992

Winters KC, Henly GA: Personal Experience Inventory and Manual. Los Angeles, CA, Western Psychological Services, 1989

Winters KC, Henly GA: Adolescent Diagnostic Interview Schedule and Manual. Los Angeles, CA, Western Psychological Services, 1993

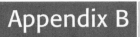

Clinical Information
Resources

Assessment Resources

Print resource	Publisher
Guide to Risk Factor and Outcome Instruments for Youth Substance Abuse Prevention Program Evaluations	DHHS Publication No. 99-3279 Center for Substance Abuse Prevention, Rockville, MD
Handbook of Psychiatric Measures, 2nd Edition, by J.A. Rush, M.B. First, and D. Blacker	American Psychiatric Publishing, Washington, DC, 2007
Screening and Assessing Adolescents for Substance Use Disorders	CSAT TIP 31 Center for Substance Abuse Treatment, Rockville, MD, 1999

Website	URL
Alcohol and Drug Abuse Institute, University of Washington	http://depts.washington.edu/adai
Assessing Alcohol Problems: A Guide for Clinicians and Researchers	http://pubs.niaaa.nih.gov/silk/ publications/Assessing%Alcohol/ index.htm
Buros Institute of Mental Measurements Tests in Print Mental Measurements Yearbook	http://www.unl.edu/buros
ERIC/AE Test Locator	http://www.ericae.net/testcol.htm
PsycINFO	http://www.apa.org/pubs/databases/ psycinfo/index.aspx
Simple Screening Instruments for Outreach for Alcohol and Other Drug Abuse Treatment	CSAT TIP 11 Center for Substance Abuse Treatment, Rockville, MD, 1994

Evidence-Based Treatment Resource

Website	URL
National Registry of Evidence-based Programs and Practices	www.nrepp.samhsa.gov

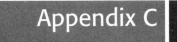

Appendix C

Parent Information Resources

Website	URL	Description
4 Parents	http://www.4parents.gov	Parent resources cover a broad range of youth mental and physical health issues, with a heavy focus on how to talk to a child about health and choices.
Join Together	http://www.jointogether.org	This community-focused drug prevention website focuses on mobilizing community groups to take action to promote substance abuse prevention and treatment.
Parents. The Anti-Drug	http://theanti-drug.com	Created by the National Youth Anti-War Media Campaign, this program serves as a drug prevention information center, and a supportive community for parents to interact and learn from each other.
The Partnership for a Drug-Free America	http://www.drugfree.org/Parent	A very comprehensive resource that includes a parent tool kit, a blog site, resources on teenage brain development, and treatment resources.
Too Smart To Start	http://www.toosmarttostart.samhsa.gov	This site provides research-based strategies and materials to professionals and parents to help them address the problem of underage drinking by young teenagers.

Websites for Self-Help, Alcoholics Anonymous, and Narcotics Anonymous

General Information on Self-Help

http://helpguide.org/mental/drug_abuse_addiction_rehab_treatment.htm
http://www.treatment4addiction.com

How to Find a Local Alcoholics Anonymous Meeting

http://www.aa.org/lang/en/meeting_finder.cfm

How to Find a Local Narcotics Anonymous Meeting

http://web.na.org

Index

Page numbers printed in **boldface** *type refer to tables or figures.*

465

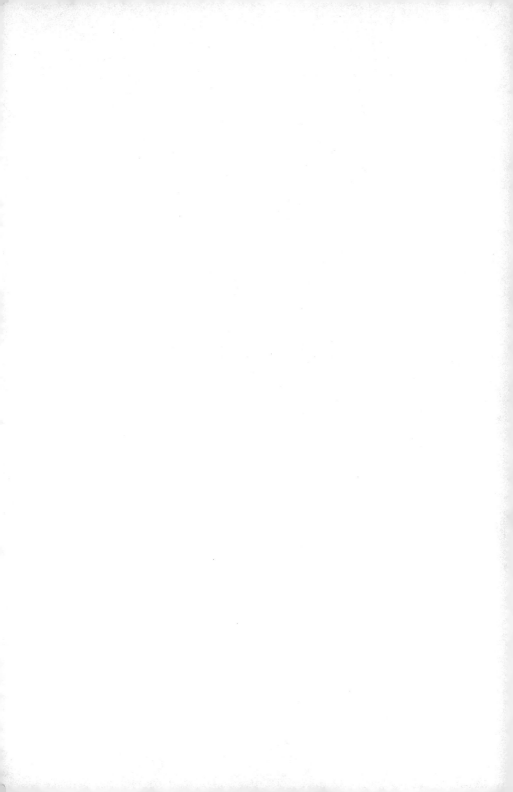